FUNDAMENTALS OF

Skeletal Radiology

Second Edition

Clyde A. Helms, M.D.

Professor of Radiology
Department of Radiology
School of Medicine
University of California, San Francisco

W.B. SAUNDERS COMPANY

A Division of Harcourt Brace & Company
Philadelphia   London   Toronto   Montreal   Sydney   Tokyo

W.B. SAUNDERS COMPANY

A Division of
Harcourt Brace & Company

The Curtis Center
Independence Square West
Philadelphia, PA 19106

Library of Congress Cataloging-in-Publication Data

Helms, Clyde A.
    Fundamentals of skeletal radiology / Clyde A. Helms.—2nd ed.
       p.   cm.
    Includes bibliographical references and index.
    ISBN 0-7216-4680-8
    1. Human skeleton—Radiography. 2. Human skeleton—Diseases—
—Diagnosis.   I. Title.
    [DNLM: 1. Bone and Bones—radiography.   WE 141 H481f 1995]
  RC930.5.H45   1995
  616.7′10757—dc20
  DNLM / DLC
                                94-17893

FUNDAMENTALS OF SKELETAL RADIOLOGY   ISBN 0-7216-4680-8

Printed in the United States of America

Last digit is the print number: 9 8 7 6 5 4 3

This book is dedicated to my children:

Caroline

Jeremy

Allyson

Jason

Benjamin

Like interns and residents they love to learn,
and they are a joy to teach.

And to
Nancy Marie Major,
my wife, my friend, and my most reliable and trusted critic.
She helped make this book better than it was before,
and she did the same with me.

Foreword

Clyde Helms, as a radiologist in training during the mid 70s, was, in many ways, the ideal radiology resident. Able, perceptive, informed, and responsible, he progressed through the various stages of residency training in superb fashion. On the other hand, he was different. Whereas the traditional "best resident" always had at hand exhaustive lists of differential diagnoses, Dr. Helms quietly ignored the trivial, the esoteric, and the information that was not likely to serve him in his work as a radiologist in the "real world," sometimes to the discomfiture of the radiology faculty of the University of California, San Francisco (of which I was then a junior member). Whereas the traditional "best resident" was suitably in awe of the faculty (many of whom were truly awesome), Dr. Helms fearlessly challenged what he perceived as unsupportable dogma. Not one to sit still for pretension, he poked gentle (and sometimes not so gentle) fun at the faculty. Occasional pranks were perpetrated, sometimes at the expense of members of the faculty. No one was immune, no matter how lofty his status. Dr. Helms, as the Sinatra song goes, did it his way. Irreverent, witty, occasionally outrageous, and a superb radiologist, he completed his residency and went on to fulfill his military commitment.

He returned to UCSF 3 years later as a faculty member in the skeletal radiology section. That he had not changed was immediately apparent. Faculty meetings are disrupted by his irreverent remarks, frequently hilarious. Now a mentor, his teaching reflects the same realistic, nontraditional approach he used as a resident. He emphasizes not the exotic or esoteric but the practical, the information that is critical in the day-to-day practice of radiology. Incorporated into his teaching method are mnemonics, one or two of which might not be recommended for family viewing. On the other hand, if they work, why not use them? An increasingly large number of young radiologists (his residents and former residents) will attest that, indeed, they do work. The teaching may be unorthodox, but the learning is real and substantial.

This volume is also unorthodox. Several excellent, superbly researched and crafted treatises on skeletal radiology are available to the radiology resident and practicing radiologist. This volume is not intended as an exhaustive compendium of skeletal radiology. Rather it is, as indicated by the title, an exposition of the *basics* of skeletal radiology. In keeping with his personalized, unusual approach to teaching, he begins with a discussion of radiologic examinations that should *not* be performed. The remainder of the book deals with skeletal conditions that radiologists are likely to encounter any day of the week. The reader who wishes to become familiar with Scheie syndrome or tricho-rhinophalangeal dysplasia Type II must look elsewhere.

Rather than the usual, formal language found in other radiology texts, the reader will encounter the vernacular used by all radiologists when they discuss their work with other radiologists. The text is much like Dr. Helms himself—witty, irreverent, unpretentious, and fast-paced. The reader will find the book refreshing, eminently readable, and highly informative.

The ideal condition
Would be, I admit, that men should be right by instinct;
But since we are all likely to go astray,
The reasonable thing is to learn from those who can teach.
               Sophocles

Clyde Helms can teach!

Hideyo Minagi, M.D.

Preface

The first edition of this work has served many radiology residents as a simplified text for learning the basics of skeletal radiology. However, it is clearly out of date in that it contains little magnetic resonance (MR) instruction, particularly as it is used in imaging the joints and the spine. The fundamentals of skeletal radiology must now encompass not only the plain film knowledge that was once all that was necessary for a bone radiologist but also MR imaging of the musculoskeletal system. This second edition attempts to rectify that shortcoming. In keeping with the style of the first edition, I have attempted to retain a casual, if not flippant, attitude. It is my opinion that most academicians are pretentious and take themselves too seriously. This attitude, for many of us, is intimidating and actually impedes learning. There is no reason you can't learn and have fun, too. This book allows both fun and learning to co-exist, as should most good residency programs.

I have deliberately not included basic physics or MR physics for two reasons: one, I don't feel you have to know them in depth to interpret images; and two, I don't know any physics. I have also not included precise MR imaging sequences (TR/TE), as it doesn't make any difference for most cases. I simply indicate T1 or T2 usually.

I would like to thank the many individuals who brought to my attention errors in the first edition. Also, thanks to all who gave suggestions for improving the first edition. Special thanks are due to Ferris Hall who gave me a detailed critique with suggestions for improvement, almost all of which are in this second edition. Thanks to my favorite radiology resident, Nancy Major, who is now my wife, for her hours of proofreading every chapter. Her help and support have been invaluable.

Clyde A. Helms

Contents

Unnecessary Examinations

Before beginning to learn how to interpret pathologic skeletal films, it is important to briefly consider unnecessary skeletal radiographic examinations. Dr. Ferris Hall from Boston first brought to my attention the idea that just because we *could* x-ray something didn't mean that we *should*. His article entitled "Overutilization of Radiologic Examinations" in the August 1976 issue of *Radiology*[1] details many examples of overuse and misuse of radiologic examinations. This article and a similar one by Dr. Herbert Abrams in the *New England Journal of Medicine*[2] should be mandatory reading for every intern before he or she begins to order examinations. Much of what follows is from Dr. Hall's article.

There are many reasons why it is undesirable to have unnecessary radiologic examinations: excess cost, excess radiation, waste of patient's time, waste of technician's and radiologist's time, false hopes and expectations based on the outcome of the examination, and, not least of all, they indicate a breakdown in the logical thought pattern concerning the patient's workup.

Many examinations are ordered because of so-called medicolegal considerations. It is believed that if a certain finding is not documented (e.g., a broken rib), the doctor could be sued. In fact, few, if any, examples of medicolegal "covering yourself" types of examinations are valid. With the move toward greater consumer awareness, lawsuits in the future are more likely to result from unnecessary radiation exposure because of needless examinations rather than from too few examinations. One study shows that up to "30 per cent of the total x-rays ordered are related to the physician concern for potential malpractice threats and are not primarily designed to assist the patient."[3] This is a sad state of affairs, and it is hoped that more common sense will prevail in the future.

EXAMPLES OF UNNECESARY EXAMINATIONS

Skull Series. Except for a depressed skull fracture or the presence of intracranial metallic fragments, there is no reason to order a skull series for trauma. This is one of the most abused examinations in radiology, costing millions of dollars per year unnecessarily. There is virtually no finding on a skull series that will alter the next step in the patient's workup. Presence or absence of a fracture should not influence whether or not the patient receives a computed tomography (CT) scan. A CT scan is obtained for other reasons: continued unconsciousness or focal neurologic signs. The plain films only delay the eventual diagnosis, and in a patient with a subdural or an epidural hematoma, that delay could be fatal.[4] The mortality from intracranial bleeds is significantly increased as the time to surgical decompression is increased; therefore, any delay caused by obtaining unnecessary examinations (skull films) is potentially harmful. There are no findings on a plain skull series to indicate (or not indicate) subdural or epidural hematoma (Fig. 1–1). Fewer than 10 per cent of patients with fractures have subdural or epidural hematomas, and up to 60 per cent of patients with subdural or epidural bleeds have no fractures.[5,6] Therefore, why order the examinations? Medicolegal reasons? On the contrary! It is well documented that

1

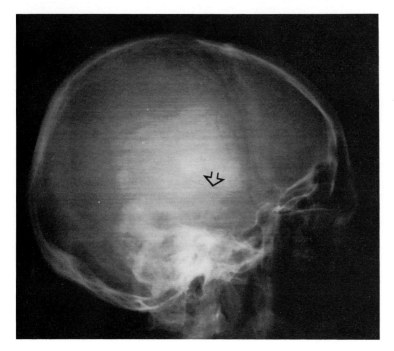

FIGURE 1–1 Skull fracture. A thin radiolucent line characteristic of a skull fracture is noted (arrow) extending obliquely across the temporal bone. A fracture in this area is often associated with an epidural hematoma because the middle meningeal artery lies here. This finding by itself, however, has little or no significance and must be correlated with clinical findings.

delays in diagnosis in this setting can be fatal, so ordering unnecessary examinations might in fact be asking for a lawsuit!

Sinus Series. It is true that an opaque sinus and/or an air-fluid level can be seen with sinusitis. But often the patient with these findings is asymptomatic, and just as often in another patient the sinus series is interpreted as normal when the patient has typical clinical findings of sinusitis. Both of these patients are treated based on their clinical, not radiographic, presentation, which is appropriate. Therefore, the information from the sinus series is ignored. If that is the way you practice—and many recommend that as being proper—don't order the sinus series: treat the patient. Reserve the sinus series for the patient who doesn't respond to treatment, or has an unusual presentation. Also, if it is only sinusitis you are concerned with, most times a simple upright Water's view (Fig. 1–2) to examine the maxillary and frontal sinuses, rather than a full sinus series, will suffice, saving money and decreasing patient exposure.[7]

Nasal Bone. A nasal series is often requested to see if a patient has suffered a broken nose after trauma to the face. So what if the nasal bone is fractured? It won't be casted. It won't be reduced. In other words, no treatment will be given regardless of what the x-ray shows. Therefore, don't order the films in the first place. Occasionally a nasal bone is displaced badly enough to warrant intervention, but even then an acute, posttraumatic x-ray adds nothing for the patient except expense and radiation exposure. A facial series to search for additional fractures might be in order but not a nasal series.

Rib Series. Fractured ribs are commonly seen in any radiologic practice. The significance of the finding of a fractured rib or ribs is not well appreciated by most physicians. If the truth be known, the finding of a rib fracture after trauma has almost no clinical significance and does not alter treatment. One must rule out a pneumothorax and even a lung contusion, both of which are uncommon and are best done on chest films, not a rib series. In older patients with chest wall pain and rib fractures from undetermined causes, it is extremely difficult and often impossible to differentiate a pathologic rib fracture through a metastatic focus from a posttraumatic rib fracture. Hence, x-raying a patient with focal rib pain to find a fracture serves little purpose other than to find a cause for the pain. Most rib series can be eliminated without loss of information.

Coccyx. Although not a common x-ray examination, we receive occasional requests to x-ray the coccyx to rule out a fracture. As with the nasal bone and ribs, a fracture in this location will not be casted or reduced. Also, this examination involves significantly more gonadal radiation dose than a rib or nasal series. Because no treatment is predicated on the x-ray results, don't order the x-ray for routine trauma to the coccyx.

Lumbar Spine. Plain films of the lumbar spine are probably the most abused examinations in radiology. They give the highest gonadal ra-

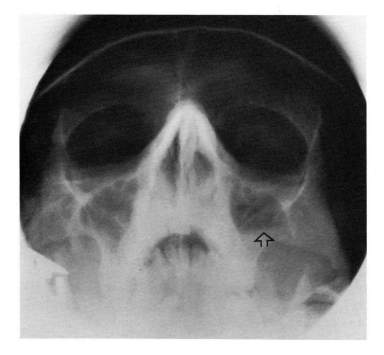

FIGURE 1-2 **Water's view of the sinuses.** This film is obtained with the patient's head slightly tilted upward (as if he were drinking water—apologies to Dr. Water). It is an excellent film to obtain when the maxillary sinuses need to be seen. When done in an upright position, air-fluid levels can be seen (arrow).

diation dose of any plain film examination, and in most cases they offer no diagnostic information that will be acted on by the physician. A significant number of lumbar spine films are done in a population under the age of 40 with acute onset of back pain after lifting or straining. There is virtually no plain film x-ray finding in this patient subgroup that can be responsible for the acute problem or that can be treated. Even the severest spondylolisthesis cannot unequivocally be said to be the origin of the symptoms. Disc herniation cannot be identified. Tumors and infections are not clinical considerations in this setting. Treatment invariably consists of rest, perhaps traction, generally relaxing the muscle groups, and then flexion and extension exercises to strengthen the muscles. Radiographs have nothing to offer unless the pain is very atypical or the clinical picture is clouded by other considerations (such as intravenous drug use, in which case infection must be ruled out).

The gonadal radiation dose from a lumbar spine film is the same as that from a daily chest x-ray for 6,[8] 16,[9] or 98 years,[10] depending on which study you choose to believe. These studies were based on a three-view lumbosacral spine series and do not include the oblique views routinely obtained in many practices. Subtle osseous changes found on oblique views are thought by many orthopedists to be insignificant in most cases anyway.

So when should a lumbosacral spine series be ordered? In cases of severe trauma, possible primary or metastatic tumor, and possible infection. Acute low back pain with radicular signs is no indication for a spine series. A CT scan or magnetic resonance (MR) imaging will show disc herniation and would be the preferred examination over plain films, if clinically warranted.

Metabolic Bone Survey. Many institutions routinely order metabolic bone surveys in patients with hyperparathyroidism or renal osteodystrophy to look for Looser's fractures, brown tumors, and subperiosteal bone resorption. Most institutions have replaced the bone survey with hand films, which is preferable in regard to patient expense and radiation dose. Subperiosteal bone resorption is seen earliest and easiest on the middle phalanges, radial sides (Fig. 1-3), and is virtually pathognomonic for hyperparathyroidism. Looser's fractures are rare and not treated anyway. Brown tumors are uncommon and also are not treated. Therefore, if no treatment is based on the x-ray findings, the survey only satisfies curiosity and is not worth the patient's money or radiation exposure.

Metastatic Bone Survey. Little useful information is obtained from the majority of metastatic bone surveys. Occult lesions that are not found on radionuclide bone scans are seldom encountered. Radionuclide scans are more effective at picking up most metastatic lesions and could be substituted for bone surveys with less cost and better diagnostic yield.[11] Many investigators believe that searching for bone metastases is not warranted in every patient with a primary tumor

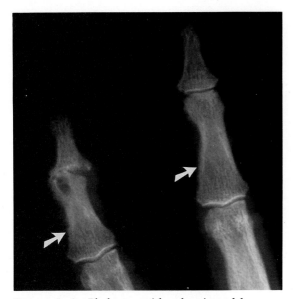

FIGURE 1–3 Phalanges with subperiosteal bone resorption. Subperiosteal bone resorption is seen as a subtle irregularity or interruption of the cortex. It is best seen on the radial aspect of the middle phalanges (arrows) and is pathognomonic for hyperparathyroidism.

unless finding metastatic disease (mets) will obviate surgery or otherwise change the patient's therapy. Radionuclide bone scans with x-rays of questionable or clinically suspicious areas makes more sense than a complete metastatic bone survey. An exception to this is in patients with multiple myeloma. Radionuclide bone scans are often negative in multiple myeloma even with marked skeletal involvement, hence a plain film bone survey is warrented in these patients.

Ankle Series. A significant percentage of all emergency department films are obtained for ankle trauma. Ligamentous injuries can easily be clinically differentiated from significant fractures. One study showed a 50% reduction of ankle films with no fractures missed if the radiology resident would simply examine the patient.[12] Another study revealed that if the patient were able to walk three steps immediately after the injury or during the examination in the emergency room there was almost zero chance of a fracture.[13] Small bony avulsions receive the same treatment as ligament tears, and are often difficult to differentiate from accessory ossicles (Fig. 1–4). Therefore, in most cases the x-ray is not a factor in determining the patient's treatment and could be skipped.

Lumbar Myelograms. One of the most painful radiologic examinations extant is the lumbar myelogram, in which a spinal needle is placed into the subarachnoid space of the lumbar spine and contrast medium is injected (Fig. 1–5). Al-

though this is done for tumors, it is most commonly performed in the workup of lumbar disc disease. Many studies show that CT or MR imaging of the lumbar spine is more accurate than myelography in diagnosing disc disease and emphasize that CT or MR imaging should be the study of choice. Many surgeons, however, still request myelograms in addition to the CT or MR imaging study when only the CT or MR imaging need be performed. In addition to being painful, the myelogram produces side effects in some people that can be pronounced and debilitating; the myelogram occasionally necessitates overnight hospitalization; the radiation dose from the myelogram is higher overall than with CT; and, perhaps most important, the myelogram is not as accurate and does not give as complete a picture of additional back structures as the CT or MR imaging examination (Fig. 1–6). We can hope that the myelogram will go the way of the pneu-

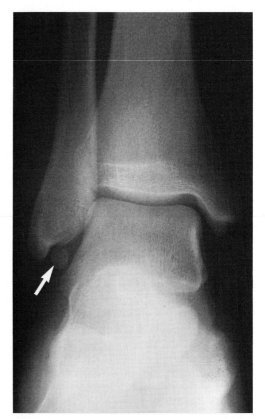

FIGURE 1–4 Ankle after trauma. Calcific densities around the ankle that can be mistaken for avulsions are often seen (arrow). When rounded and smoothly corticated, as in this example, they are either accessory ossicles or old avulsions. An acute avulsion is best diagnosed clinically by noting point tenderness at ligament insertion sites. Because a ligament can avulse with or without a fragment of bone being attached, the x-ray finding will not influence the patient's treatment.

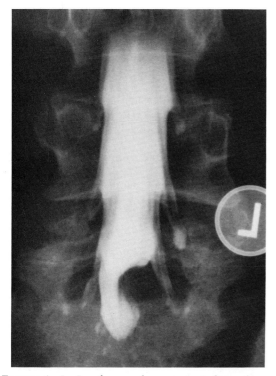

FIGURE 1–5 **Lumbar myelogram.** An iodinated contrast medium has been injected into the subarachnoid space by way of a spinal needle. A large extradural defect is seen that is caused by a disc herniation. A tumor could have a similar appearance. This examination can be quite painful, has occasional long-lasting complications, and gives no information that could not be obtained with a plain CT examination. In some institutions it requires an overnight stay in the hospital as well. For these reasons a majority of doctors prefer a CT scan or an MR imaging exam to a myelogram.

moencephalogram and the epidural venogram.

So far as choosing between a CT scan and MR imaging of the lumbar spine for disc disease and spinal stenosis, either one will suffice. There is very little to be gained from one exam over the other unless it is a postoperative spine, in which case MR imaging is definitely the exam of choice. It must be kept in mind that MR imaging is generally more expensive than CT.

Cervical Spine (C-Spine). Many emergency rooms routinely order C-spine films on all trauma patients, primarily because of the horrible consequences of not stabilizing a fractured neck. This is ridiculous. It has been demonstrated in numerous publications that patients who are alert and have no C-spine pain have almost zero chance of having a fracture.[14] If the patient is unconscious, obtunded for whatever reason, not able to communicate, or has a significant fracture elsewhere, all bets are off. But, if the patient is alert and has no pain with motion on clinical exam of the neck, no C-spine film need be performed.

TECHNICAL CONSIDERATIONS

Avoiding unnecessary examinations constitutes only one way to decrease unnecessary radiation exposure in the general population. Another way to significantly diminish exposure is to collimate the x-ray beam tighter. One study reported that if collimation were limited just to the size of the film, the radiation dose could be reduced by one third.[15] Exposure could be further reduced by having proper filtration, fast screen-film combination, and adequate gonadal shield-

FIGURE 1–6 **Lumbar CT scan.** An axial scan at the L5–S1 level reveals a large right-sided disc herniation (arrows) with some associated calcification or osteophytosis. In addition to the presence of a disc, the neuroforamen, central canal, ligamentum flavum, and facet joints can be evaluated. This makes the CT scan a more complete examination than a myelogram.

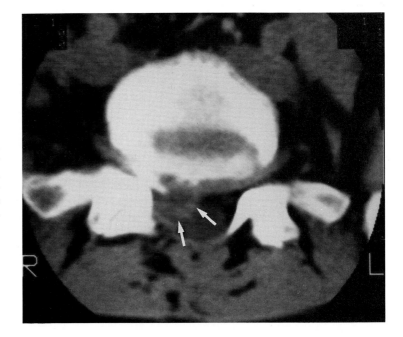

ing. Certainly having properly trained technicians and properly functioning equipment will diminish the number of retakes. These should be high-priority goals for all radiologists to make our specialty more cost-effective and to provide better service to both the referring clinician and the patient. It should be part of every radiologist's responsibility to help educate and guide the unknowing clinician in obtaining the appropriate imaging exams while eliminating those which are unnecessary.

REFERENCES

1. Hall F: Overutilization of radiological examinations. Radiology 1976;120:443–448.
2. Abrams HL: The "overutilization" of x-rays: Sounding board. N Engl J Med 1979;300:1213–1216.
3. Twine EH, Potchen EJ: A dynamic systems analysis of defensive medicine. Thesis, MIT, June 1973.
4. Seelig JM, Becker DP, Miller JD, et al: Traumatic acute subdural hematoma. N Engl J Med 1981;304:1511–1518.
5. Rogers LF: Radiology of Skeletal Trauma. New York, Churchill Livingstone, 1982, p. 187.
6. Masters JS, McClean PM, Arcarese JS, et al: Skull x-ray examinations after head trauma. N Engl J Med 1987;316:84–91.
7. Williams JJ, Roberts L, Distell B, Simel D: Diagnosing sinusitis by x-ray: Comparing a single Waters view to 4-view paranasal sinus radiographs. J Gen Intern Med 1992;7:481–485.
8. Webster EW, Merrill OE: Radiation hazards: II. Measurements of gonadal dose in radiologic examinations. N Engl J Med 1957;257:811–819.
9. Antoku S, Russell WJ: Dose to the active bone marrow, gonads, and skin from roentgenography and fluoroscopy. Radiology 1957;101:669–678.
10. Andron GM, Crooks HE: Gonad radiation dose from diagnostic procedures. Br J Radiol 1957;30:295–297.
11. Mall JC, Bekerman C, Hoffer PB, et al: A unified radiological approach to the detection of skeletal metastases. Radiology 1976;118:323–329.
12. Auletta A, Conway W, Hayes C, et al: Indications for radiography in patients with acute ankle injuries: Role of the physical examination. AJR 1991;157:789–791.
13. Stiell I, Greenberg G, McKnight R: Decision rules for the use of radiography in acute ankle injuries. JAMA 1993;269:1127–1132.
14. Mirvis S, Diaconis J, Chirico P: Protocol-driven radiologic evaluation of suspected cervical spine injury: Efficacy study. Radiology 1989;170:831–834.
15. Morgan RH: Hearings before the Committee on Commerce, Science and Transportation. U.S. Senate, an oversight of radiation health and safety. 95th Congress, 1st session, June 1977, pp. 241–266.

2

Benign Cystic Lesions

A benign, bubbly cystic lesion of bone is probably one of the most common skeletal findings a radiologist encounters. The differential diagnosis can be quite lengthy and is usually given on an "Aunt Minnie" basis (I know that's Aunt Minnie because she *looks* like Aunt Minnie); in other words, the differential diagnosis is structured on how the lesion looks to the radiologist, using his or her experience as a guide. This method, called "pattern identification," certainly has merit, but it can lead to many erroneous conclusions if not tempered with some logic. For instance, most radiologists would justifiably miss the diagnosis of a rare presentation of a primary malignant neoplasm that initially looks benign. Many of these radiologists would subsequently insist on including primary malignant neoplasms in their benign cystic differential even though the rare malignancy is "1 in a million." If every differential is geared to cover even the long shots, there would be a lot of extremely long differentials, and the clinicians wouldn't get much useful information from us. We might as well give the clinician the index to a multivolume bone book as give a differential that will never miss anything.

Then again, you don't want a differential diagnosis list that is wrong half the time. You could almost do better with a coin flip. I'm willing to accept a differential that is accurate (that is, one that contains the correct diagnosis) 95 per cent of the time. This is acceptable to me for most skeletal entities; however, I would be remiss if I were willing to accept a 1-out-of-20 miss rate for fractures and dislocations. Nevertheless, for most of the entities in this book I will accept a 95 per cent accuracy differential and would expect most

radiologists to concur. If you want to be more accurate than that, you simply add more diagnoses to the list of differential possibilities.

The shorter the differential diagnosis list, the handier it is to remember and apply. As the differential list gets longer, it generally gets more accurate, but it can be difficult to remember and often falls into disuse. Mnemonics are helpful in recalling long lists of information, and I will pass on many that I use; many people, however, do not like to use mnemonics (for no good reason that I've been able to ascertain) and will just have to use whatever method that works for them to remember the differentials. The list of entities that cause benign cystic lesions is quite long, and therefore a mnemonic is helpful in recalling them.

I was a flight surgeon in the Air Force before my radiology residency, and I would spend a half day a week or so with the radiologist, trying to pick up some pearls. This radiologist was Ivan Barrett and he did me a great favor. He taught me the mnemonic FEGNOMASHIC, which is made up from the first letter of each of the entities in the differential of benign cystic lesions of bone. For instance, the *F* stands for fibrous dysplasia, the *E* for enchondroma, and so on, as I will show. I diligently learned what each letter stood for, even though I had no idea what most of the processes were or looked like on an x-ray. Before I could learn another mnemonic from Ivan (I was a slow learner), I moved away to begin residency.

Sure enough, the first week of residency, in a formal conference with 15 to 20 residents present, I was chosen as the sacrificial lamb among the first-year residents to take an unknown case. It happened to be a benign cystic lesion, which I proceeded to expound on with a list of 12 to 15 differential possibilities. The conference room got quiet, I was thanked cordially but a little frostily, and the conference was adjourned. One of the first-year residents, whom I barely knew at the time, asked how I knew so many of the possibilities on that case, since the staff man showing the case (who was a chest radiologist) didn't even know that many. I explained, with a straight face, that those just seemed like the logical things to mention. I was trying to be matter-of-fact and not come off as too much of a show-off, but I couldn't help laughing. I then told the resident how I had learned a single mnemonic and by getting lucky it made me seem to know a lot more than I really did. He and the rest of my fellow residents were relieved and quickly learned the mnemonic themselves. I became hopelessly addicted to mnemonics from that day on.

FEGNOMASHIC

FEGNOMASHIC is defined in "Funk and Wagner's" unabridged dictionary, 13th edition, as "one who uses mnemonics." It serves as a nice starting point for discussing possibilities that appear as benign cystic lesions in bone. That mnemonic has been in general use for many years, but I have never heard a claim as to who first coined it. The first mention of it that I saw in print was in 1972 in a radiology article by Gold and Margulis. By itself it is merely a long list—about 14 entities—and needs to be coupled with other criteria to shorten the list into manageable form for each particular case. For instance, if the lesion is epiphyseal, only three to five entities, depending on how accurate you care to be, need to be mentioned. If multiple lesions are present, only half a dozen entities need to be discussed. Ways of narrowing the differential are discussed later in this chapter.

The next step after learning the names of all the lesions is getting some idea of what each one looks like. This is where experience becomes a factor. For the medical student or first-year resident it's difficult to go beyond saying that they all look cystic or bubbly and benign. However, the third-year resident should have no trouble

---

TABLE 2–1 Differential Criteria for Benign Lytic Bone Lesions

Mnemonic: Fegnomashic

F   *Fibrous Dysplasia* = No periosteal reaction; if in tibia, mention adamantinoma

E   *Enchondroma* = Must have calcificaton, except in phalanges; no periostitis

     Eosinophilic Granuloma (EG) = Must be under 30

G   *Giant Cell Tumor (GCT)* = (1) Epiphyses must be closed; (2) must be epiphyseal *and* abut the articular surface; (3) eccentric; (4) well-defined but nonsclerotic border

N   *Nonossifying fibroma (NOF)* = Must be under 30; no periostitis

O   *Osteoblastoma* = Mentioned whenever ABC is mentioned, even if over 30

M   *Mets and Myeloma* = Must be over 40

A   *Aneurysmal Bone Cyst (ABC)* = Must be under 30; expansile

S   *Solitary Bone Cyst* = Must be centrally located; under age 30

H   *Hyperparathyroidism (Brown Tumor)* = Must have other evidence of hyperparathyroidism

I   *Infection* = If adjacent to a joint, must involve the joint (weak)

C   *Chondroblastoma* = Must be under 30; epiphyseal

     Chondromyxoid Fibroma = Mention when considering nonossifying fibroma

Less Than 30	No Periostitis or Pain	Epiphyseal	Multiple
EG	Fibrous dysplasia	Chondroblastoma	(Mnemonic: FEEMHI)
ABC	Enchondroma	Infection	Fibrous dysplasia
NOF	NOF	GCT	EG
Chondroblastoma	Solitary bone cyst	Geode	Enchondroma
Solitary bone cyst		(EG and ABC are optional)	Mets and Myeloma
			Hyperparathyroidism
			Infection

differentiating between a unicameral bone cyst and a giant cell tumor because he or she has seen examples of each many times before and knows what each looks like. The third-year resident may have a hard time verbalizing the differences but should be able to tell them apart.

A novice can quickly gain experience by looking at the examples of each of these lesions in a major skeletal radiology text. In fact, I highly recommend that you compare my description and differential points on each lesion with multiple examples in other books. Some of these lesions can only be diagnosed radiologically on a "pattern identification" or "Aunt Minnie" basis. In other words, there are no hard and fast criteria to differentiate some of the lesions from the others.

After getting a feel for what each lesion looks like radiographically, and overcoming the frustration that builds when you realize that many of them look alike, you should try to learn ways to differentiate each lesion from the others. I have developed a number of keys that I call "discriminators" that will help to differentiate each lesion. These discriminators are 90 to 95 per cent useful (I will mention when they are more or less accurate, in my experience) and are by no means meant to be absolutes or dogma. They are guidelines but have a high confidence rate.

Textbooks rarely tell you that a finding "always" or "never" occurs. They temper their descriptions with "virtually always," or "invariably," or "usually," or "characteristically." I have tried to pick out findings that come as close to "always" as I can, realizing that I will usually only be 95 per cent accurate. That's good enough for me. If it's not good enough for you, you'll have to get your own differential criteria or discriminators. Try these and see if they work for you. If they don't modify them as necessary. But whatever you do, develop *reasons* for including things in your differential. Have concrete criteria of some kind for including or excluding each entity.

I will give a brief description of each entity, as complete descriptions are readily available in any skeletal radiology text. What I will dwell on, however, are the points that are unique for each entity, thereby enabling differentiation from the others. Table 2–1 is a synopsis of these discriminators.

FIBROUS DYSPLASIA

It is unfortunate that this differential starts with fibrous dysplasia because fibrous dysplasia can look like almost anything. It can be wild-looking, a discrete lucency, patchy, sclerotic, expansile, multiple, and a host of other descriptions.

It is, therefore, difficult to look at a bubbly lytic lesion and unequivocally say it is or is not fibrous dysplasia. When assessing such a lesion, radiology residents usually say, "I suppose it *could* be fibrous dysplasia, but I'm not sure." The resident is feeling insecure and becomes defensive right off, setting the tone for the entire differential diagnosis. It would be better if the differential started on a positive note, say, with giant cell tumor or chondroblastoma, where there are some hard and definite criteria. That way the resident would set the tone of self-assurance and decisiveness rather than appear wishy-washy.

How do you know whether to include or exclude fibrous dysplasia if it can look like almost anything? Experience is the best guideline. In other words, look in a few texts and find as many different examples as you can; get a feeling for what fibrous dysplasia looks like. A few examples are shown here (Figs. 2–1 to 2–6), but pouring

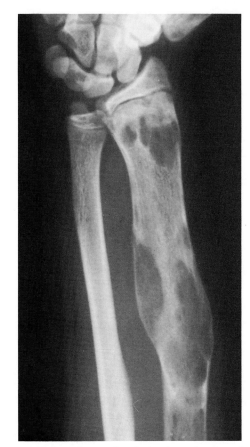

FIGURE 2–1 Fibrous dysplasia. A predominantly lytic lesion with some sclerosis and expansion is seen in the distal half of the radius in a child. A long lesion in a long bone typifies fibrous dysplasia. Although parts of this lesion indeed have a ground-glass appearance, most of it does not. Expansion and bone deformity like this is commonly seen in fibrous dysplasia.

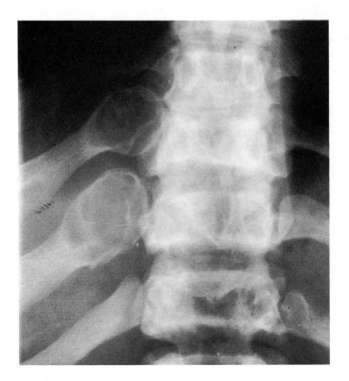

FIGURE 2–2 **Fibrous dysplasia.** The ribs are often involved with fibrous dysplasia, as in this example. When the posterior ribs are involved the process is often a lytic expansile lesion, whereas when the anterior ribs are involved it is commonly a sclerotic process.

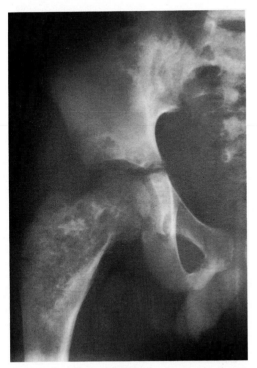

FIGURE 2–3 **Fibrous dysplasia.** An expansile mixed lytic/sclerotic process in the proximal femur is a common pattern for fibrous dysplasia. Note that the supra-acetabular region is also involved. The ipsilateral proximal femur is invariably affected when the pelvis is involved with fibrous dysplasia.

over another text for 10 to 15 minutes will be time well spent.

Fibrous dysplasia will not have periostitis associated with it; therefore, if periostitis is present, you can safely exclude fibrous dysplasia. It would be possible to have a pathologic fracture through an area of fibrous dysplasia, which then had periostitis, but I have never seen this occur. Fibrous dysplasia virtually never undergoes malignant degeneration and should not be a painful lesion in the long bones unless there is a fracture.

Fibrous dysplasia can be either monostotic (most commonly) or polyostotic and has a predilection for the pelvis, proximal femur, ribs, and skull. When it is present in the pelvis, it is invariably present in the ipsilateral proximal femur (Figs. 2–3 and 2–4). I have seen only one case in which the pelvis was involved with fibrous dysplasia and the proximal femur was spared. The proximal femur, however, may be affected alone, without involvement in the pelvis (Figs. 2–5 and 2–6).

The classic description of fibrous dysplasia is that it has a ground-glass or smoky appearing matrix. This description confuses people rather than helps them, and I do not recommend using "ground-glass appearance" as a buzz word for fibrous dysplasia. Fibrous dysplasia is often purely lytic and becomes hazy or takes on a ground-glass look as the matrix calcifies. It can go on to calcify quite a bit, and then it presents

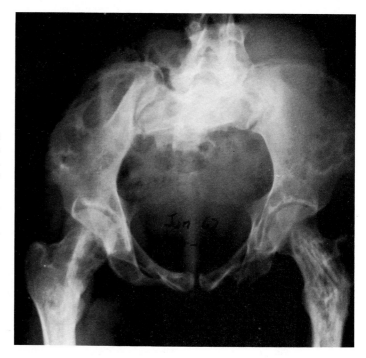

FIGURE 2–4 **Fibrous dysplasia.** The entire pelvis and proximal femurs are diffusely involved with polyostotic fibrous dysplasia. The pelvis is severely deformed with predominantly lytic lesions. The proximal femurs are involved with both lytic and sclerotic lesions.

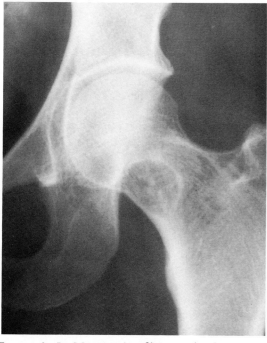

FIGURE 2–5 **Monostotic fibrous dysplasia.** The proximal femur is a common place for monostotic fibrous dysplasia. This presentation is typical and should not be confused with an infection. Some speckled calcification is noted within the lesion that should not be misconstrued as chondroid calcification in an enchondroma.

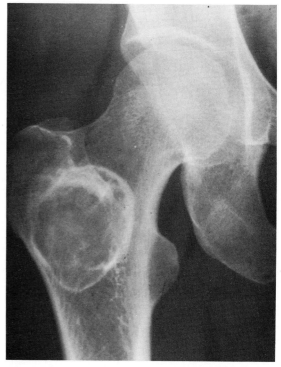

FIGURE 2–6 **Monostotic fibrous dysplasia.** Another example of proximal femur involvement that shows a lytic lesion with a thick sclerotic border reminiscent of a chronic infection. This is characteristic of fibrous dysplasia in the hip.

as a sclerotic lesion. Also, I often see other lytic lesions that have a distinct ground-glass appearance; therefore the ground-glass quality can be misleading.

When a lesion in the tibia that has fibrous dysplasia in the differential diagnosis is encountered, an adamantinoma should also be mentioned (Fig. 2–7). An adamantinoma is a malignant tumor that radiographically and histologically resembles fibrous dysplasia. It occurs almost exclusively in the tibia and the jaw (for unknown reasons) and is rare. Because it is rare you may choose not to include it in your memory bank— you won't miss more than one or two in your life, even if you're a busy radiologist.

Polyostotic fibrous dysplasia occasionally occurs in association with café au lait spots on the skin (dark-pigmented, freckle-like lesions) and precocious puberty. This complex is called McCune-Albright syndrome. The bony lesions in this syndrome, and even in the simple polyostotic

form, often occur unilaterally (that is, in one half of the body). This doesn't happen often enough to be of any diagnostic use in differentiating fibrous dysplasia from other lesions. The presence of multiple lesions in the jaw has been termed cherubism, which relates to the physical appearance of the affected child. Such children present with puffed out cheeks, producing an "angelic" look. The jaw lesions in cherubism regress in adulthood.

Discriminator:
No periosteal reaction.

ENCHONDROMA AND EOSINOPHILIC GRANULOMA
Enchondroma

The most common benign cystic lesion of the phalanges is an enchondroma (Fig. 2–8). Enchondromas occur in any bone formed from cartilage and may be central, eccentric, expansile, or nonexpansile. They invariably contain calcified chondroid matrix (Fig. 2–9A) except when in the phalanges. If a cystic lesion is present without calcified chondroid matrix anywhere except in the phalanges, I will not include enchondroma in my differential.

Often it is difficult to differentiate between an enchondroma and a bone infarct. Although some of the following criteria are helpful in separating an infarct from an enchondroma, they are not foolproof. An infarct usually has a well-defined, densely sclerotic, serpiginous border, whereas an enchondroma does not (Fig. 2–9B). An enchondroma often causes endosteal scalloping, whereas a bone infarct will not.

It is difficult, if not impossible, to differentiate an enchondroma from a chondrosarcoma. Clinical findings (primarily pain) serve as a better indicator than radiographic findings, and indeed pain in an apparent enchondroma should warrant surgical investigation. Periostitis should not be seen in an enchondroma either. Trying to differentiate an enchondroma from a chondrosarcoma histologically is also difficult, if not impossible at times. Therefore, biopsy of an apparent enchondroma should not be performed routinely for histologic differentiation.

Multiple enchondromas occur on occasion, and this condition has been termed Ollier's disease (Fig. 2–10A). It is not hereditary and does not have an increased rate of malignant degeneration. The presence of multiple enchondromas associated with soft tissue hemangiomas is known as Maffucci's syndrome (Fig. 2–10B). This syndrome also is not hereditary; however, it is characterized by an increased incidence of malignant degeneration of the enchondromas.

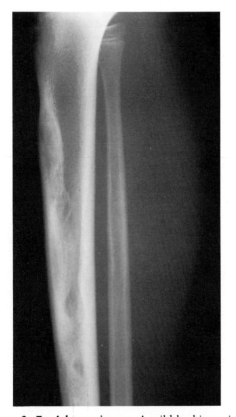

FIGURE 2–7 **Adamantinoma.** A wild-looking mixed lytic and sclerotic lesion in the tibia that resembles fibrous dysplasia is classic for an adamantinoma. This lesion occurs only in the tibia and in the jaw and has some malignant potential. An adamantinoma should always be considered when a lesion resembling fibrous dysplasia is seen in the tibia.

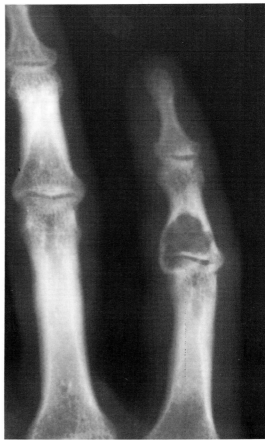

FIGURE 2–8 **Enchondroma.** A benign lytic lesion in the hand is an enchondroma until proved otherwise. This is a common presentation of an enchondroma. Enchondromas in any other part of the body should contain some calcified chondroid matrix before they are included in the differential. However, calcified chondroid matrix is unusual in the phalanges.

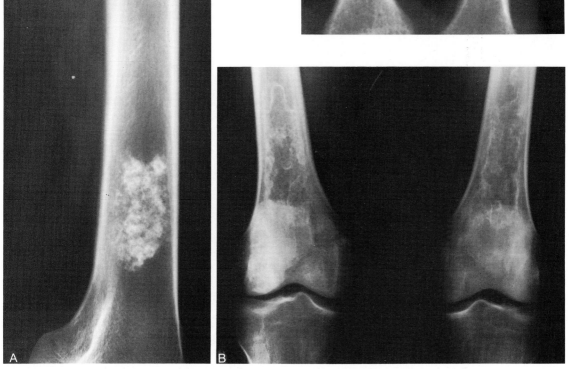

A

B

FIGURE 2–9 *(A)* **Enchondroma.** A lesion in the distal femur is seen with irregular speckled calcification typical of chondroid matrix. This is virtually pathognomonic of an enchondroma. A chondrosarcoma could have an identical appearance but requires clinical symptomatology for consideration in the differential diagnosis. A bone infarct can be similar in appearance to an enchondroma. *(B)* **Bone infarcts.** Bilateral lytic lesions in the femurs are noted with a densely calcified serpiginous border characteristic of bone infarcts. Compare these lesions with *(A)*, which does not have a well-defined serpiginous border. Often the differentiation between bone infarcts as in this example and an enchondroma *(A)* is not so clear-cut. (Case courtesy of Dr. Hideyo Minagi.)

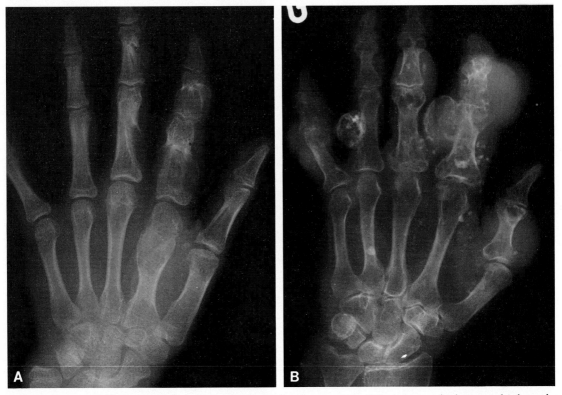

FIGURE 2–10 *(A)* **Ollier's.** Multiple lytic lesions in the hand are seen in this patient, which are multiple enchondromas. This is known as Ollier's disease. *(B)* **Maffucci's.** Multiple enchondromas associated with soft tissue hemangiomas are seen in the hand in this patient. This is Maffucci's syndrome. Note the multiple rounded calcifications in the soft tissues, which are phleboliths in the hemangiomas.

Discriminators:

1. Must have calcification (except in phalanges).
2. No periostitis.

Eosinophilic Granuloma

Eosinophilic granuloma (EG) is a form of histiocytosis X, the other forms being Letterer-Siwe disease and Hand-Schüller-Christian disease. Although these forms may be merely different phases of the same disease, most investigators categorize them separately. The bony manifestations of all three disorders are similar and are discussed in this text simply as eosinophilic granuloma, or EG.

EG, unfortunately for radiologists, has many appearances. It can be lytic or blastic; it may be well defined or ill defined (Figs. 2–11 and 2–12); it may or may not have a sclerotic border; and it may or may not elicit a periosteal response.[1]

The periostitis, when present, is typically benign in appearance (thick, uniform, wavy) but can be lamellated or amorphous. EG can mimic Ewing's sarcoma and present as a permeative (multiple small holes) lesion.

How, then, can one distinguish EG from any of the other lytic lesions in this differential? Let me say right out that it is difficult to exclude EG from almost any differential of a bony lesion. Although some authorities say that up to 20 per cent of EG occurs in patients over the age of 30, others claim that it is rare in older age-groups. I have seen only one or two cases of EG in someone over the age of 30 and have seen at least 100 cases in children and young adults. Therefore, I find the 30 years' cutoff point quite useful and am willing to exclude the diagnosis of EG in anyone over the age of 30. (I accept the fact that I will miss the diagnosis in older age-groups, but I hate to clutter up *every* differential with EG.)

EG is most often monostotic, but it can be

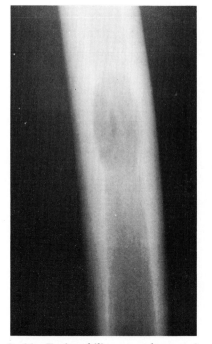

FIGURE 2–11 **Eosinophilic granuloma.** A well-defined lytic lesion in the midshaft of a femur in a child. At biopsy this was shown to be eosinophilic granuloma. This is an entirely nonspecific pattern that could easily represent a focus of infection or one of several other processes. Because the lesion is present in a child, eosinophilic granuloma must be included in the differential diagnosis.

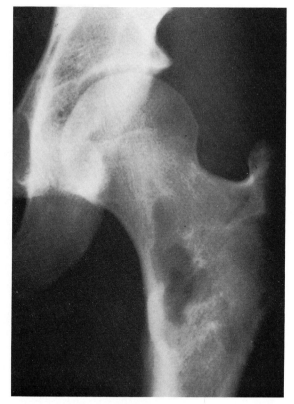

FIGURE 2–12 **Eosinophilic granuloma.** A predominantly lytic process with some sclerosis is seen in the proximal femur in a child. Again, this case would have a long differential diagnosis. Eosinophilic granuloma must be mentioned because the patient is under the age of 30. In this example the zone of transition is narrow and the lesion appears benign, but eosinophilic granuloma can have an aggressive appearance and mimic a sarcoma.

polyostotic and thus has to be included whenever multiple lesions are present.

EG may or may not have a soft tissue mass associated with it, so the presence or absence of a soft tissue mass will not help in the differential diagnosis. In fact, I know of no entity in which presence or absence of an associated soft tissue mass will warrant inclusion or exclusion of a process from a differential. It is important to note the presence of a soft tissue mass (or its absence), but it will do little to narrow your differential diagnosis.

EG occasionally has a bony sequestrum (Fig. 2–13). Only three other entities have been described that, on occasion, have bone sequestra: osteomyelitis, lymphoma and fibrosarcoma. Therefore, when a sequestrum is identified, these four entities should be considered (Table 2–2). (Another entity, osteoid osteoma, can sometimes have an appearance that mimics a sequestrum—this is discussed in Chapter 8, Miscellaneous Conditions.)

Clinically, EG may or may not be associated with pain; therefore, clinical history is noncontributory for the most part.

Discriminator:
Must be under age 30.

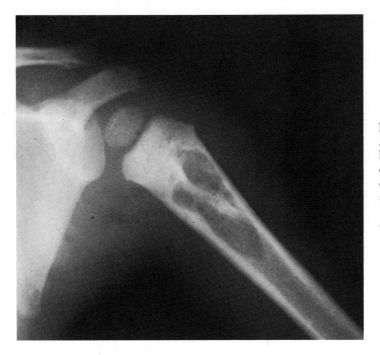

FIGURE 2–13 **Eosinophilic granuloma.** A well-defined lytic lesion with a dense bony sequestrum in the proximal humerus of a child should conjure up the diagnosis of an infection. Eosinophilic granuloma also occasionally has a bony sequestrum (as in this example) and must be considered.

TABLE 2–2 **Entities That Can Present with a Sequestration**

Osteomyelitis
Eosinophilic granuloma
Fibrosarcoma (includes malignant fibrous histiocytoma and desmoids)
Lymphoma
(Osteoid osteoma mimics a sequestration)

GIANT CELL TUMOR

Giant cell tumor (GCT) is a somewhat controversial lesion with several schools of thought as to its radiographic appearance. I subscribe to the most widely used approach and will only briefly mention the other viewpoints.

First, it is important to realize that one is unable to tell, regardless of its radiographic appearance, if a GCT is benign or malignant. In fact, histologically, a GCT cannot be divided into either a benign or a malignant category. Most surgeons curettage and pack the lesions and consider them benign unless they recur. Even then they can still be benign and recur a second or third time. About 15 per cent of GCTs are thought to be malignant, based on their recurrence rate.

I use four radiographic criteria for diagnosing GCTs (Figs. 2–14 and 2–15). If any of these criteria are not met when looking at a lesion, I discard GCT from my differential diagnosis.

Number one: Giant cell tumor occurs only in patients with closed epiphyses; this is valid at least 98 to 99 per cent of the time and is extremely useful. I will not entertain the diagnosis of GCT in a patient with open epiphyses.

Number two: The lesion must be epiphyseal and abut the articular surface. There is disagreement over whether GCTs begin in the epiphysis or metaphysis, or from the physeal plate itself; however, except for rare cases, when radiologists see the lesions, they are epiphyseal and are flush against the articular surface. The metaphysis also has some of the tumor in it because the lesions are generally very large. I'm not terribly interested in the embryogenesis of a lesion when I'm looking at it as an unknown and a handful of surgeons are breathing down my neck wanting a differential diagnosis. I (and they) want to be able to intelligently say what it is or is not. Therefore, I don't get caught up in the argument of where the lesion began. When you see a GCT, it will be epiphyseal. Perhaps more important, it should be flush against the articular surface of the joint. This occurs in 98 to 99 per cent of GCTs[2]; therefore, if I have a lesion that is separated from the articular surface by a definite margin of bone, I will not include GCT in the diagnosis.

Number three: These lesions are said to be eccentrically located in the bone, as opposed to being centrally placed in the medullary cavity. I don't find this to be a terribly helpful description, but it is one of the classic "rules" of a GCT. It is accurate; however, occasionally the lesion is so

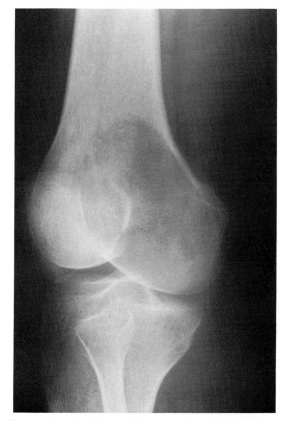

FIGURE 2–14 **Giant cell tumor.** A well-defined lytic lesion in the distal femur that has all four criteria typical for a giant cell tumor: (1) a well-defined but non-sclerotic zone of transition, (2) the epiphyses are closed, (3) the lesion is eccentrically placed in the bone, and (4) the lesion is epiphyseal and abuts the articular surface. If any one of these criteria were *not* adhered to, I would not include giant cell tumor in my differential.

ossifying fibromas, will usually have a sclerotic margin, but it doesn't occur enough to include as a differential point). No other lesion must always abut the articular surface, and no other lesion has the classic description of being eccentrically placed (although several lesions, including non-ossifying fibroma and chondromyxoid fibroma, are in fact eccentric in greater than 98 per cent of cases).

So although these four criteria work nicely for GCT, they don't work at all for any other lesions. Residents have a tendency to apply these criteria to every lytic lesion encountered for the simple reason that they've learned the four criteria. Once one of the criteria is violated, the remainder don't even have to be used to eliminate a GCT. For instance, if a lytic lesion is found in the mid-diaphysis of a bone, GCT can be excluded. There's no need to check further to see if it's eccentric, if it has a nonsclerotic margin, or if the epiphyses are closed.

Again, these "rules" will be greater than 95 per cent effective and, in my experience, close to 99 per cent effective. If one or two cases are found that don't fit the criteria, another pathologist should probably review the slides. Many pathologists refer to aneurysmal bone cysts as GCTs; hence they have "giant cell tumors" that don't

large that it's difficult to tell whether or not it is really eccentric.

Number four: The lesion must have a sharply defined zone of transition (border) that is not sclerotic. This is a very helpful finding in GCT. The only places this does not apply is in flat bones, such as the pelvis, and the calcaneus.

Using these four "rules" will allow one to eliminate GCT from a list of differential possibilities with accuracy and assurance, when otherwise it would have to be included. Unwarranted inclusion of a lesion in a differential tends to clutter up the list and make it unnecessarily long.

It is important to realize that the four criteria for a GCT apply only to GCTs and to no other lesion. For instance, I know of no other lesion that is dependent on whether the epiphyses are open or closed. No other lesion in any of my lists can be defined by whether or not the zone of transition is sclerotic (many lesions, such as non-

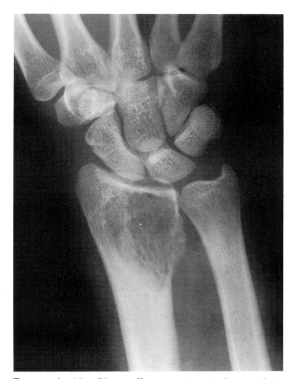

FIGURE 2–15 **Giant cell tumor.** A typical example in the distal radius, which is a common location for giant cell tumor.

obey *any* of the criteria. These pathologists may be correct, but they are not in the mainstream of what most people use for GCT criteria, both radiographically and histologically.

Discriminators:

1. Epiphyses must be closed.
2. Must abut the articular surface.
3. Must be well defined with a nonsclerotic margin.
4. Must be eccentric.

NONOSSIFYING FIBROMA

A nonossifying fibroma (NOF) is probably the most common bone lesion encountered by radiologists. It reportedly occurs in up to 20 per cent

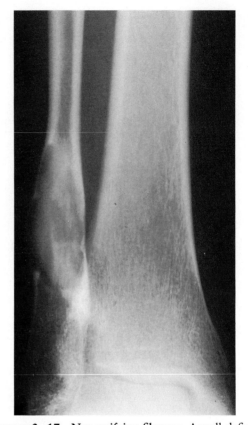

FIGURE 2–17 Nonossifying fibroma. A well-defined expansile lytic lesion in the distal fibula is noted, which is characteristic for a nonossifying fibroma. The patient was asymptomatic, and the lesion was an incidental finding. The faint sclerosis seen in the lesion is secondary to the partial calcification or ossification of the matrix, which in a few years time will be complete as the lesion disappears.

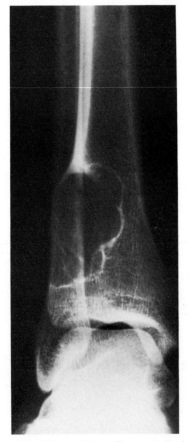

FIGURE 2–16 Nonossifying fibroma. A classic example of a nonossifying fibroma that is slightly expansile and lytic and has a scalloped, well-defined sclerotic border. The location in the metaphysis is characteristic. The fact that the cortex is not well seen should not imply cortical destruction but rather that the cortex has been replaced with benign fibrous tissue. This was an incidental finding in a patient who was asymptomatic.

of children and usually spontaneously regresses so as to be seen only rarely after the age of 30. "Fibrous cortical defect" is a common synonym, although some people divide the two lesions on the basis of size, with fibrous cortical defect being smaller than 2 cm in length and NOF being larger than 2 cm. Histologically, these lesions are identical; therefore, it seems illogical to subdivide the lesion by its size.

NOFs are benign, asymptomatic lesions that typically occur in the metaphysis of a long bone emanating from the cortex (Figs. 2–16 to 2–18). They classically have a thin, sclerotic border that is scalloped and slightly expansile; however, this is a general description that probably applies to only 75 per cent of the lesions. They do not have to have expansion or a scalloped or sclerotic border, and they are not limited to the metaphyses. Then how will you recognize them? The best way is, again, familiarize yourself with their general

FIGURE 2–18 Nonossifying fibroma. A multilocular, expansile, well-defined lytic lesion in a long bone of a child who is asymptomatic. There is no need to do a biopsy for diagnosis because this is an obviously benign lesion and characteristic of a nonossifying fibroma.

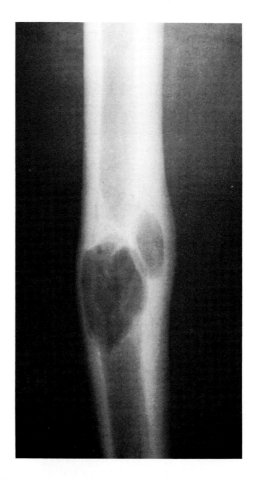

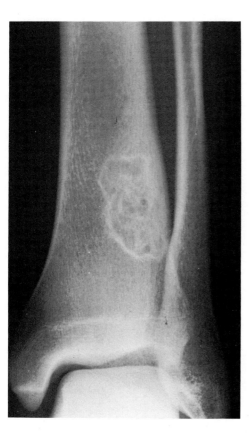

FIGURE 2–19 Healing nonossifying fibroma. A lesion in a young adult, characteristic of a nonossifying fibroma that is beginning to disappear or "heal." As these lesions are typically not seen in patients over the age of 30, it is thought that they ossify and then blend into the normal bone.

appearance by looking at examples in textbooks. That can be done in 15 minutes. It's important to recognize these lesions because they are what I call "don't touch" lesions; that is, the radiologist's diagnosis should be the final word and thereby supplant a biopsy (see Chapter 4, "Don't Touch" Lesions). These lesions are so characteristic that no logical differential diagnosis should be entertained, although a few entities can indeed occasionally simulate them.

I use age 30 as a cutoff point for NOFs. If the patient is over 30 years of age, I will not include NOF in the differential diagnosis. The lesions must be asymptomatic and exhibit no periostitis, unless there is an antecedent history of trauma. NOFs routinely "heal" with sclerosis and even-

tually disappear (Figs. 2–19 and 2–20). During this "healing" period they can appear hot on a radionuclide bone scan because there is osteoblastic activity. Computed tomography (CT) scan can show apparent cortical breakthrough, which is really only fibrous tissue replacing cortex (Fig. 2–21). These lesions can occasionally get quite large (Fig. 2–22); therefore, growth or change in size will not alter the diagnosis. They are most commonly seen about the knee but can occur in any long bone.

Discriminators:

1. Must be under age 30.
2. No periostitis or pain.

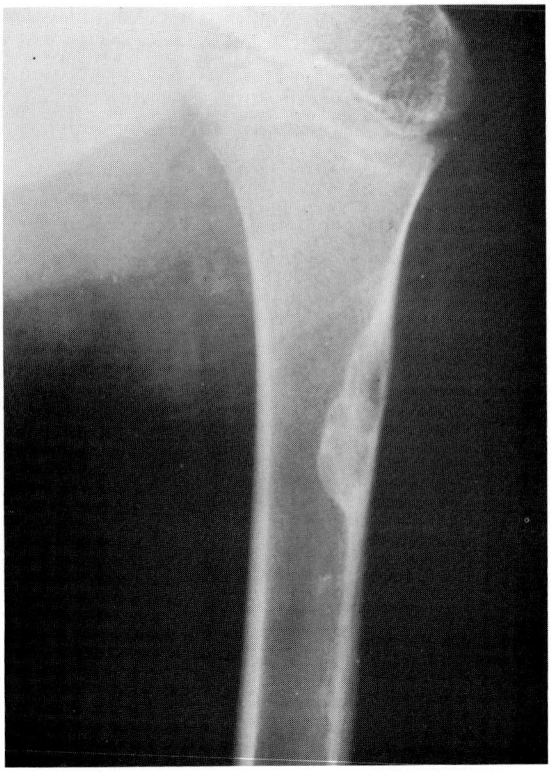

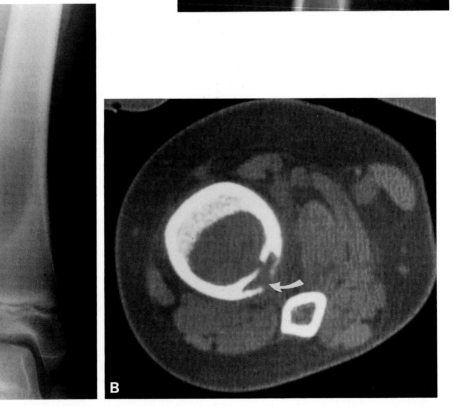

FIGURE 2–20 **Healing nonossifying fibroma.** A typical nonossifying fibroma in the proximal humerus of a child that is beginning to ossify. In a few years time this lesion will essentially be nonexistent.

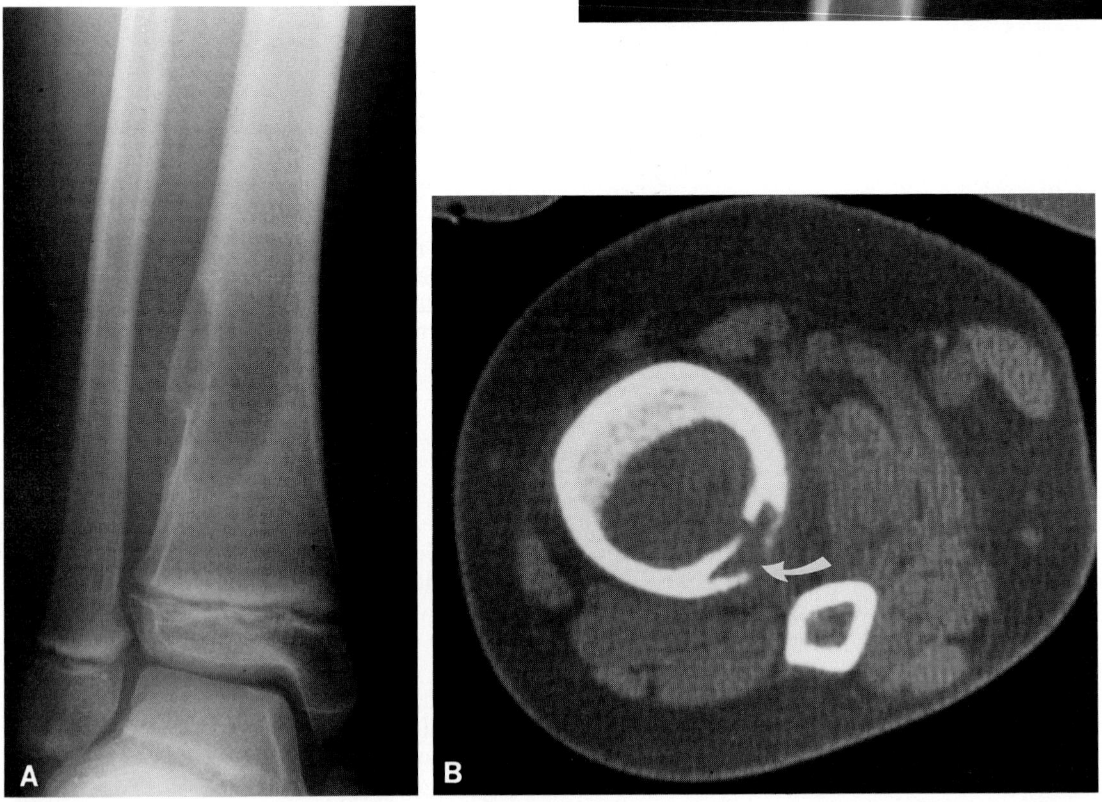

FIGURE 2–21 **CT of nonossifying fibroma.** An AP plain film *(A)* shows an expansile lytic lesion that was seen when this child had x-rays obtained for a sprained ankle. This is typical for a nonossifying fibroma. A CT scan was obtained through this lesion (for no good reason) *(B);* it shows some disruption of the cortex (arrow), which was felt to represent "cortical destruction." The lesion was therefore biopsied and found to be a nonossifying fibroma. This cortex is not destroyed but rather replaced with benign fibrous tissue.

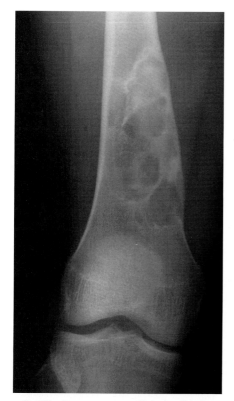

FIGURE 2–22 Large nonossifying fibroma. This large, expansile, well-defined lytic lesion was noted in an asymptomatic 16-year-old and biopsied because it had grown over a several year follow-up. It was found to be a nonossifying fibroma. There is little justification for biopsying this lesion, even though it is larger than most nonossifying fibromas.

OSTEOBLASTOMA

Osteoblastomas are rare lesions that could justifiably be excluded from this differential without the fear of missing a diagnosis more than once in your lifetime. Why, then, include them? The mnemonic FEGNOMASHIC would not have nearly the same ring without the extra vowel, so osteoblastoma remains.

Osteoblastomas have two appearances: (1) They look like large osteoid osteomas and are often called giant osteoid osteomas. Because osteoid osteomas are sclerotic lesions and do not resemble bubbly lytic lesions, this is not the type of osteoblastoma we are concerned with in this differential. (2) They simulate aneurysmal bone cysts (ABCs). They are expansile, often having a soap bubble appearance (Fig. 2–23). If an ABC is being considered, so should an osteoblastoma. They most commonly occur in the posterior elements of the vertebral bodies, and about half of the cases demonstrate speckled calcifications. A classic radiology differential is that of an expan-

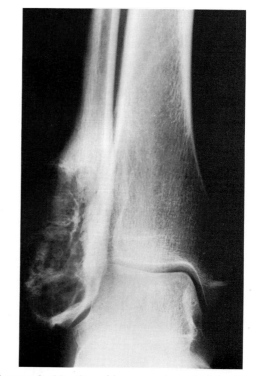

FIGURE 2–23 Osteoblastoma. A well-defined, expansile, lytic lesion in a 35-year-old patient that looks like an aneurysmal bone cyst. This is only one appearance of this very rare lesion (the other appearance being a sclerotic lesion similar to an osteoid osteoma, although considerably larger).

TABLE 2–3 Differential Diagnosis of Expansile, Lytic Lesion in Posterior Elements of Spine

Aneurysmal bone cyst
Osteoblastoma
Tuberculosis

sile lytic lesion of the posterior elements of the spine, and it includes osteoblastoma, ABC, and tuberculosis (Table 2–3).

Discriminator:

Mentioned when ABC is mentioned.

METASTATIC DISEASE AND MYELOMA

Metastatic disease (mets) should be considered for any lytic lesion—benign or aggressive in appearance—in a patient over the age of 40. Mets can appear perfectly benign radiographically (Fig. 2–24), so it is not valid to say, "Since this lesion

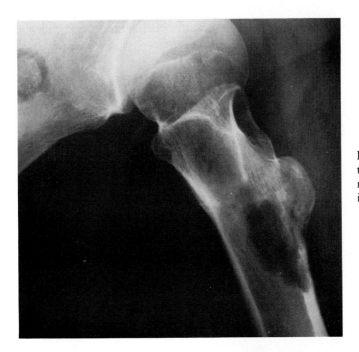

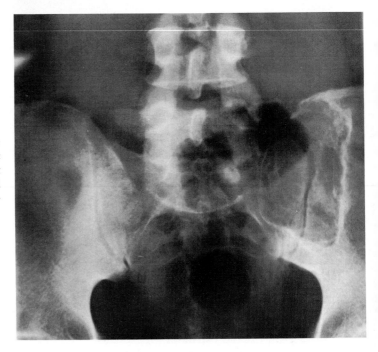

FIGURE 2–24 Metastatic disease. A typical renal metastasis is seen as a benign lytic lesion in the proximal femur in this patient.

FIGURE 2–25 Plasmacytoma. A large lytic lesion with a well-defined sclerotic border is seen in the left ilium in a patient with multiple myeloma. The ilium and sacrum are common sites for plasmacytomas.

looks benign, it should not be a met." Most mets have an aggressive appearance and won't be in the FEGNOMASHIC differential, but a significant number appear benign.

For statistical purposes I will not mention mets in a patient under the age of 40. I'll be correct more than 99 per cent of the time using 40 as a cutoff age. Otherwise, mets would have to be mentioned in every single case of a lytic lesion, and I'm trying to find ways to limit the list of differential possibilities. I'm not saying that mets

don't occur in patients under the age of 40, only that I'm willing to miss them (unless I'm given a history of a known primary neoplasm).

Myeloma can present as either solitary or multiple lytic lesions, which are more correctly called plasmacytomas (Fig. 2–25). I try to mention plasmacytoma separately from metastatic disease because it can occur in a slightly younger population (35 years is my cutoff) and can precede clinical or hematologic evidence of myeloma by 3 to 5 years. In general, there is no harm in lumping all

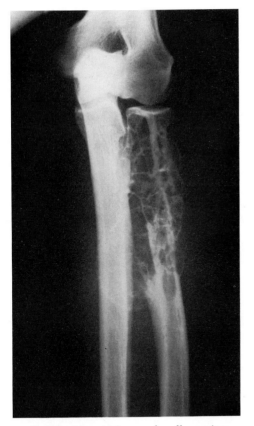

FIGURE 2–26 **Metastatic renal cell carcinoma.** A bubbly expansile lesion of the proximal radius is noted that is typical for renal cell carcinoma metastasis. It is similar in appearance to an aneurysmal bone cyst.

metastatic disease, including myeloma, into one group and using greater than age 40 as the limiting factor.

Virtually any metastatic process can present as a lytic, benign-appearing lesion; therefore, it serves no purpose to try to guess the source of the met from its appearance. In general, lytic expansile mets tend to come from thyroid and renal tumors (Fig. 2–26). The only metastatic lesion that is said to always be lytic is renal cell carcinoma.

Discriminator:

Must be over age 40.

ANEURYSMAL BONE CYST

ABCs are the only lesions I know of that are named for their radiographic appearance. They are virtually always aneurysmal or expansile (Figs. 2–27 and 2–28). Rarely an ABC will present before it is expansile but that is unusual enough to not worry about. ABCs primarily occur in patients who are under the age of 30, although occasionally one will be encountered in

older patients. I use expansion and below the age of 30 as fairly rigid guidelines and seldom miss the diagnosis of ABC.

ABCs have a characteristic appearance on MR imaging exam with multiple fluid-fluid levels (Fig. 2–29). Although other entities can have fluid-fluid levels and ABCs don't always have them, the appearance is nevertheless so characteristic for an ABC that it is almost pathognomonic.

ABCs are, like GCTs, somewhat controversial. There are apparently two types of ABCs: a primary type and a secondary type. The secondary type occurs in conjunction with another lesion or from trauma, whereas a primary ABC has no known cause or association with other lesions. Secondary ABCs have been described to occur with GCTs, osteosarcomas, and almost any other lesion you can name. I have seen dozens of ABCs and have yet to see one in association with another lesion, so I doubt that this occurs very often. As to occurring after trauma, I don't understand why they would be age-limited if trauma were

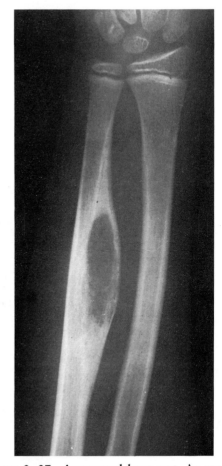

FIGURE 2–27 **Aneurysmal bone cyst.** An expansile lesion in the diaphysis of the ulna in a young child that is typical for an aneurysmal bone cyst.

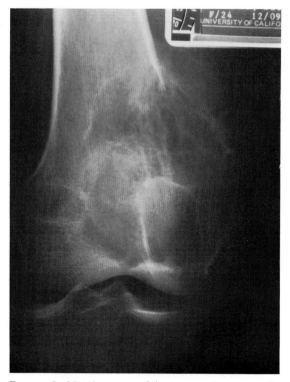

FIGURE 2–28 Aneurysmal bone cyst. An expansile lytic lesion in a 25-year-old that is typical for an aneurysmal bone cyst. At first glance one might consider this typical for a giant cell tumor. However, note the sclerotic margins and the fact that it does not abut the articular surface.

the cause. Also, malignant tumors were once thought to occur after trauma because of the frequent antecedent history of trauma with malignant bone tumors. This is not seriously considered today and is thought to be coincidental. I suspect that ABCs and trauma are also coincidental, but this is mere speculation. This history of prior trauma should not make you think more or less of the proper diagnosis; therefore, it makes no difference when addressing an unknown lesion. Even in cases of myositis ossificans (a lesion known to be caused by trauma), a history of antecedent trauma is elicited only half the time.

ABCs typically present because of pain. They occasionally can occur in the epiphyses, but there is no location in which they should be given more weight in the differential. As with osteoblastoma, they often occur in the posterior elements of the spine.

Discriminators:

1. Must be expansile.
2. Must be under age 30.

SOLITARY BONE CYST

Solitary bone cysts are also called simple bone cysts or unicameral bone cysts. They are not necessarily unicameral (one compartment), however. This is the only lesion in FEGNOMASHIC that

FIGURE 2–29 Aneurysmal bone cyst (MR imaging). An axial proton-density MR image through an expansile lytic lesion involving the posterior elements of a thoracic vertebral body reveals several fluid-fluid levels (arrows). This appearance is classic for an aneurysmal bone cyst.

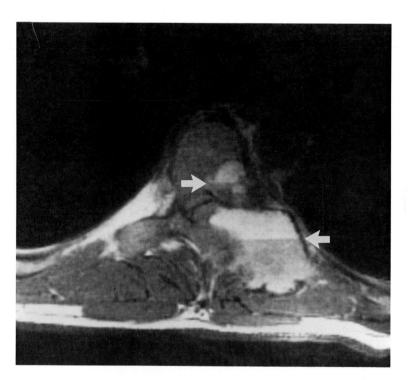

FIGURE 2–30 **Solitary bone cyst.** A centrally placed lesion in the proximal femur that is classic for a solitary bone cyst.

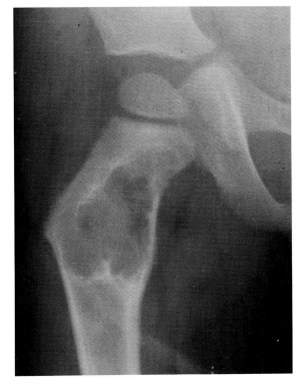

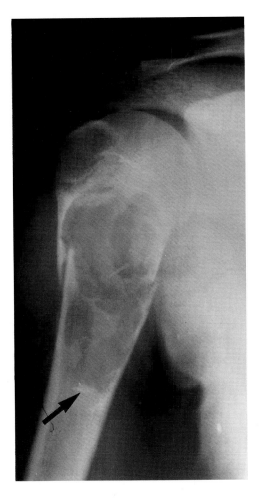

FIGURE 2–31 **Solitary bone cyst.** A pathologic fracture has occurred through this lesion in the proximal humerus. Its location and appearance are typical for a solitary bone cyst. Note the cortical fragments (arrow) produced from the fracture that have sunk to the bottom of this fluid-filled lesion. This is termed a "fallen fragment sign." No other lesion has been reported to have a fallen fragment sign; therefore, this is virtually pathognomonic.

is always central in location (Fig. 2–30). Many of the other lesions may be central, but a solitary bone cyst can be excluded if it is not. It is one of the few lesions that doesn't occur most commonly around the knees. Two thirds to three fourths of these lesions occur in the proximal humerus and proximal femur. By itself this fact isn't that helpful, or one third to one fourth of the lesions would be missed.

Solitary bone cysts are usually asymptomatic unless fractured—a common occurrence (Fig. 2–31). Even when pathologic fractures occur,

they rarely form periostitis. They usually occur in young patients, and it is unusual to see one in a patient over the age of 30. Although long bones are most commonly involved, solitary bone cysts have been described in almost every bone in the body. They begin at the physeal plate in long bones and grow into the shaft of the bone; therefore, they are not epiphyseal lesions. They can, however, extend up into an epiphysis after the plate closes, but this is unusual. A fairly common location is in the calcaneus, where they have a characteristic triangular appearance (Fig. 2–32).

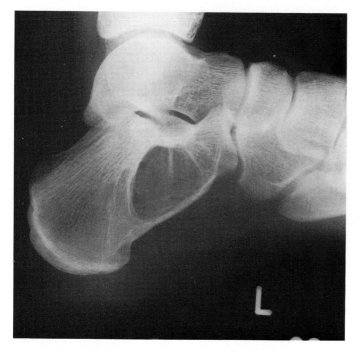

FIGURE 2–32 **Solitary bone cyst.** A classic appearance of a solitary bone cyst in the calcaneus. This lesion in the calcaneus occurs only in this position (anterior to the midportion of the calcaneus and on the inferior border). Although other lesions could occur in this location, a solitary bone cyst of the calcaneus virtually never occurs away from this spot.

Discriminators:

1. Must be central.
2. Must be under age 30.

HYPERPARATHYROIDISM (BROWN TUMORS)

Brown tumors of hyperparathyroidism (HPT) can have almost any appearance, from a purely lytic lesion to a sclerotic process (Fig. 2–33). Generally, when the patient's HPT is treated, the brown tumor undergoes sclerosis and will eventually disappear. If a brown tumor is going to be considered in the differential, additional radiographic findings of HPT should be seen. Subperiosteal bone resorption is pathognomonic for HPT and should be searched for in the phalanges (particularly the radial aspect of the middle phalanges), distal clavicles (resorption), medial aspect of the proximal tibias, and sacroiliac joints (it has the appearance of bilateral SI joint erosive disease). Osteoporosis or osteosclerosis might suggest that renal osteodystrophy with secondary HPT is present, but subperiosteal resorption must be present; otherwise brown tumor can be excluded from the differential.

Most authorities believe that brown tumors occur most commonly in primary HPT; however, because we see so many more patients with secondary HPT, more brown tumors are seen in patients with secondary rather than primary HPT.

Discriminator:

Must have other evidence of HPT.

INFECTION

Unfortunately there is no reliable way to radiographically exclude a focus of osteomyelitis (Figs. 2–34 and 2–35). It has a protean radiographic appearance and can occur at any location and in a patient of any age. It may or may not be expansile, have a sclerotic or nonsclerotic border, or have periostitis associated with it. Soft tissue findings such as obliteration of adjacent fat planes are notoriously unreliable and even misleading, as tumors and eosinophilic granuloma can do the same thing.

When osteomyelitis occurs near a joint, if the articular surface is abutted, invariably the adjacent joint will be involved and show either cartilage loss or an effusion, or both (Fig. 2–36). This finding is not particularly helpful, since any lesion can cause an effusion, but it's the best I can come up with.

When a sclerotic margin is present, infection usually causes the sclerotic margin to be thick and ill-defined or fuzzy on its outermost portion, but these findings are by no means always present and are only of limited usefulness.

If a bony sequestrum is present, osteomyelitis should be strongly considered. As previously mentioned, the only lesions described that demonstrate sequestra are infection, EG, lymphoma,

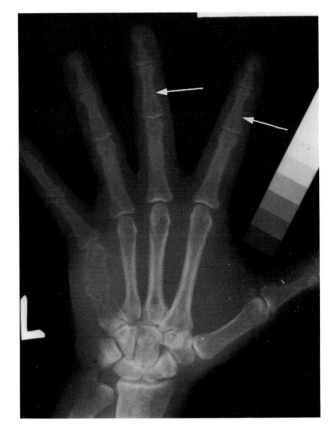

FIGURE 2–33 Brown tumor. An expansile lytic lesion in the fifth metacarpal that would have an extremely long differential diagnosis. Barely discernible is subperiosteal bone resorption on the radial aspect of the middle phalanges (arrows). A second, smaller lytic lesion is seen at the proximal portion of the fourth proximal phalanx. It has a different appearance than the other lytic lesion, emphasizing how brown tumors can have almost any appearance. The multiplicity is typical for a brown tumor and limits the differential diagnosis. However, the finding of subperiosteal bone resorption makes any other diagnosis unlikely.

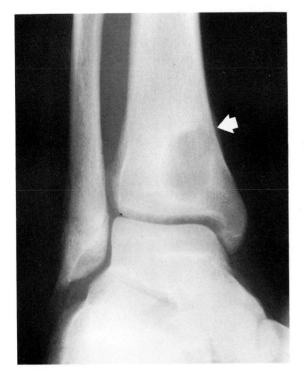

FIGURE 2–34 Brodie's abscess. A focus of infection that was chronic in this patient is seen in the distal tibia. The differential diagnosis for this lesion would be quite long if the subtle periostitis (arrow) and the clinical history of pain were not noted. Although this is a typical appearance for a chronic osteomyelitis (Brodie's abscess), infection can resemble almost anything.

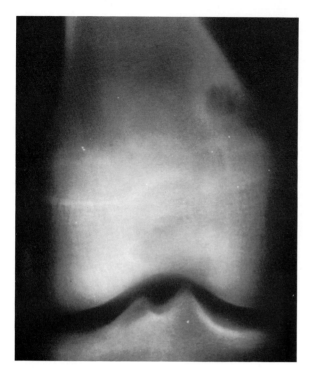

FIGURE 2–35 **Fungal infection.** A lytic lesion with faintly seen sclerotic margins is noted in the distal femoral metaphysis and was found on biopsy to be blastomycosis.

FIGURE 2–36 **Osteomyelitis with pyoarthritis.** A plain film of the shoulder *(A)* in this child with shoulder pain shows a well-defined lytic lesion.

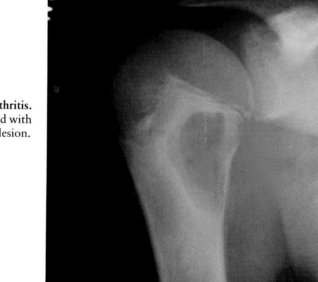

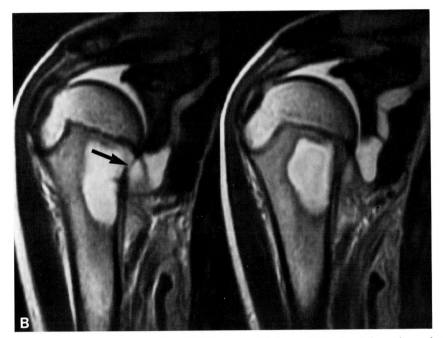

FIGURE 2–36 *Continued*   Coronal T2-weighted MR imaging *(B)* shows high signal throughout the lesion, which extends through the cortex (arrow) into the joint. This is a typical appearance for osteomyelitis with extension into the joint.

and fibrosarcoma. Most cases of osteomyelitis, however, do not have sequestra, so this feature is also of limited use. Therefore, infection will be in almost every differential diagnosis of a lytic lesion, which is all right, since it is one of the most common lesions encountered.

Discriminators:

None.

CHONDROBLASTOMA

Chondroblastomas are among the easiest lesions to deal with because they occur only in the epiphyses (a handful of cases have been reported in the metaphyses—they're rare), and they occur almost exclusively in patients under the age of 30 (Fig. 2–37). What could be easier? Anywhere from 40 to 60 per cent demonstrate calcification, so absence of calcification is not helpful. Presence of calcification is helpful so long as you can be sure that it's not detritus or sequestra from infection or EG (both of which can occur in the epiphyses). Because I can never be certain about the calcification, I don't worry about it.

The differential diagnosis of a lytic lesion in the epiphysis of a patient under the age of 30 is short and simple: (1) infection (most common), (2) chondroblastoma, and (3) GCT (it has its own

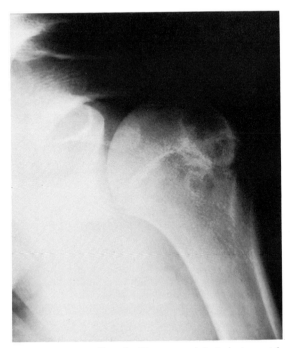

FIGURE 2–37   **Chondroblastoma.** A lytic lesion with a well-defined sclerotic margin in the proximal humeral epiphysis extending slightly across the epiphyseal plate. This is a typical appearance of a chondroblastoma. Almost half of all chondroblastomas have a small portion of the lesion extending across the physeal plate.

diagnostic criteria so it can usually be definitely ruled out or in). This is an old, classic differential and probably takes care of 98 per cent of epiphyseal lesions. If you want to be 99 per cent certain, you must add two more lesions—ABC (be certain it is expansile) and EG—and add mets and myeloma if the age is over 40. I no longer recommend using the longer differential as it just seems to cause confusion. Residents remember that there are three entities in the epiphyseal differential and then pick from the longer list of five entities, often leaving out the main things while including EG and ABC. Most of you have too much to commit to memory already without trying to stuff in a few rare presentations that will not be seen very often.

A caveat on epiphyseal lesions is to always consider the possibility of a subchondral cyst or geode, which has been described in four disease processes: (1) degenerative joint disease (must have joint space narrowing, sclerosis, and osteophytes), (2) rheumatoid arthritis, (3) CPPD (calcium pyrophosphate dihydrate) or pseudogout, and (4) avascular necrosis. Be certain no joint pathology that might indicate one of these processes is present, or an unnecessary biopsy of a geode might be performed based on your differential of an epiphyseal lesion (see Chapter 4, "Don't Touch" Lesions).

The carpal bones, the tarsal bones, and the patella have a tendency to behave like epiphyses as far as their differential diagnosis of lesions is concerned. Therefore, a lytic lesion in these areas has a similar differential as an epiphyseal lesion (Fig. 2–38).

Discriminators:
1. Must be under age 30.
2. Must be epiphyseal.

CHONDROMYXOID FIBROMA

Like osteoblastoma, the chondromyxoid fibroma is such a rare lesion that failure to mention it is probably not going to result in missing more than one in your lifetime. Why include it then? I recommend not including it, but it's part of the classic differential. If you do mention it, at least know what it looks like. Basically, chondromyxoid fibromas resemble NOFs (Fig. 2–39). Unlike NOFs, however, they can be seen in patients of any age. They can present with pain also, which will not occur with an NOF. They have been reported to progress from a benign process to an aggressive and even malignant lesion, but this is extremely rare.

Discriminator:
Mention when an NOF is mentioned.

ADDITIONAL POINTS

That, in essence, is my differential for a benign cystic lesion of bone. It is probably 98 per cent accurate, which is good enough for me. To increase the accuracy to 99 per cent it would be

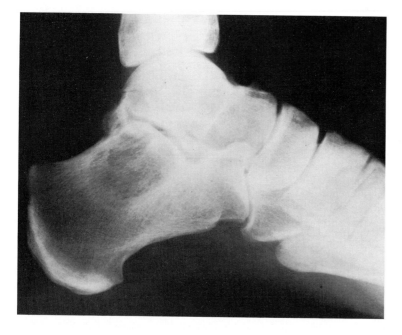

FIGURE 2–38 Chondroblastoma. A lytic lesion in the calcaneus that abuts the superior portion of the calcaneus has a fairly short differential diagnosis. The differential is essentially the same as in an epiphysis. On biopsy this lesion was found to be a chondroblastoma.

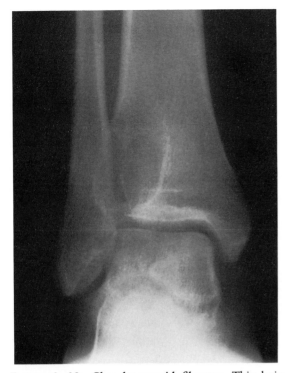

FIGURE 2–39 **Chondromyxoid fibroma.** This lytic lesion in the distal tibia with a well-defined sclerotic margin should have been a nonossifying fibroma. The differential diagnosis for this lesion would include several other entities, all of which are benign. Although a biopsy of this lesion probably should not have been done in this asymptomatic patient, it was performed, and the lesion was found to be a chondromyxoid fibroma.

necessary to add a host of uncommon or rare lesions, and the whole process would become too confusing for most residents to learn. If you have a favorite lesion that is not in this list, by all means add it. Likewise, if the list is already too cumbersome, forget about osteoblastoma and chondromyxoid fibroma. I'm unable to make it much simpler than that and still be reasonably accurate.

Some of the lesions I have purposefully omitted are intraosseous ganglion, pseudotumor of hemophilia, hemangioendothelioma, ossifying fibroma, intraosseous lipoma, glomus tumor, neurofibroma, plasma cell granuloma, and schwannoma. Others could be added to this list, of course, but are best left to the pathologist—not the radiologist—for the diagnosis.

There are several features that are somewhat useful in separating out the various lesions in FEGNOMASHIC (Table 2–1). For instance, if the patient is under the age of 30, be sure to consider EG, chondroblastoma, NOF, ABC, and

solitary bone cyst. This is not a differential diagnosis to list when faced with a lytic lesion in a patient less than 30; several other lesions should be included in that differential. This means don't mention those five lesions in a patient over 30. If the patient is over 30, those five lesions can probably be excluded.

If periostitis or pain is present (assuming no trauma, which can be a foolhardy assumption), you can exclude fibrous dysplasia, solitary bone cyst, NOF, and enchondroma. If the lesion is epiphyseal, the classic differential is infection, GCT, and chondroblastoma. ABC and EG could be added to that differential too but are not mandatory. If the patient is over 40 years of age, add mets and myeloma and remove ABC, chondroblastoma, and EG from the epiphyseal list. Don't forget to consider a subchondral cyst or geode in epiphyseal lesions.

The epiphyseal differential tends to work also for the tarsal bones (especially the calcaneus), the carpal bones, and the patella. In the calcaneus, a unicameral bone cyst should also be considered and has a characteristic appearance and location (see Fig. 2–32). Apophyses are "epiphyseal equivalents" and have the same differential as epiphyses. The difference between an epiphysis and an apophysis is that epiphyses contribute to the length of a bone, whereas apophyses serve as ligamentous attachments.

A few findings that just don't seem to narrow the differential diagnosis are presence or absence of a soft tissue mass, expansion of the bone (except must be present in an ABC), a sclerotic or nonsclerotic border (except must be nonsclerotic in GCT), presence or absence of bony struts or compartments in the lesion, and size of the lesion.

There are a few lesions which I call "automatics." That is, they need to be included automatically in almost every case. In patients less than 30 EG and infection must be included in every differential of a lytic bone lesion. In fact, they should be mentioned in any case except for trauma or arthritis because they can have virtually *any* appearance—lytic, sclerotic, mixed, benign, aggressive, etc. Hence they can mimic almost any bone lesion. I recommend mentioning EG and infection for every bone lesion in patients under the age of 30. Make sure you give a thoughtful pause after inspecting the film—as if you really considered the pros and cons of mentioning them. This is gamesmanship, but it adds to your credibility. In patients over the age of 40 mets and infection are "automatics." No consideration for the lesion's appearance or location needs to be made when using the automatics—simply find a lesion.

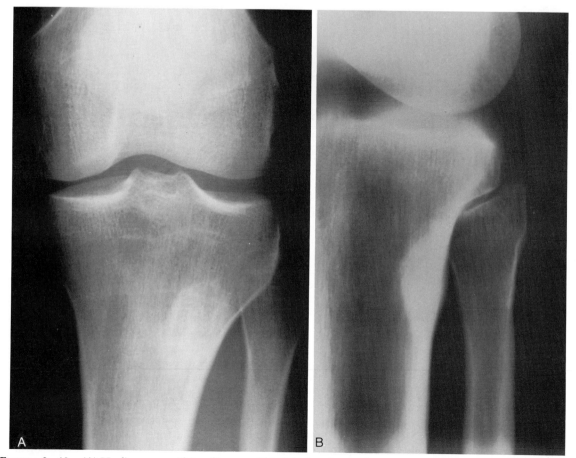

FIGURE 2–40 *(A)* **Healing nonossifying fibroma.** This faintly sclerotic lesion in the proximal tibia of a 30-year-old asymptomatic patient is characteristic for a healing or disappearing nonossifying fibroma. Prior films showed a typical lytic nonossifying fibroma. *(B)* **Healing nonossifying fibroma.** This densely sclerotic lesion in the posterior proximal tibia in a young asymptomatic patient was thought to represent an osteoid osteoma or osteomyelitis. Even though the patient was asymptomatic, a biopsy was performed. It revealed a nonossifying fibroma that had ossified. In a patient over the age of 40, metastatic disease would need to be considered.

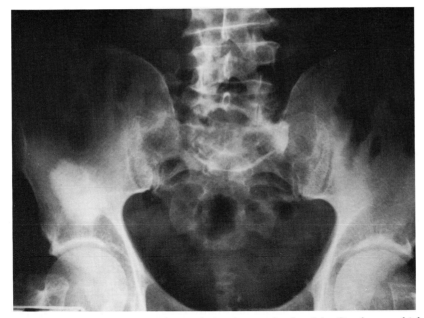

FIGURE 2–41 Giant bone island. A large sclerotic lesion is seen in the right iliac bone, which could easily be mistaken for a focus of metastatic disease in a patient over the age of 40. This is a giant bone island and has the typical pattern of irregular "feathered" margins with the trabecula blending into the normal bone. The axis of the lesion is in the long axis of the bone or in the direction of the primary weight-bearing trabecula.

DIFFERENTIAL DIAGNOSIS OF A SCLEROTIC LESION

Many lytic lesions spontaneously regress and are not usually seen in patients over the age of 30. When these lesions regress, they often fill in with new bone and have a sclerotic or blastic appearance. Therefore, when a sclerotic focus is identified in a 20- to 40-year-old patient, especially if it is an asymptomatic, incidental finding, the following lesions should be considered: NOF (Fig. 2–40), EG, solitary bone cyst, ABC, chondroblastoma. Several other lesions should be included that can also appear sclerotic: fibrous dysplasia, osteoid osteoma, infection, brown tumor (healing), and perhaps a giant bone island (Fig. 2–41). In any patient over the age of 40 the number one possibility should be metastatic disease (now that I've passed 40, I'm seriously considering moving the age to 50).

REFERENCES

1. David R, Oria R, Kumar R, et al: Radiologic features of eosinophilic granuloma of bone. Pictorial essay. AJR 1989;153:1021–1026.
2. Dahlin D: Giant cell tumor of bone: Highlights of 407 cases. AJR 1985;144:955–960.

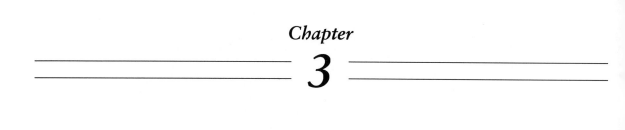

Chapter

3

Malignant Bone Tumors

Radiology residents have difficulty diagnosing malignant bone tumors, and the difficulty gets worse in the years after residency. This is simply because malignant bone tumors, thankfully, are not very common. Nevertheless, every radiologist will encounter one or two a year in most practices and should be able to recognize them and give a good differential diagnosis.

First, how do you recognize a malignant tumor and differentiate it from a benign process? This can be difficult and oftentimes it is impossible. Recognizing that it is *aggressive* is usually easy, but saying that it is *malignant* is another matter altogether. Processes such as infection and eosinophilic granuloma can mimic malignant tumors and are, of course, benign. They will often be included in the differential diagnosis of an aggressive lesion along with malignant tumors.

DIFFERENTIATION OF MALIGNANT FROM BENIGN

What radiologic criteria are useful for determining malignant versus benign? Standard textbooks and the literature give four aspects of a lesion to be examined: (1) cortical destruction, (2) periostitis, (3) orientation or axis of the lesion, and (4) zone of transition.

Let me expound on each of these criteria and show why only the last one—the zone of transition—is accurate to a 90 per cent plus rate.

Cortical Destruction

Often cortical bone is replaced by part of the noncalcified matrix (fibrous matrix or chondroid matrix) of benign fibro-osseous lesions and car-

tilaginous lesions. This can give the false impression of cortical destruction on plain films (Fig. 3–1) or computed tomography (CT). Also, benign processes such as infection and eosinophilic granuloma can cause extensive cortical destruction and mimic a malignant tumor. Aneurysmal bone cysts are known to cause such thinning of the cortex as to make it radiographically undetectable (Fig. 3–2). For these reasons I find cortical destruction to occasionally be misleading. Cortical destruction makes one think of a malignant lesion when using the Gestalt approach, but the lesion must also have other criteria for a malignant process, such as a wide zone of transition.

Periostitis

Periosteal reaction occurs in a nonspecific manner whenever the periosteum is irritated, whether it is irritated by a malignant tumor, a benign tumor, infection, or trauma. Callus formation in a fracture is actually just periosteal reaction of the most benign type. Periosteal reaction occurs in two types: benign (Fig. 3–3A and B) and aggressive (Fig. 3–3C and D). The difference between the two is based more on the timing of the growth of the irritation than on whether the process causing the periostitis is malignant or benign. For example, a slow-growing benign tumor will cause thick, wavy, uniform, or dense periostitis because it is a low-grade chronic irritation that gives the periosteum time to lay down thick new bone and remodel into more normal cortex. A malignant tumor causes a periosteal reaction that is high grade and more acute; hence the periosteum does not have time to consolidate. It appears lamellated (onion skinned) or

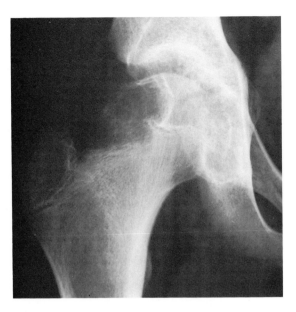

FIGURE 3–1 Apparent cortical destruction. This benign chondroblastoma has noncalcified chondroid tissue replacing cortical bone in the proximal femur, which gives the lesion a destructive appearance. This is an example of cortical replacement rather than of cortical destruction, which can be very confusing if one uses cortical destruction as an aggressive or malignant key in differential diagnosis. Note that the zone of transition is narrow, as one would expect in a benign lesion such as this.

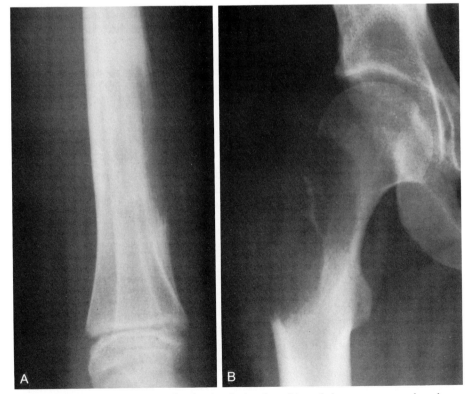

FIGURE 3–2 *(A)* **Aneurysmal bone cyst.** This benign lesion has thinned the cortex to such a degree as to make it imperceptible on a plain radiograph. As in Figure 3–1, this can be misconstrued as cortical destruction, giving the false impression of a malignant or very aggressive lesion. *(B)* **Giant cell tumor.** This lesion in the proximal femur has expanded and thinned the cortex to such a degree that it is imperceptible on the plain film.

Continued

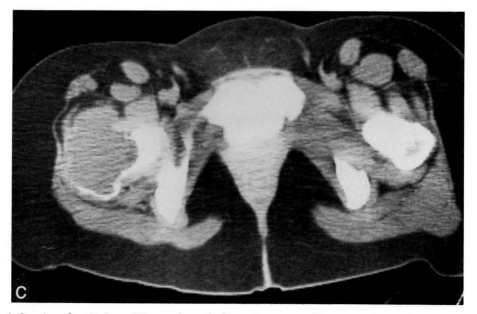

FIGURE 3–2 *Continued* *(C)* On a CT scan through this region a very thin cortex that was greatly expanded was identified. This giant cell tumor originated from the greater trochanter, which is an epiphyseal equivalent. Note that it has a well-defined but nonsclerotic zone of transition, as all giant cell tumors in long bones do.

amorphous, or even sunburst. If the irritation stops or diminishes, the aggressive periostitis will solidify and appear benign. Therefore, when periostitis is seen, the radiologist should try to characterize it into either a benign (thick, dense, wavy) type or an aggressive (lamellated, amorphous, sunburst) type.

Unfortunately, judging the lesion by its periostitis can be misleading. First, it takes considerable experience to accurately characterize periostitis because many times the reaction is not clearly benign or aggressive. Second, many benign lesions cause aggressive periostitis, such as infection, eosinophilic granuloma, aneurysmal bone cysts, osteoid osteomas, and even trauma. Seeing

benign periostitis, however, can be helpful because malignant lesions will not cause benign periostitis. Some investigators with great experience in dealing with malignant bone tumors state that the only way benign periostitis can occur in a malignant lesion is if there is a concomitant fracture or infection. I have seen a few exceptions, but overall I think it is a valid statement.

Orientation or Axis of the Lesion

The orientation or axis of the lesion is a poor determinant of benign versus aggressive and seldom helps me to decide into which category the lesion should be placed. It has been said that if

FIGURE 3–3 **Benign periostitis.** *(A)* An osteoid osteoma in the midshaft of the tibia has caused thick, wavy, dense periostitis, which is classic for benign type of periostitis. Malignant lesions are incapable of forming this type of periostitis and should not be considered in the differential. This type of periostitis is basically indistinguishable from callus formation in a fracture. *(B)* Thick, wavy periostitis (arrows) along the ilium in a child with a permeative lesion in the pelvis is characteristic for infection or eosinophilic granuloma. Ewing's sarcoma was initially considered in the differential; however, the benign periostitis would make a malignant lesion very unlikely. Biopsy showed this lesion to be eosinophilic granuloma. *(C)* Aggressive periostitis. Amorphous, sunburst periostitis with a Codman's triangle (arrows) in a patient with a mixed lytic-sclerotic lesion of the humerus, which on biopsy was shown to be Ewing's sarcoma. Although this type of periostitis is characteristic for a malignant lesion, it could also be seen with benign processes such as eosinophilic granuloma or infection. *(D)* Lamellated, or onion-skinned, periostitis is characteristic of an aggressive process, such as in this patient with Ewing's sarcoma of the femur. Again, this aggressive type of periostitis could conceivably occur in a benign process such as infection or eosinophilic granuloma.

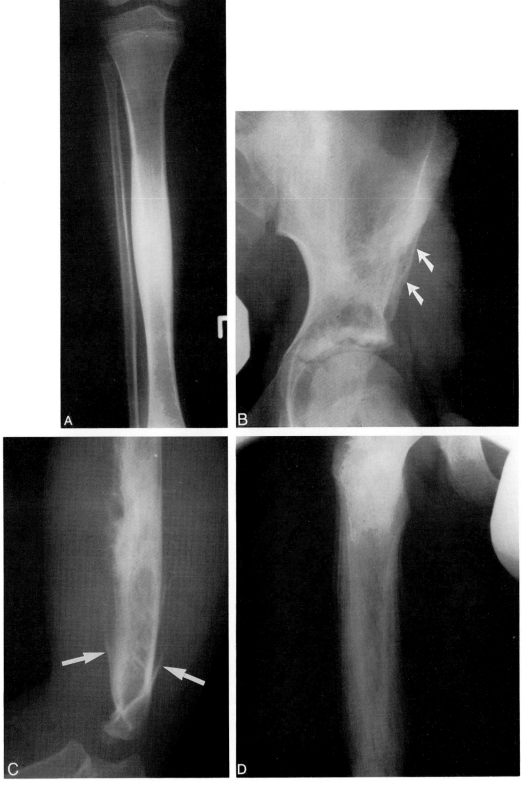

Figure 3–3 *For legend see opposite page.*

a lesion grows in the long axis of a long bone, rather than being circular, it is benign. Nonsense! Ewing's sarcoma, an extremely malignant lesion, usually has its axis along the shaft of a long bone. Conversely, many fibrous cortical defects are circular yet totally benign. I see no reason to even consider the axis of a lesion as part of its radiologic evaluation.

Zone of Transition

Without question the zone of transition is the most reliable indicator in determining benign versus malignant lesions. Unfortunately it also has some drawbacks, which I will elucidate.

The zone of transition is the border between the lesion and the normal bone. It is said to be narrow if it is so well defined that it can be drawn with a fine-point pen (Fig. 3–4). If it is imperceptible and cannot be clearly drawn, it is said to be wide (Fig. 3–5). Obviously all shades of gray lie in between, but most lesions can be characterized as having either a narrow or a wide zone of transition. If the lesion has a sclerotic border, it, of course, has a narrow zone of transition.

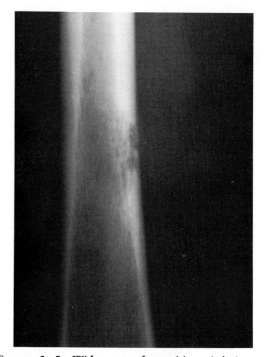

FIGURE 3–5 **Wide zone of transition.** A lytic permeative process is seen in the midshaft of the femur in this patient. On biopsy it was found to be a malignant fibrous histiocytoma. The zone of transition in this lesion is said to be wide, as it cannot be easily drawn with a fine-point pen. A permeative lesion such as this, by definition, has a wide zone of transition.

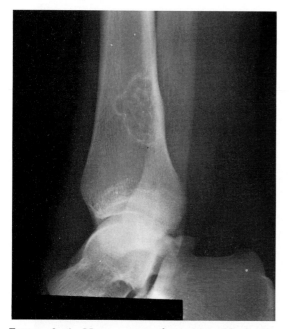

FIGURE 3–4 **Narrow zone of transition.** The border of normal bone with a lesion is known as the zone of transition. When, as in this example of a nonossifying fibroma, the border can be drawn with a fine-point pen it is said to be a narrow zone of transition, which is characteristic of a benign lesion. A narrow zone of transition may or may not have a sclerotic border.

If a lesion has a narrow zone of transition, it is a benign process. The exceptions to that are rare, and I'm willing to miss them. If a lesion has a wide zone of transition, it is aggressive. Notice that I said aggressive and not malignant. As with aggressive periostitis, many benign lesions, as well as malignant lesions, can have a wide zone of transition. A few of the same processes that can cause aggressive periostitis, and thereby mimic a malignant tumor, can cause a wide zone of transition (i.e., infection and eosinophilic granuloma). They are aggressive in their radiographic appearance because they are fast-acting, aggressive lesions. The zone of transition is usually easier to characterize than the periostitis, plus it is always there to evaluate (or you wouldn't see a lesion), whereas many lesions, benign and malignant, have no periostitis. For these reasons the zone of transition is the most useful indicator of whether a lesion is benign or malignant.

A lesion that consists of multiple small holes is said to be permeative. It has no perceptible border and therefore has a wide zone of transi-

FIGURE 3–6 **Permeative pattern.** A permeative pattern is defined as multiple, small, irregular holes in bone and indicates an aggressive process. Ewing's sarcoma typically has a permeative pattern; however, infection and eosinophilic granuloma, as in this example, can also have a permeative pattern. This is a fine-detailed film of the same case shown in Figure 3–3B.

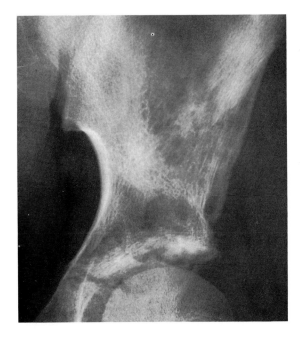

tion. Round cell tumors such as multiple myeloma, reticulum cell sarcoma (primary lymphoma of bone), and Ewing's sarcoma are typical of this type of lesion. However, infection and eosinophilic granuloma (Fig. 3–6) can have the same appearance.

The zone of transition only applies to lytic or predominantly lytic lesions. A blastic or sclerotic lesion will always appear to have a narrow zone of transition and may erroneously get into the benign differential even if it is malignant.

It is critical to be aware that the zone of transition is a plain film finding and cannot be used with MR imaging. Most malignant tumors will appear to have narrow zones of transition on MR imaging exams and can mislead one into thinking a benign lesion is present (Fig. 3–7). The zone of transition can only be used with lytic lesions and on plain films.

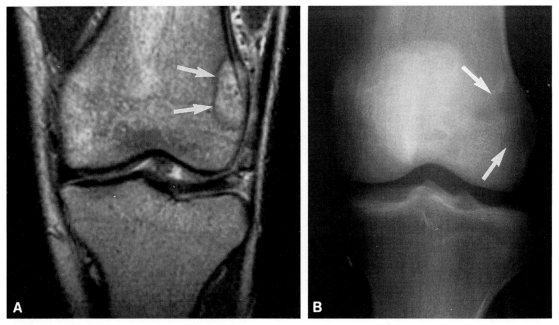

FIGURE 3–7 **Zone of transition on MR imaging.** *(A)* A T2-weighted MR imaging of the knee in this child with knee pain shows a well-defined lesion (arrow) with a low signal border suggesting a narrow zone of transition with a sclerotic border. Because the knee pain was described as probably related to the menisci, this lesion was felt to be an incidental, benign process, such as a nonossifying fibroma. However, the plain film *(B)*, obtained later, shows a barely discernible lytic lesion with a wide zone of transition (arrow). This lesion was, in fact, painful, and the differential diagnosis, based solely on the plain film, would include osteosarcoma—the eventual histologic diagnosis. The zone of transition can only be used on plain films—it is invalid on MR imaging.

DIFFERENTIATING TYPES OF TUMORS

Once it has been decided that a particular lesion is probably malignant, the differential is fairly straightforward. First of all, the list of malignant tumors is relatively short, and second, most tumors follow somewhat strict age groupings. Jack Edeiken, a famed skeletal radiologist, evaluated 4,000 malignant bone tumors and found that they could be correctly diagnosed 80 per cent of the time just by using the patient's age! He basically divides the tumors into decades of when they will affect a patient; for example, osteosarcoma and Ewing's sarcoma are the only childhood primary malignant tumors of bone, and after the age of 40 only metastatic disease (mets), myeloma, and chondrosarcoma are common (Table 3–1). Although there are certainly outliers that are uncommon, these age guidelines are extremely useful. It is inappropriate to mention Ewing's sarcoma in a 40-year-old or mets in a 15-year-old. Obviously, if a 15-year-old has a known primary tumor, then mets must be considered—in fact, *any* bone lesion, regardless of its appearance, could be a met and would be suspicious in a patient with a known primary tumor.

MR imaging should be routinely employed in the workup of malignant tumors. MR imaging will show the full bony and soft tissue extent and can identify the position of the larger adjacent vessels, making angiography unnecessary. Routine use of Gd-DTPA with tumors does not appear to be justified, as it currently seems to give no additional information over non–contrast-enhanced studies.

Rather than give a description of characteristics of every malignant tumor, which is available in any of the leading skeletal radiology texts, let me make a few points on many of the primary malignant tumors of bone that I think may be helpful in their diagnosis.

Osteosarcoma

The most common malignant primary bone tumor is an osteosarcoma. Although it typically occurs toward the end of a long bone, it may occur anywhere in the skeleton with enough frequency so that location is not a helpful discriminator. Osteosarcomas are usually destructive, with obvious sclerosis present from either tumor new bone or reactive sclerosis (Figs. 3–8 and 3–9); however, on occasion they can be entirely lytic (Fig. 3–10). These are usually so-called telangiectatic osteosarcomas. There are many types and classifications of osteosarcomas, but it serves little purpose to the radiologist to try to distinguish between most of them.

These tumors occur almost exclusively in patients under the age of 30. Although some texts claim there is a second peak of osteosarcomas in

TABLE 3–1 Malignant Tumors and
Patient Age

Age	Tumor
1–30	Ewing's
	Osteosarcoma
30–40	Fibrosarcoma and malignant fibrous histiocytoma
	Malignant giant cell tumor
	Reticulum cell sarcoma
	Parosteal sarcoma
40+	Mets
	Myeloma
	Chondrosarcoma

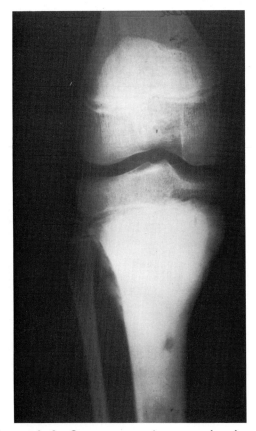

FIGURE 3–8 Osteosarcoma. An extremely sclerotic lesion in the proximal tibia of a child is noted, which is characteristic for an osteogenic sarcoma.

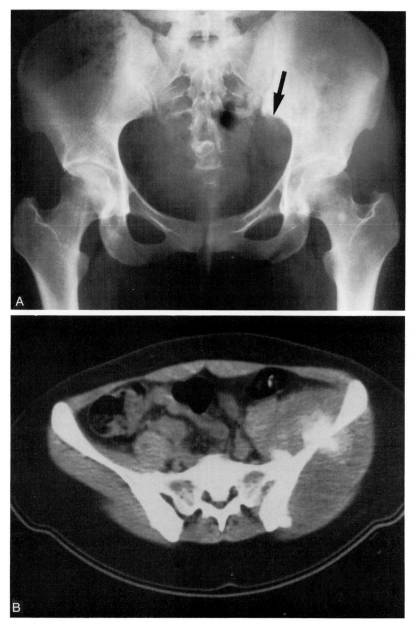

FIGURE 3–9 **Osteosarcoma.** *(A)* A subtle sclerotic lesion is seen in the left ilium adjacent to the sacroiliac joint that was initially diagnosed as osteitis condensans ilii, a benign entity. Because of persistent pain the patient returned for a follow-up visit, and a small amount of cortical destruction on the pelvic brim was noted (arrow). *(B)* A CT scan was performed, which showed a large soft tissue mass and tumor new bone around the ilium, which is characteristic for an osteogenic sarcoma.

patients around age 60, I, and others, do not believe this to be correct. Some osteosarcomas occur in older patients who have malignant degeneration of Paget's disease, and some occur secondary to prior irradiation; but de novo osteosarcomas in the older age group are distinctly rare.

Parosteal Osteosarcoma

A type of osteosarcoma that should be distinguished, however, from the central osteosarcoma is the parosteal osteosarcoma. The parosteal osteosarcoma originates from the periosteum of the bone and grows outside the bone (Fig. 3–11). It often wraps around the diaphysis without break-

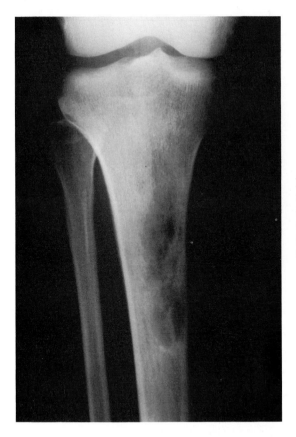

FIGURE 3–10 **Lytic osteosarcoma.** An ill-defined lytic lesion was noted in the proximal tibia of a 20-year-old with pain. The lesion had a differential diagnosis of EG, infection, Ewing's sarcoma, and osteogenic sarcoma. Biopsy showed it to be a lytic osteogenic sarcoma.

ing through the cortex. It occurs in an older age-group than the central osteosarcomas and is not as aggressive. Treatment used to consist of merely shaving the tumor off the bone it originated from; however, recurrence rates were so high that now wide-bloc excisions are performed. Once a parosteal osteosarcoma violates the cortex of the adjacent bone, it is considered to be as aggressive as a central osteosarcoma and is treated in a similar fashion (i.e., amputation or radical excision). Therefore, the radiologist needs to evaluate the lesion for invasion of the adjacent cortex to help determine treatment and prognosis. This is best done with CT or MR imaging (Fig. 3–11*B* and *C*).

A common location for parosteal osteosarcomas to arise is from the posterior femur, near the knee. A lesion that can mimic an early parosteal osteosarcoma in this location is a so-called cortical desmoid (Fig. 3–12). A cortical desmoid is an avulsion injury that is totally benign but can appear somewhat aggressive. Unfortunately it can appear malignant histologically, so biopsy can lead to disastrous consequences. Amputations for benign cortical desmoids being mistaken for malignancies have occurred. (See Chapter 4 for further points on cortical desmoids.) Another

lesion that can be mistaken for a parosteal osteosarcoma is an area of myositis ossificans (Fig. 3–13). Like cortical desmoids, areas of myositis ossificans can be histologically mistaken for malignancies with disastrous consequences. Therefore, differentiation is vital. Fortunately differentiation between parosteal osteosarcoma and myositis ossificans is fairly easily done radiographically. (See Chapter 4 for differential points between parosteal osteosarcoma and myositis ossificans.)

Another type of osteosarcoma that often gets mentioned by residents in their differential of a parosteal osteosarcoma is a periosteal osteosarcoma. It should not get such attention. First, it's extremely rare, with fewer than 50 such lesions reported in the literature. Second, and most significantly, periosteal osteosarcomas do not resemble parosteal osteosarcomas (Fig. 3–14). Therefore, mentioning both of these lesions in the same differential is inappropriate and simply means that the resident doesn't know what a periosteal osteosarcoma looks like. It's such a rare lesion that I teach residents not to worry about it—don't mention it. Radiology is hard enough without remembering all the rare lesions that might be seen once in a lifetime—if at all.

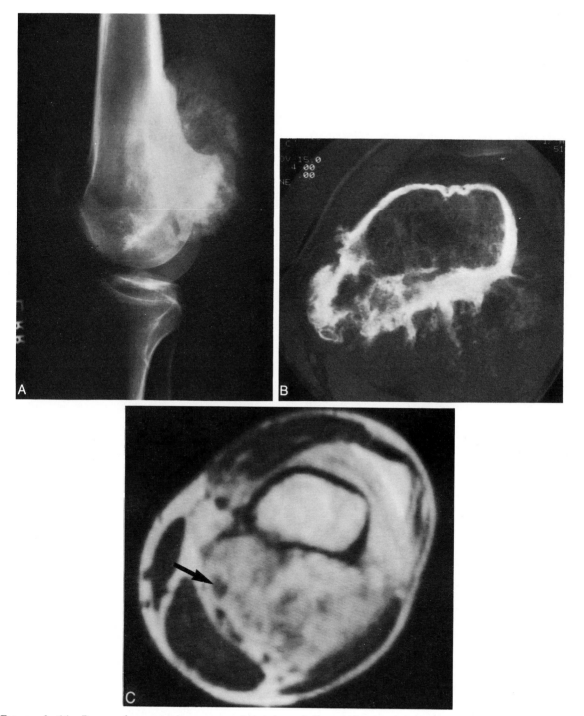

FIGURE 3–11 Parosteal osteogenic sarcoma. *(A)* A lateral film of the distal femur shows a large calcific mass with an ill-defined, fluffy, calcific periphery growing off the posterior femur. The location and appearance are characteristic for a parosteal osteogenic sarcoma. *(B)* A CT scan through this lesion shows cortical and medullary involvement, which indicates a more sinister lesion, with treatment and prognosis similar to that of a central osteogenic sarcoma. Without intramedullary involvement, a parosteal sarcoma has a favorable prognosis. *(C)* A proton density MR image in another patient with a parosteal osteosarcoma shows how the vessels (arrow) can be easily identified in relation to the tumor. In this example the vessels are displaced posteriorly by the tumor.

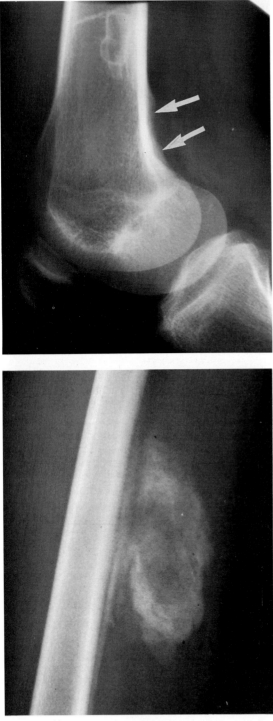

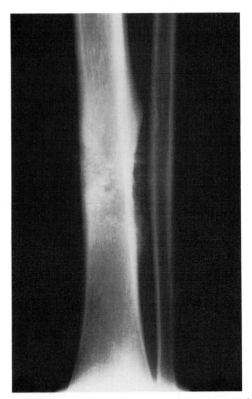

FIGURE 3–12 **Cortical desmoid.** Irregular periostitis (arrows) off the medial supracondylar ridge of the distal femur is pathognomonic for a small avulsion of the adductor muscles and is called a cortical desmoid. Biopsy of this lesion can easily result in a mistaken diagnosis of a sarcomatous lesion and should, therefore, be avoided. A cortical desmoid should not be confused with an early parosteal osteogenic sarcoma on radiographs, as it will then lead to an unnecessary biopsy, perhaps with dire consequences. An incidental finding is a nonossifying fibroma seen just proximal to the cortical desmoid.

FIGURE 3–13 **Myositis ossificans.** This lesion is often confused with parosteal osteogenic sarcoma, since at first glance it has a close resemblance. However, myositis ossificans, as in this example, will demonstrate calcification that is densest in the periphery and well defined, whereas parosteal osteogenic sarcoma has calcification that is most concentrated centrally and ill defined in the periphery. Myositis ossificans is another lesion that can be confused with a malignant lesion on biopsy and, therefore, should be radiographically rather than surgically diagnosed.

FIGURE 3–14 **Periosteal osteogenic sarcoma.** Unlike the parosteal osteosarcoma, the periosteal osteogenic sarcoma does not have large amounts of calcification in soft tissues. It typically has a saucerized configuration with periostitis that resembles hair on end or is sunburst, as in this example. Although this lesion is very malignant, it inexplicably will not invade the medullary space. Although parosteal and periosteal sarcomas originate from the same point and have similar names, they do not have a similar radiographic appearance.

Ewing's Sarcoma

The classic Ewing's sarcoma is a permeative (multiple small holes) lesion in the diaphysis of a long bone in a child (Fig. 3–3D). However, only about 40 per cent of these tumors occur in the diaphysis, with the remainder being metaphyseal or diametaphyseal or in flat bones. They do tend to be found primarily in children and adolescents, although a significant number occur in patients who are in their 20s, especially in flat bones. Although most often permeative in appearance, they can elicit reactive new bone, which can give the lesion a partially sclerotic or "patchy" appearance (Figs. 3–3C, 3–15, and 3–16). Ewing's sarcomas often have an onion-skinned type of periostitis, but they can also have periostitis that is sunburst or amorphous in character (Fig. 3–16). Rarely, if ever, will a Ewing's sarcoma have benign-appearing periostitis (thick, uniform, or wavy). If benign periostitis is present, other lesions should be considered instead, such as infection or eosinophilic granuloma.

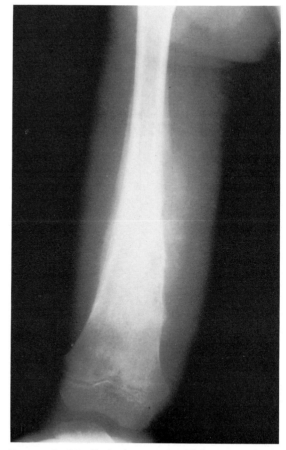

FIGURE 3–16 **Ewing's sarcoma.** This is a predominantly sclerotic process with large amounts of sunburst periostitis in the diaphysis of a femur that, on biopsy, was found to be Ewing's sarcoma.

A knee jerk differential diagnosis for a permeative lesion in a child should be Ewing's sarcoma, infection, and eosinophilic granuloma. These three entities can appear radiologically identical. I exclude Ewing's sarcoma from the differential if I can see definite benign periostitis or if I can see a definite sequestrum of bone. In this differential list only eosinophilic granuloma and infection can have benign periostitis or a sequestrum. Presence or absence of a soft tissue mass is not helpful in distinguishing between these three lesions. Presence of symptoms is not helpful, as all three entities can be symptomatic; however, it would be unusual to find an asymptomatic Ewing's sarcoma.

Chondrosarcoma

Chondrosarcomas have a number of appearances that at times make them difficult to diagnose with any assurance. They most frequently occur in patients over age 40. An eminent bone radiologist once told me that if a pathologist

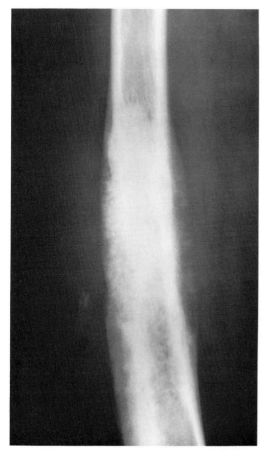

FIGURE 3–15 **Ewing's sarcoma.** A mixed lytic-sclerotic lesion in the femur of a child with periostitis that is amorphous and sunburst, such as in this example, is characteristic of a Ewing's sarcoma.

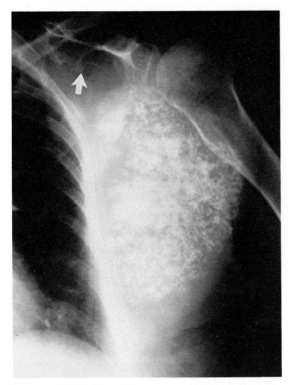

FIGURE 3–17 **Chrondrosarcoma.** A large soft tissue mass with typical chondroid matrix is seen in this young adult with a history of multiple osteochromatosis. A sessile osteochondroma is seen off the proximal humerus, and another osteochondroma is seen protruding off the scapula (arrow). The chrondrosarcoma in the axilla presumably arose from a prior benign osteochondroma that has undergone malignant degeneration.

makes the diagnosis of chondrosarcoma in a child, get another pathologist. Although it is very uncommon, chondrosarcomas occasionally occur in children; usually they are from malignant degeneration of an osteochondroma (Fig. 3–17) but do not have to be. I reserve the diagnosis of a chondrosarcoma for patients over the age of 40 unless they have an obvious enchondroma or osteochondroma that is painful or has a destructive appearance.

Probably the most difficult lesion for a pathologist to deal with is an enchondroma. It can be extremely difficult histologically to differentiate a low-grade chondrosarcoma from an enchondroma. Because low-grade chondrosarcomas do not metastasize, some pathologists call them "active enchondromas." The diagnosis of chondrosarcoma usually initiates radical excision and therapy, although it is debatable (and somewhat controversial) as to whether a low-grade chondrosarcoma is even a malignant tumor. For these reasons I usually reserve the diagnosis of "possible chondrosarcoma" for those lesions that are painful or show definite aggressive characteristics, such as periostitis and destruction. The truth of the matter is that neither radiologists nor pathologists can distinguish between enchondromas and many chondrosarcomas (Fig. 3–18).

Chondrosarcoma should be considered in the diagnosis anytime there is a lytic, destructive lesion with amorphous, snowflake calcification in an older patient (over 40) (Fig. 3–19). Without the presence of the calcified chondroid matrix the lesion is indistinguishable from any other aggressive lytic lesion, such as metastatic disease,

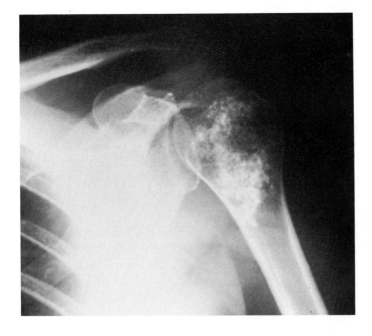

FIGURE 3–18 **Chondrosarcoma.** Typical snowflake, punctate, amorphous calcification in the proximal humerus is seen, which is typical of an enchondroma. The patient, however, had pain associated with this lesion, and on biopsy it was found to be a chondrosarcoma. (Courtesy of Dr. Tomas Jimenez-Robinson.)

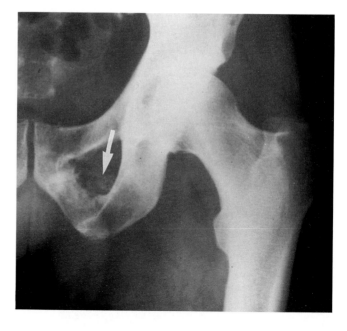

FIGURE 3–19 **Chondrosarcoma.** An amorphous, irregular calcification is seen in a lesion arising in the ischium (arrow). This is fairly typical for a chondrosarcoma.

plasmacytoma, fibrosarcoma, malignant fibrous histiocytoma (MFH), or infection. Usually the radiologist can only give a long differential diagnosis such as this, which is entirely acceptable. A biopsy of the lesion will have to be performed at any rate, so it is not necessary for the radiologist to make the diagnosis. This is the case with most malignant tumors. The radiologist does play an important role, however, in suggesting additional lesions that might masquerade as malignancies and in imaging the lesion to show such features as the full extent, the presence of a soft tissue component, and metastases. As mentioned earlier, MR imaging plays an invaluable role in this regard and should be performed on every potential malignant bone lesion.

Malignant Giant Cell Tumor

Approximately 15 per cent of giant cell tumors are malignant. Unfortunately there does not seem to be any way to foretell which giant cell tumor will become malignant. Benign and malignant giant cell tumors appear radiologically identical (see Chapter 2). They also are histologically the same. So how is the diagnosis made? If metastases (usually to the lung) occur, or if a previously resected giant cell tumor recurs, the tumor is considered malignant. Malignant giant cell tumors tend to occur primarily in the fourth decade of life.

Fibrosarcoma

Fibrosarcomas are lytic malignant tumors that do not produce osteoid or chondroid matrix.

They usually do not elicit reactive new bone and, therefore, are almost always lytic in appearance. This lytic appearance may take any form, from permeative to moth-eaten (Fig. 3–20) to a fairly well-defined area of lysis (Fig. 3–21). This can make radiographic diagnosis very difficult.

The age range for fibrosarcomas is quite broad, but they tend to predominate in the fourth decade. Fibrosarcoma (and its cousins—MFHs and desmoids) and lymphoma are the only malignant tumors that can, on occasion, have a bony sequestrum.

Also, fibrosarcomas, desmoids, and MFHs tend to be the only tumors which are not consistently high in signal on T2-weighted MR images.

Malignant Fibrous Histiocytoma

Originally classified as fibrosarcoma by most pathologists, MFH has come into its own grouping in the past few decades. Radiologically they appear identical to fibrosarcomas—lytic lesions with variations extending from permeative (Fig. 3–22) to fairly well defined. Like fibrosarcomas, they may, on occasion, have a bony sequestrum. Anytime fibrosarcoma is mentioned, MFH should be included, as they can look identical radiographically.

Desmoid

A desmoid tumor (not to be confused with a cortical desmoid—see Chapter 4) is a half-grade fibrosarcoma. It has also been called a desmoplastic fibroma or aggressive fibromatosis. These

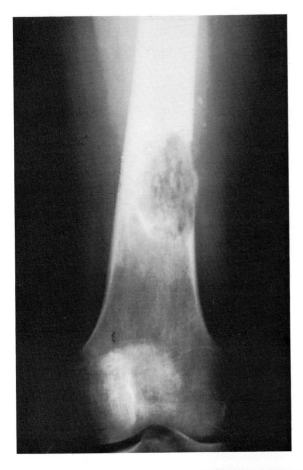

FIGURE 3–20 **Fibrosarcoma.** An ill-defined lytic lesion that is permeative or moth-eaten is seen in the diaphysis of the femur. On biopsy it was shown to be a fibrosarcoma.

FIGURE 3–21 **Fibrosarcoma.** A large, fairly well-defined destructive process of the entire right iliac wing is noted. On biopsy this was shown to be a fibrosarcoma. Fibrosarcomas can be very slow growing and will occasionally have a narrow zone of transition, such as this.

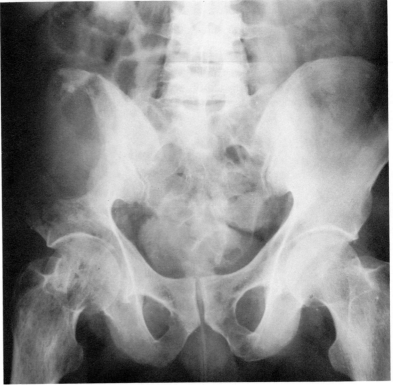

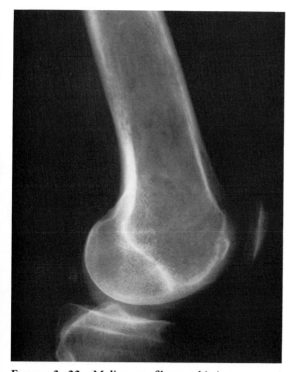

FIGURE 3–22 Malignant fibrous histiocytoma. A moth-eaten or permeative process in the distal femur, with some involvement of the posterior cortex, is seen on this lateral radiograph. In a patient under the age of 30 a Ewing's sarcoma, eosinophilic granuloma, or infection would be the differential diagnosis. In a patient over the age of 30 infection and MFH would be more common. A reticulum cell sarcoma could have a similar appearance.

lesions, like fibrosarcoma, are lytic but are usually fairly well defined because of their slow growth. They often have benign periostitis present that has thick spicules, or "spikes," and normally have a multilocular appearance with thick septa (Figs. 3–23 and 3–24). They are slow growing and seldom metastasize, but they can exhibit inexorable tumor extension into surrounding soft tissues with disastrous results. Like fibrosarcoma and MFHs, these lesions can exhibit a bony sequestrum (Fig. 3–23).

Reticulum Cell Sarcoma (Primary Lymphoma of Bone)

A rare neoplasm, reticulum cell sarcoma has a radiologic appearance identical to that of Ewing's sarcoma (i.e., a permeative or moth-eaten pattern) (Fig. 3–25). It tends to occur in an older age-group than does Ewing's sarcoma, and whereas the Ewing's sarcoma patient is typically systemically symptomatic, the reticulum cell sar-

coma patient is usually asymptomatic. In fact, reticulum cell sarcoma is the only malignant tumor that can involve a large amount of bone while the patient is systemically asymptomatic.

Metastatic Disease

Metastatic lesions must be included in *any* differential diagnosis of a bone lesion in a patient over the age of 40. They can have virtually any appearance: they can mimic a benign lesion (see Chapter 2) or a primary bone tumor. Judging the origin of the tumor from the appearance of the metastatic focus can be difficult—if not impossible—although some appearances are fairly characteristic. For instance, multiple sclerotic foci in a male are probably prostatic metastases (Fig. 3–26), although lung, bowel, or almost any other organ tumor could present in the same way. In a female the same picture would probably result from breast metastases. The only primary tumor that virtually never presents with blastic mets is renal cell carcinoma. Typically, an expansile lytic metastasis should be either renal or thyroid in origin (Fig. 3–27).

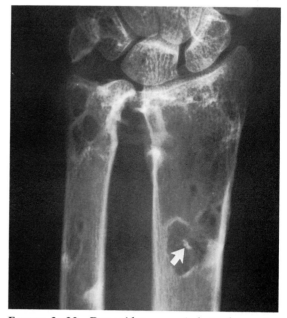

FIGURE 3–23 Desmoid tumor. A lytic destructive process involving both bones of the distal forearm is noted, with at least one portion demonstrating a sequestrum (arrow). A desmoid tumor is a fibrosarcoma-like lesion, and fibrosarcomas are known to occasionally demonstrate bony sequestra in the same manner as will osteomyelitis, lymphoma, and eosinophilic granuloma.

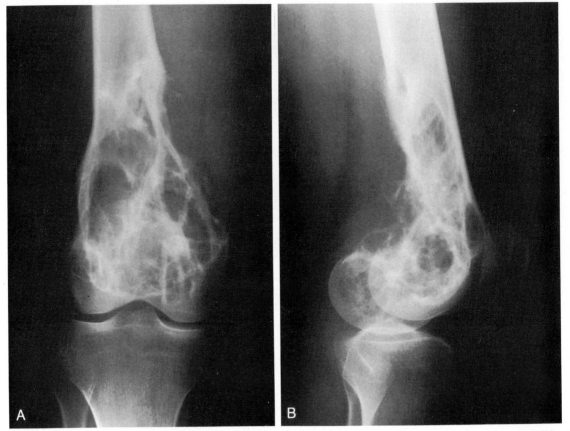

FIGURE 3–24 Desmoid tumor. *(A and B)* A multilocular, heavily septated, destructive lytic lesion of the distal femur is noted, which is fairly characteristic for a desmoid tumor. The thick septa and narrow zone of transition are characteristic of a benign process, whereas the Codman's triangle and the large amount of bony destruction indicate an aggressive process.

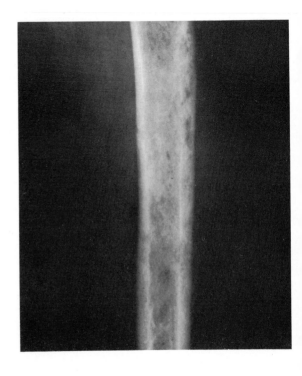

FIGURE 3–25 Reticulum cell sarcoma. A diffuse permeative pattern throughout the humerus in this 35-year-old patient is characteristic of reticulum cell sarcoma.

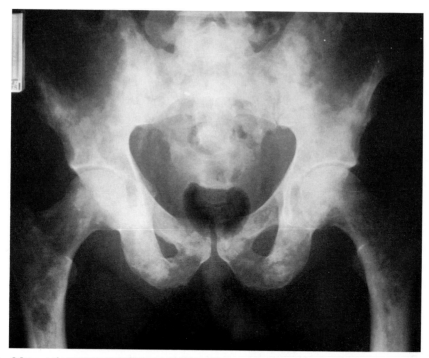

FIGURE 3–26   **Metastatic prostate carcinoma.** Diffuse blastic metastases are seen throughout the pelvis and proximal femurs, with a lytic destructive lesion seen in the right proximal femur. Prostate metastases tend to be blastic, but as shown here they can occasionally be lytic.

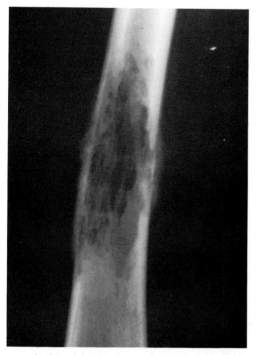

FIGURE 3–27   **Metastatic renal cell carcinoma.** A lytic lesion in the diaphysis of the femur is noted, which is characteristic for renal cell carcinoma. Up to one third of renal cell carcinomas initially present with a bony metastasis. Renal cell carcinoma virtually never presents with a blastic metastatic focus.

Myeloma

Like metastases, myeloma should be considered only in a patient over the age of 40, although some radiologists use age 35 for the lower limits of myeloma. Myeloma typically has a diffuse permeative appearance that can mimic a Ewing's sarcoma or a reticulum cell sarcoma (Fig. 3–28). It frequently involves the calvarium (Fig. 3–29). Because of the age criteria, Ewing's sarcoma and myeloma are not in the same differential, however. Rarely, myeloma can present with multiple sclerotic foci that resemble diffuse mets. Myeloma is one of the only lesions that is not characteristically "hot" on a radionuclide bone scan; therefore, radiologic "bone surveys" are performed instead of radionuclide bone scans when evidence of myeloma is found clinically.

Occasionally myeloma will present with a lytic bone lesion called a plasmacytoma. This lesion can mimic any lytic bone lesion, benign or aggressive, in its appearance; it can precede other evidence of myeloma by up to 3 years.

Myeloma has two different appearances in the spine on CT scans. Acute myeloma appears as one would imagine—it has a "Swiss cheese" pattern of multiple holes (Fig. 3–30). Chronic or long-standing myeloma, however, has a wild-looking pattern of dense, thick bony struts that resembles Paget's disease (Fig. 3–31). This is a characteristic "Aunt Minnie" on CT but is not

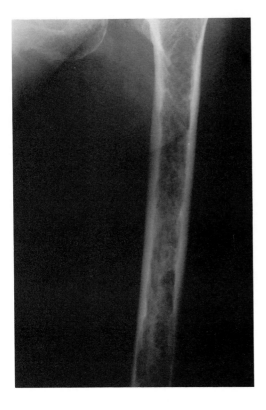

FIGURE 3–28   **Multiple myeloma.** A diffuse moth-eaten pattern is seen throughout the diaphysis of the femur in this 45-year-old patient, which is characteristic for myeloma. Reticulum cell sarcoma could have a similar appearance.

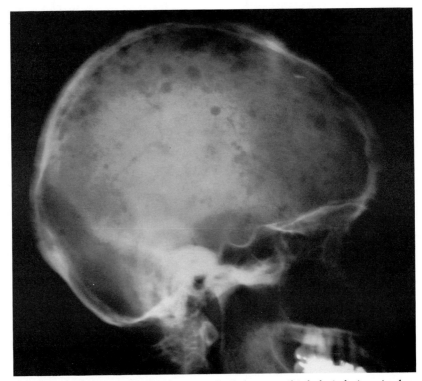

FIGURE 3–29   **Multiple myeloma.** A lateral view of the skull shows multiple lytic lesions in the calvarium, which is a characteristic appearance of multiple myeloma.

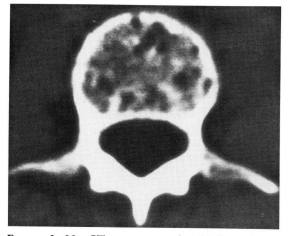

FIGURE 3–30 **CT appearance of multiple myeloma.** An axial CT image through a vertebral body in a patient with multiple myeloma shows a "Swiss-cheese" appearance typical for this disease in the acute stages.

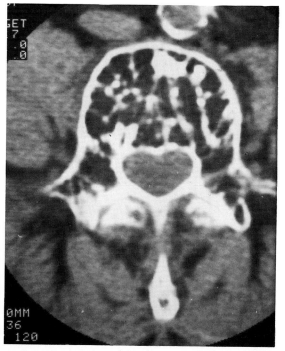

FIGURE 3–31 **CT appearance of chronic multiple myeloma.** An axial CT image through a vertebral body in a patient with long-standing multiple myeloma shows the typical appearance of hypertrophied bony struts giving a wild-looking pattern somewhat resembling Paget's disease.

appreciated on plain films—both the acute and chronic myeloma simply appear osteopenic on plain films.

Soft Tissue Tumors

Most radiology residents feel uneasy when faced with the differential diagnosis of a soft tissue tumor. They will give elaborate description with plenty of pertinent and not-so-pertinent negatives, such as "no calcifications are seen," "no bony destruction is noted," and "no obliteration of fat planes is apparent." Then, when faced with finally giving a differential, few can give an authoritative list of the possibilities. The reason for this is quite simple: there is no authoritative, useful differential for soft tissue tumors, whether or not there is calcification, bony destruction, fat plane involvement, or whatever. You can play the odds and mention the two most common soft tissue tumors, fibrosarcoma and liposarcoma, as the best candidates, but any cell type can produce a benign or malignant tumor and mimic any other soft tissue tumor. A lipoma can be separated out by the appearance of fat, but a liposarcoma may or may not have fat present. Therefore, we are left to give descriptions of size and extent, and let the pathologist tell us the rest. Most of us are uncomfortable with this approach because our training has been to derive an answer—or at least a listing of probable lesions. This is just not possible for soft tissue tumors.

A few words about soft tissue tumors that may be helpful: as mentioned earlier, liposarcomas do not have to have fat visible in the tumor. There are at least three subtypes of liposarcomas, two of which have only small amounts of fat present. Synovial sarcomas, or synoviomas, only rarely originate in a joint. They are often adjacent to joints but probably arise from synovial tissue in tendon sheaths rather than in joints themselves. There are no malignant tumors that routinely need to be considered in the differential diagnosis of joint lesions. Synovial osteochondromatosis is a benign joint lesion that probably occurs from metaplasia of the synovium and leads to multiple calcific loose bodies in a joint. This can histologically mimic a chondrosarcoma; therefore, it is best diagnosed radiographically, since it has a pathognomonic radiographic appearance (Fig. 3–32). Up to 30 per cent of the time, however, the loose bodies do not calcify, and the lesion then can mimic pigmented villonodular synovitis. This also is a benign synovial soft tissue process that causes joint swelling and pain and, occasionally, joint erosions (Fig. 3–33). Calcifications are virtually never associated with it. Hemangiomas often have phleboliths associated with

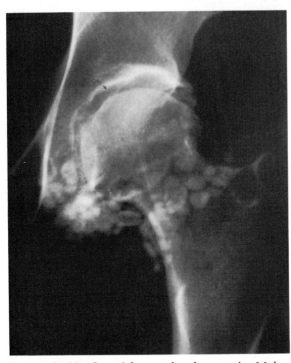

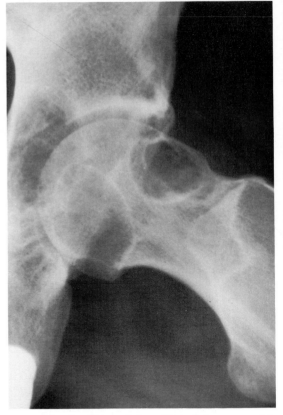

FIGURE 3–32 Synovial osteochondromatosis. Multiple calcific loose bodies in a hip joint such as this are virtually pathognomonic for synovial osteochondromatosis. Notice the erosions in the acetabulum. In up to 30 per cent of cases the loose bodies are nonossified. When nonossified this process is indistinguishable from pigmented villonodular synovitis.

FIGURE 3–33 Pigmented villonodular synovitis. Large erosions in the femoral head and acetabulum are characteristic for pigmented villonodular synovitis; however, nonossified synovial osteochondromatosis could present like this.

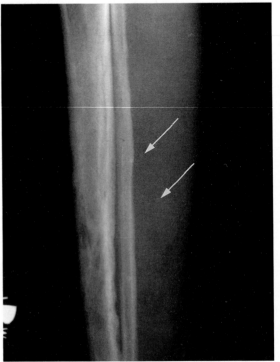

FIGURE 3–34 Hemangioma. Multiple, irregular lytic lesions, predominantly cortical in nature, are seen in the tibia in this patient with a soft tissue mass. Cortical holes such as this occur almost exclusively in radiation and soft tissue hemangioma. Note the phleboliths in the posterior soft tissues (arrows), which are often seen in hemangioma and make this an easy diagnosis.

them and often cause "cortical holes" in adjacent bone that mimic a permeative pattern (Fig. 3–34). The permeative pattern of round cell lesions occurs in the intramedullary or endosteal part of the bone and can be differentiated from "cortical holes" by the intact cortex (see Chapter 7, Metabolic Bone Disease). Atypical synovial cysts, such as Baker's cysts around the knee, can present as a soft tissue mass and result in an unnecessary biopsy. On CT these lesions may not be appreciated as fluid-filled lesions, and their association with a joint can be easily overlooked. MR imaging will demonstrate a very high-signal intensity with T2 weighting and may show some fluid in the adjacent joint with an identical signal (Fig. 3–35). Differentiation of a solid mass from a ganglion is one of the few uses of Gd-DTPA in musculoskeletal MR imaging. A solid tumor will diffusely enhance with gadolinium, whereas a ganglion will have rim enhancement only.

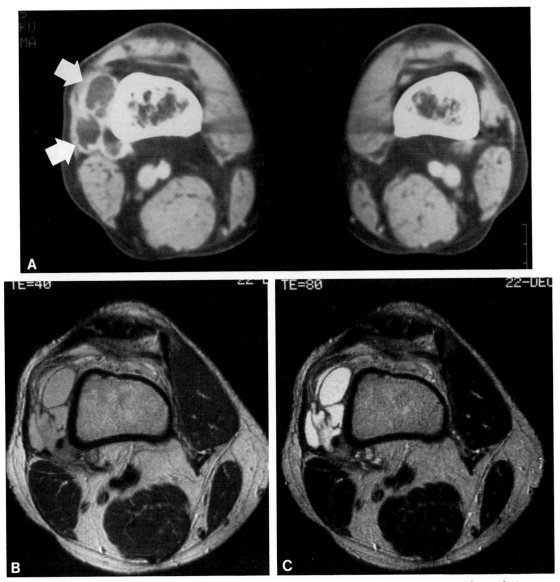

FIGURE 3–35 Atypical synovial cyst. *(A)* CT scan through the distal femurs in a patient with a soft tissue mass around the right knee shows a multilocular soft tissue tumor adjacent to the distal right femur (arrows). *(B)* An MR imaging scan with T1 weighting through the same area as imaged in *(A)* shows intermediate-intensity signal in a multilocular soft tissue mass. *(C)* An MR imaging scan with T2 weighting shows high-intensity signal in the lesion, which is characteristic for fluid. This was an atypical synovial cyst arising from the knee joint.

4

"Don't Touch" Lesions

Skeletal "don't touch" lesions are those processes that are so radiographically characteristic that a biopsy or additional diagnostic tests are unnecessary. Not only does the biopsy result in unnecessary morbidity and cost, but in some instances, as mentioned later, a biopsy also can be frankly misleading and lead to additional unnecessary surgery.

Most of our radiology training teaches us to give a differential diagnosis of a lesion, leaving it up to the clinician to decide between the various entities. For the "don't touch" lesions, however, a differential list is inappropriate, as that often makes the next step on the decision tree a biopsy. Because a biopsy of these lesions is not required for a final diagnosis, a radiologic diagnosis should be made without a list of differential possibilities. "Don't touch" lesions can be classified into three categories: (1) posttraumatic lesions, (2) normal variants, and (3) lesions that are real but obviously benign.

POSTTRAUMATIC LESIONS

Myositis ossificans is an example of a lesion on which a biopsy should not be performed because its aggressive histologic appearance can often mimic a sarcoma. Unfortunately, radical surgery has been performed based on the histologic appearance of myositis ossificans when the radiologic appearance was diagnostic. The typical radiologic appearance of myositis ossificans is circumferential calcification with a lucent center (Fig. 4–1). This is often best appreciated on computed tomography (CT) exam (Fig. 4–2). A malignant tumor that mimics myositis ossificans will have an ill-defined periphery and a calcified or ossific center (Fig. 4–3). Periosteal reaction can be seen with myositis ossificans or with a tumor. Occasionally the peripheral calcification of myositis ossificans can be difficult to appreciate; in such cases a CT scan should help, or delayed films a week or two later are recommended. Biopsy should be avoided when myositis ossificans is a clinical consideration.

Another posttraumatic entity in which a biopsy can be misleading is an avulsion injury. These injuries can have an aggressive radiographic appearance, but because of their characteristic location at insertion sites (e.g., antero-inferior iliac spine or ischial tuberosity) they should be recognized as benign (Figs. 4–4 and 4–5). Again, delayed films of several weeks will usually allow the problem case to become more radiographically and clinically clear. Biopsy can lead to the mistaken diagnosis of a sarcoma and should therefore be avoided. Any area that is undergoing healing can have a high nuclear-chromatin ratio and a high mitotic figure count, thereby occasionally simulating a malignancy.

A cortical desmoid is a process considered by many to be an avulsion off the medial supracondylar ridge of the distal femur. It occasionally simulates an aggressive lesion radiographically and on biopsy can look malignant.[1] In many instances biopsy has led to amputation for this benign, radiographically characteristic lesion (Figs. 4–6 to 4–8). Cortical desmoids occur only on the posteromedial epicondyle of the femur. They may or may not be associated with pain and can have increased radionuclide uptake on bone scan. They may or may not exhibit periosteal new bone

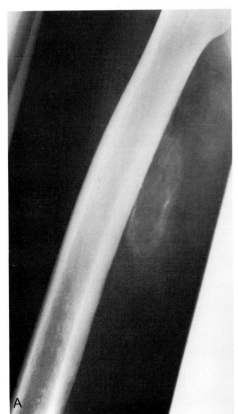

FIGURE 4–1 Myositis ossificans. *(A)* A plain film of the femur in this patient, who presented with a soft tissue mass, shows a calcific density adjacent to the posterior cortex of the femur that is calcified primarily in its periphery. From seeing the plain film alone it should not be difficult to definitely say that this is peripheral, circumferential calcification; however, the CT scan shown in *(B)* is helpful in showing that the calcification is unequivocally peripheral. This is virtually diagnostic of myositis ossificans.

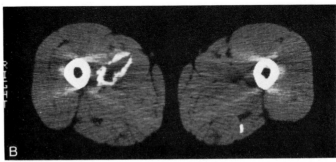

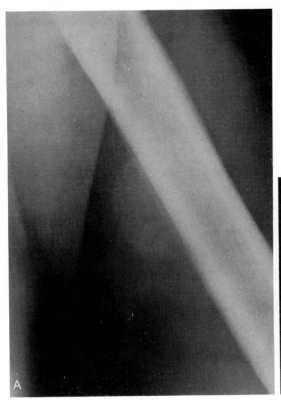

FIGURE 4–2 Myositis ossificans. *(A)* Hazy calcification is seen adjacent to the humeral shaft, with underlying periosteal reaction noted. It is difficult to ascertain whether or not the calcification is circumferential. *(B)* A CT scan through this mass shows that the calcification is unequivocally circumferential, making the diagnosis of myositis ossificans a certainty.

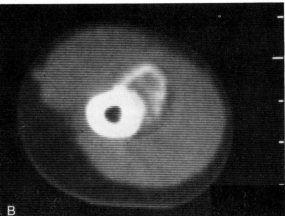

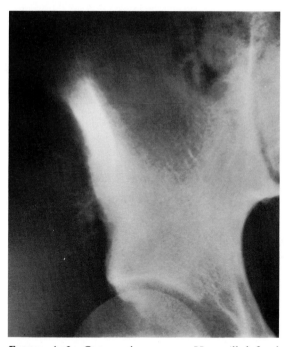

FIGURE 4–3 Osteogenic sarcoma. Hazy, ill-defined calcification is seen adjacent to the iliac wing in this patient that can be ascertained from the plain film to definitely not be circumferential. Even though a prior history of trauma was obtained in this case, myositis ossificans is not a consideration with this appearance of calcification. Biopsy showed this to be an osteogenic sarcoma.

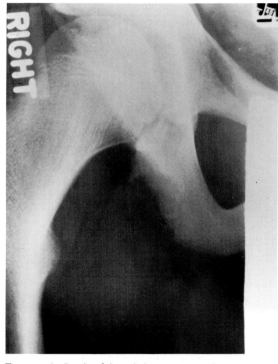

FIGURE 4–5 Avulsion injury. Cortical irregularity with a Codman's triangle of periostitis is seen along the ischial tuberosity. This was at first thought to represent a malignancy. Because of the characteristic location, an avulsion injury was considered and the lesion was observed. It healed without sequelae. (Case courtesy of Dr. John Wilson.)

FIGURE 4–4 Avulsion injury. Cortical irregularity (arrows) at the ischial tuberosity in this patient with pain over this region raises the question of possible tumor. This is a classic appearance, however, for an avulsion injury from this region, and a biopsy should be avoided.

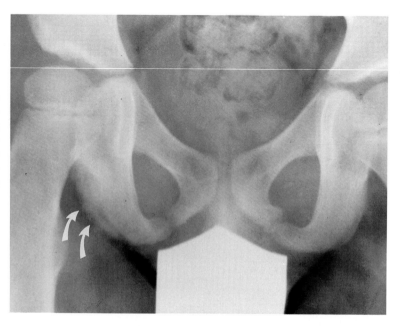

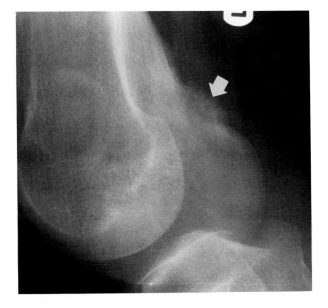

FIGURE 4–6 Cortical desmoid. A focal cortical irregularity is seen in the posterior aspect of the femur (arrow) with adjacent periostitis noted. Although a tumor such as an early parosteal osteosarcoma could perhaps have this appearance, the location and appearance are characteristic of a cortical desmoid, and a biopsy should not be performed.

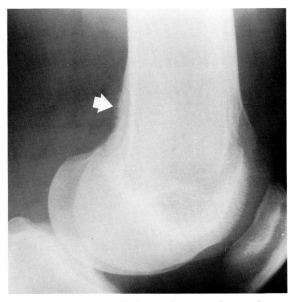

FIGURE 4–7 Cortical desmoid. Cortical irregularity with periostitis is seen in the posterior distal femur (arrow), which is characteristic in location and appearance for a cortical desmoid.

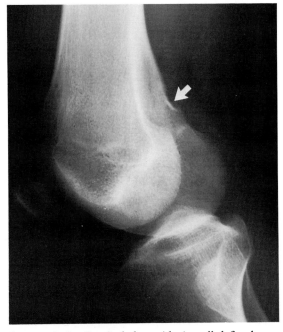

FIGURE 4–8 Cortical desmoid. A well-defined cortical defect is seen in the posterior distal femur (arrow), which is a common appearance for a fairly well-healed cortical desmoid.

and usually occur in young people. Biopsy should be avoided in all cases.

Trauma can lead to large, cystic geodes or subchondral cysts near joints that can be mistaken for other lesions, and thus a biopsy is performed. Although the biopsy specimen is not likely to mimic a malignant process, it is nevertheless

avoidable. Because geodes from degenerative disease almost always are associated with additional findings, such as joint space narrowing, sclerosis, and osteophytes, a diagnosis should be made radiographically (Figs. 4–9 and 4–10). However, on occasion the additional findings are subtle and can be missed (Fig. 4–11). Geodes can also occur

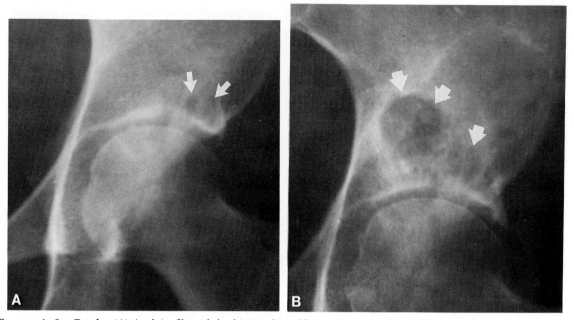

FIGURE 4–9   Geode. *(A)* A plain film of the hip in this older patient with hip pain shows a lytic lesion in the supra-acetabular region (arrow), which has a benign appearance. Mild osteoarthritis was felt to be present (when compared to the opposite hip, joint space narrowing and mimimal sclerosis were seen), hence this was felt to be a subchondral cyst or geode. *(B)* Several years later the same hip shows a large lytic lesion (arrows) that still appears benign. The osteoarthritis has increased in severity. However, because of the growth of the lesion it was biopsied and found to be a geode.

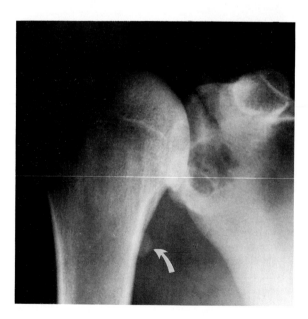

FIGURE 4–10   Geode. A large cystic lesion was found in the shoulder in this middle-aged weight lifter, and the possibility of a metastatic process was considered. Because the humeral head has sclerosis and osteophytosis as well as a loose body in the joint (arrow), the degenerative disease of the shoulder was diagnosed; this makes the cystic lesion almost certainly a geode or subchondral cyst, which made a biopsy unnecessary.

in the setting of calcium pyrophosphate dihydrate crystal disease (also known as CPPD or pseudogout), rheumatoid arthritis, and avascular necrosis.[2]

An entity that is often confused with metastatic disease to the spine is discogenic vertebral disease.

It can mimic metastatic disease radiographically and clinically, and unless the radiologist is familiar with this process, it can lead to an unnecessary biopsy.[3,4] Discogenic vertebral disease most often is sclerotic and focal (Fig. 4–12). It is adjacent to an end-plate, and the associated

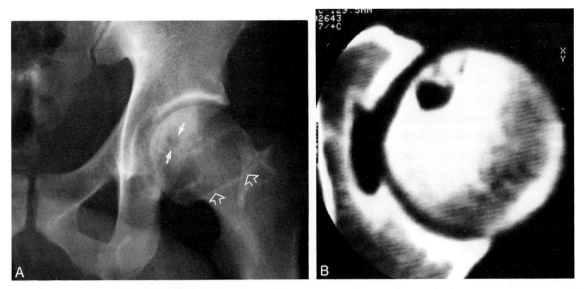

FIGURE 4–11 Geode. *(A)* A cystic lesion was noted in the femoral head (arrows) of a young male with a painful hip. *(B)* A CT scan through this area shows the subarticular nature and adjacent sclerosis. The differential diagnosis of infection, eosinophilic granuloma, and chondroblastoma was given. A ring of osteophytes (open arrow heads) was noted in retrospect on the plain film *(A)* in the subcapital region, which indicates degenerative disease of the hip. This is an extremely unusual presentation in a healthy 20-year-old male; however, it makes the lytic lesion in the femoral head almost certainly a subchondral cyst or geode. This was an active soccer player who had been playing with pain in his hip for several years after an injury that had caused the degenerative disease. Unfortunately a biopsy was performed anyway, and a subchondral cyst or geode was confirmed.

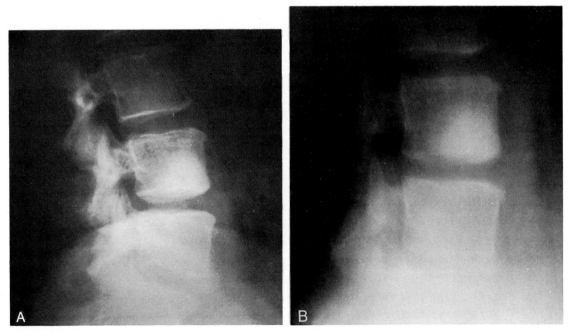

FIGURE 4–12 Discogenic vertebral sclerosis. *(A, B, C)* These films all show patients with sclerosis on the inferior portion of the L-4 vertebral body associated with minimal osteophytosis and joint space narrowing at the adjacent disc space. This is the classic appearance for discogenic vertebral sclerosis, and a biopsy to rule out metastatic disease should not be performed.

Continued

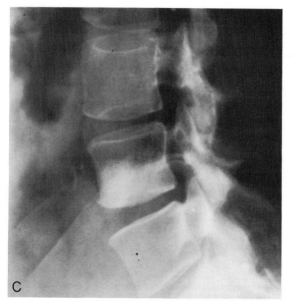

FIGURE 4–12 *Continued*

disc space should be narrow. Osteophytosis is invariably present. It really is a variant of a Schmorl's node and should not be confused with a metastatic focus. On occasion it can be lytic or even mixed lytic-sclerotic. The typical clinical setting is a middle-aged woman with chronic low back pain. Old films often confirm the benign nature of this process. In the setting of disc-space narrowing and osteophytosis, a biopsy of focal sclerosis adjacent to an end-plate should not be done.

Occasionally a fracture will be the cause of extensive osteosclerosis and periostitis, which can mimic a primary bone tumor (Fig. 4–13). Lack of immobilization can result in exuberant callus, which can be misinterpreted as aggressive periostitis or even tumor new bone. A biopsy in such a case might resemble a malignant lesion. Therefore, any case associated with trauma should be carefully reviewed for a fracture.

Another traumatic process that can be misdiagnosed radiologically, leading to inappropriate treatment and morbidity, is a pseudodislocation of the humerus (Figs. 4–14 and 4–15). This results from a fracture with hemarthrosis, which

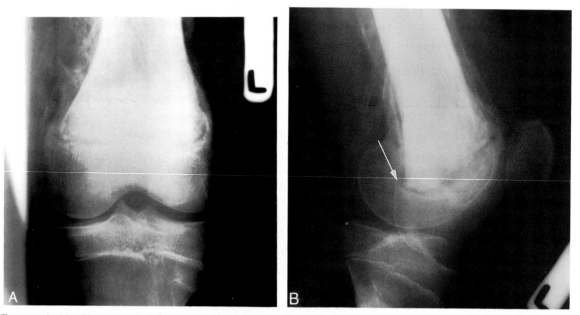

FIGURE 4–13 Fracture mimicking osteosarcoma. *(A)* This 16-year-old had experienced pain around the knee for 2 weeks before these radiographs were taken. The knee films showed diffuse sclerosis and extensive periostitis about the distal femur, which was felt to be characteristic for an osteogenic sarcoma. The periosteal reaction, however, was felt to be much too thick, dense, and wavy to represent malignant type of periostitis. *(B)* A small offset of the epiphysis can be seen (arrow), which indicates an epiphyseal slippage consistent with a Salter epiphyseal fracture. The patient had fallen off his bicycle and fractured his femur, yet continued to be active. The lack of immobility caused exuberant periostitis or callus with a large amount of reactive sclerosis, all of which mimicked an osteogenic sarcoma.

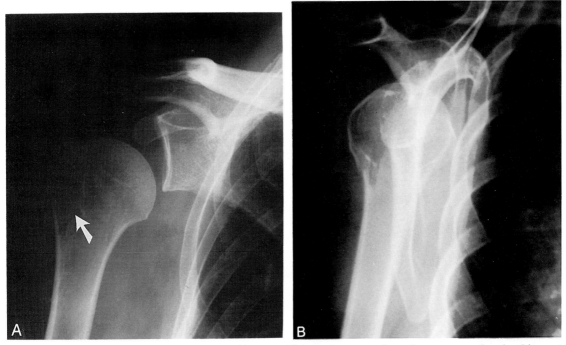

FIGURE 4–14   **Pseudodislocation of the shoulder.** *(A)* This patient experienced trauma to the shoulder, with resultant pain and immobility, and was thought to have a dislocation of the shoulder after the anteroposterior film was seen. The humeral head is inferiorly placed in relation to the glenoid; however, this is not the characteristic location of an anterior or posterior dislocation. *(B)* The transscapular view shows the humeral head to be situated normally over the glenoid without anterior or posterior dislocation. These findings are characteristic for a pseudodislocation caused by hemarthrosis, or blood in the joint, which allows the shoulder to be subluxed rather than dislocated. Aspiration of the blood will result in the humeral head returning to its normal position in relation to the glenoid; however, this is not usually necessary. When a pseudodislocation is seen, as in this example, search for an occult fracture should ensue. In this case as seen on *A* a fracture (arrow) was initially missed.

FIGURE 4–15   **Pseudodislocation of the shoulder.** The humeral head is inferiorly placed in relation to the glenoid. This is the characteristic location when a hemarthrosis is present. A minimally displaced fracture of the neck of the humerus with avulsion of the greater tuberosity has occurred, causing the hemarthrosis.

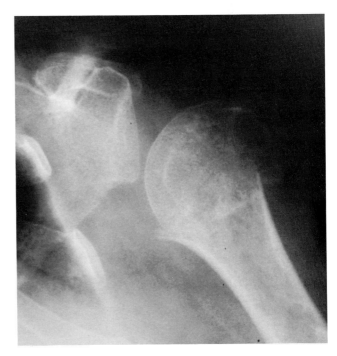

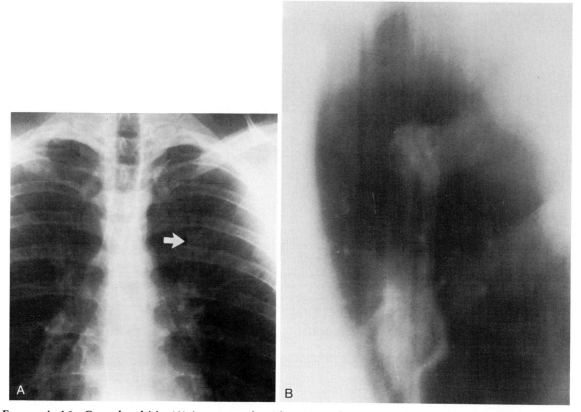

FIGURE 4–16 Costochondritis. *(A)* A young male with point tenderness over the anterior chest wall had a chest radiograph that revealed a nodular density (arrow) that appeared attached to the second rib. *(B)* Tomograms of this area show a nodular density with speckled calcification at the distal end of the rib, which was thought to possibly represent an osteochondroma. Any chondroid lesion that is painful should be suspicious for malignant degeneration, and a biopsy was planned for this patient. The clinical findings, however, were classic for costochondritis or Tietze's syndrome, which rapidly cleared; therefore, biopsy was cancelled. Costochondritis can cause periostitis and bulbous swelling of the ribs, as in this example, and a biopsy should not be performed.

causes distention of the joint and migration of the humeral head inferiorly. An axial or transscapular view shows that it is not anteriorly or posteriorly dislocated (the usual forms of shoulder dislocation) but merely inferiorly displaced. On an anteroposterior view it can mimic a posterior dislocation. Often attempts are made to "relocate" the humeral head, which are both fruitless (because it is not dislocated) and painful. A fracture is invariably present, and if not seen on the initial films should be sought after with additional views. A transscapular or an axillary view is the key to making the diagnosis of a pseudodislocation. With either of these views the humeral head can be seen to be normally positioned in relation to the glenoid, although it may appear somewhat inferiorly displaced. If necessary, the joint can be aspirated to confirm the presence of a bloody effusion and to show the normal position of the humeral head with no fluid in the joint.[5]

Costochondritis, or Tietze's syndrome, can cause a bulbous swelling of a rib (Fig. 4–16) owing to periostitis, which can mimic a rib lesion. This condition is very painful and usually easily diagnosed clinically; however, with a bony lesion seen on radiographs many clinicians may want a biopsy to rule out a malignant process. This would be a mistake, as with any posttraumatic or rapidly healing lesion it can be difficult to categorize histologically. Because Tietze's syndrome is a short-lived process, watchful waiting with repeat film in 2 to 3 weeks if the patient is not improved is probably indicated.

NORMAL VARIANTS

Numerous normal variants exist that are often confused with a pathologic process. This is best evidenced by the fact that several of the most popular radiology texts are atlases of normal variants.

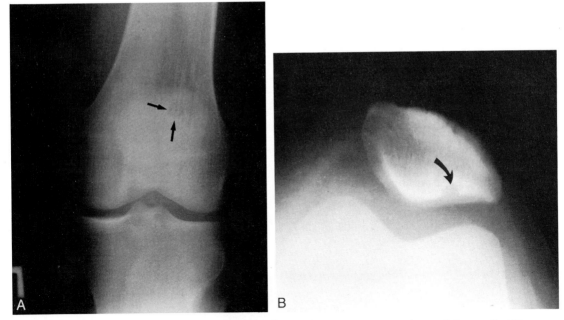

FIGURE 4–17 **Dorsal defect of the patella.** A lytic defect in the upper outer quadrant of the patella *(A)* was seen in this patient (arrows), which is characteristic for a normal variant called dorsal defect of the patella. It occurs only in the upper outer quadrant and should be asymptomatic. It lies adjacent to the articular surface as shown on the sunrise view *(B)*.

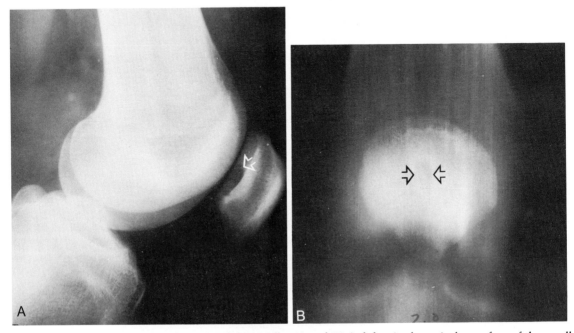

FIGURE 4–18 **Osteochondritis dissecans of the patella.** *(A and B)* A defect in the articular surface of the patella (arrows) is seen in this patient. It is centrally placed rather than in the upper outer quadrant. Because of its location, a dorsal defect of the patella is not a consideration. This was osteochondritis dissecans, which is unusual in the patella.

A normal variant that has been described in the patella is a lytic defect in the upper outer quadrant called dorsal defect of the patella (Fig. 4–17).[6] It can mimic a focus of infection, osteochondritis dissecans (Fig. 4–18), or a chondroblastoma. It is a normal developmental anomaly, however, and because of its characteristic location a biopsy of it should not be performed. It is diagnosed on magnetic resonance (MR) imaging also by its characteristic location, as the signal characteristics are similar to tumor or infection (Fig. 4–19).

Another entity often confused with a lytic pathologic process is a pseudocyst of the humerus (Fig. 4–20). This is merely an anatomic variant caused by the increased cancellous bone in the region of the greater tuberosity of the humerus, which gives this region a more lucent appearance on radiographs. With hyperemia and disuse caused by rotator cuff problems or any other shoulder disorder, this area of lucency may appear strikingly more lucent and mimic a lytic lesion. Biopsies of many of these lesions have been done mistakenly, and in several cases have been repeated (Fig. 4–20C) after the initial pathology report stated "normal bone—no lesion in speciman." Because of the associated hyperemia from the shoulder disorder (be it rotator cuff or whatever) a bone scan can show increased radionuclide uptake and thus sway the surgeon to do a biopsy of this normal variant. It is radiographically characteristic in its location and appearance,

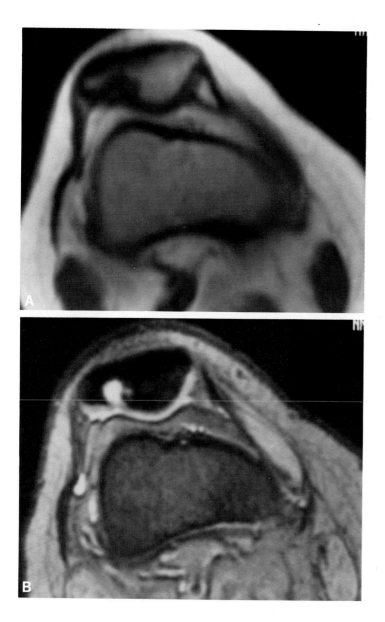

FIGURE 4–19 **MR images of dorsal defect of the patella.** *(A)* T1-weighted and *(B)* T2-weighted axial MR images through the patella in a patient with a lytic lesion in the upper outer quadrant of the patella shows low signal on the T1 image, which is high signal on T2. This is a characteristic appearance for a dorsal defect of the patella.

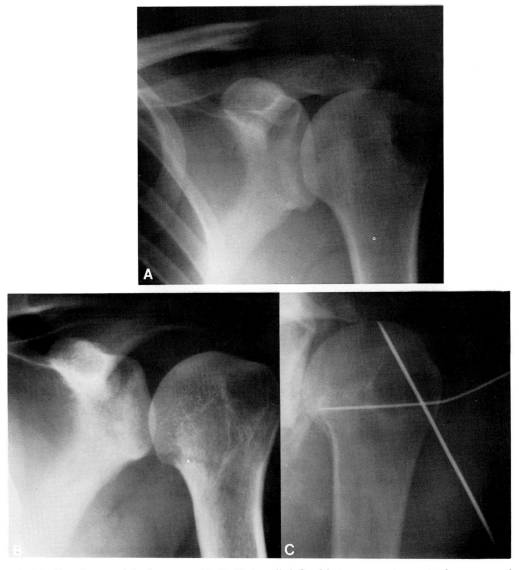

FIGURE 4–20 Pseudocyst of the humerus. *(A, B, C)* A well-defined lytic process is seen in the greater tuberosity in each of these examples. In each case it was believed to represent a lytic lesion. These patients were all symptomatic, and several had increased radionuclide uptake on isotope bone scan. The location and appearance, however, are characteristic for a pseudocyst of the humerus, which merely represents decreased cortical bone in this region. This becomes more pronounced when pain in the shoulder is present and hyperemia or disuse osteoporosis occurs. Biopsies of several of these examples were performed, and a biopsy was repeated in the example in C when the first biopsy was reported as "normal bone" and the surgeons assumed that they had missed the lesion.

and a biopsy of it should not be done.[7] Although other lesions, such as a chondroblastoma (Fig. 4–21), infection, or even a metastatic focus, could occur in a similar location, they do not have quite the same appearance as a pseudocyst of the humerus.

A normal variant of the cervical spine that may, in fact, be posttraumatic is an os odontoideum.[8] It is an unfused dens that may move anterior to the C-2 body with flexion and can mimic a fractured dens (Figs. 4–22 and 4–23). Many of these lesions require surgical fixation; some surgeons fuse every case, believing that they are all unstable. Radiologists should recognize that this process is not acute, so as to save the patient from having Crutchfield tongs applied and from possible immediate surgical intervention. Most cases are seen after trauma, and if no neurologic deficits are present, these patients can be seen electively and spared the horrors asso-

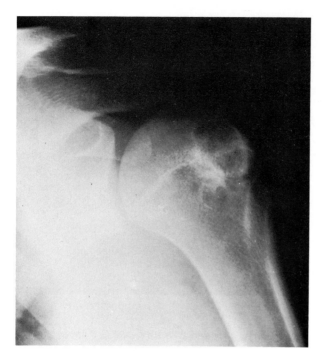

FIGURE 4–21 Chondroblastoma. A well-defined lesion in the greater tuberosity of the humerus that has a sclerotic margin is easily distinguished from the prior examples of pseudocyst of the humerus. This was found to be a chondroblastoma.

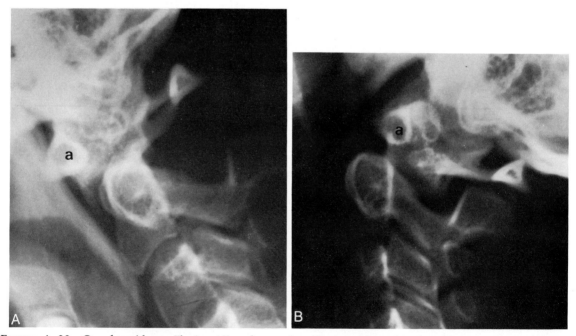

FIGURE 4–22 Os odontoideum. Flexion *(A)* and extension *(B)* views show that the anterior arch (a) of the C-1 vertebrae has moved markedly anterior in relation to the body of C-2 in flexion. The odontoid or dens is difficult to see but appears to be separated from the body of C-2. Because of the smooth borders of the separated dens and because of the cortical hypertrophy of the anterior arch of C-1, this can safely be called an os odontoideum, which is a congenital or long-standing posttraumatic abnormality rather than an acute fracture. Obviously these patients should have no neurologic problems, yet in many instances the lesions are still felt to be unstable and are surgically fused. This can be done on an elective basis.

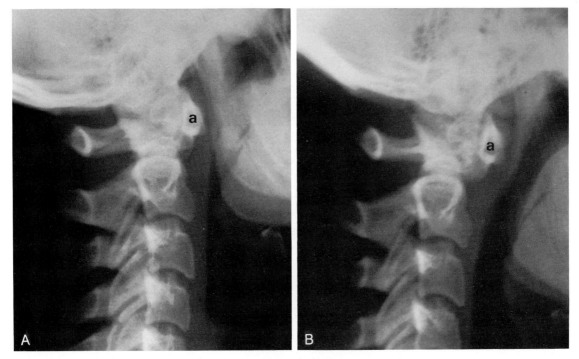

FIGURE 4–23 Os odontoideum. Extension *(A)* and flexion *(B)* show extreme motion of the anterior arch (a) of C-1 as compared with the C-2 vertebral body. The dens is difficult to find in this example but is certainly not attached to the C-2 body. Again, the smooth margins where the dens should be attached and the cortical hypertrophy of the anterior arch of C-1 make this a congenital or long-standing process consistent with an os odontoideum rather than an acute fracture.

ciated with treatment of the acutely fractured cervical spine. The radiologic signs for recognizing an os odontoideum are the smooth, often well-corticated inferior border of the dens and the hypertrophied, densely corticated anterior arch of C-1. This latter finding presumably represents compensatory hypertrophy and indicates a long-standing condition.[9]

Although unusual, osteopoikilosis, a benign familial process of multiple bone islands or small areas of osteosclerosis, has caused confusion by its similarity to metastatic disease (Fig. 4–24). Ordinarily osteopoikilosis has such a characteristic appearance that it will not be mistaken for another entity, and the predominance of sclerotic foci near the epiphyses should help to differentiate it from metastatic disease (Fig. 4–25).

OBVIOUSLY BENIGN LESIONS

Biopsies are frequently performed on some lesions that should be recognized radiographically as benign and left alone. These are lesions that should be diagnosed by the radiologist, not the pathologist. Listing a differential in such cases often spurs the surgeon to a biopsy, when in fact no biopsy should be necessary.

Perhaps the most commonly encountered lesion in this category is the nonossifying fibroma (NOF). It is thought to be identical to a fibrous cortical defect, but the term is usually reserved for defects larger than 2 cm. NOFs are, classically, lytic lesions that are located in the cortex of the metaphysis of a long bone which have a well-defined, often sclerotic, scalloped border with slight cortical expansion (Fig. 4–26) (also, see Chapter 2). They are almost exclusively found in patients under the age of 30, suggesting that the natural history of the lesion is involution. As they involute, they fill in with new bone (Fig. 4–27); hence they can have some increased radionuclide activity on bone scans. They are most often mistaken for an area of infection, eosinophilic granuloma, or aneurysmal bone cyst. NOFs are asymptomatic and have never been reported to be associated with malignant degeneration. On occasion a pathologic fracture can occur through these lesions, but most surgeons do not advocate prophylactic curettage to prevent fracture, as with unicameral bone cysts. NOFs can be quite large but invariably have a benign appearance

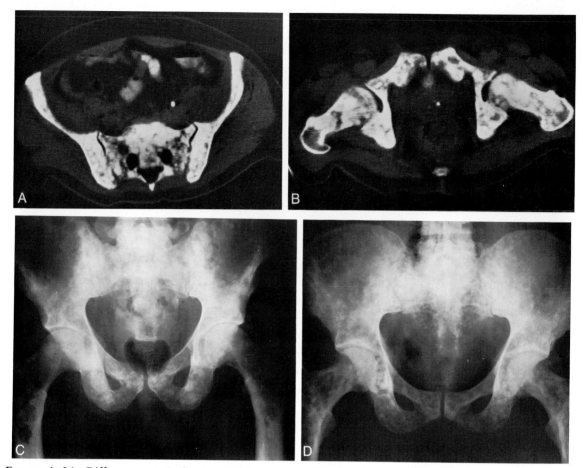

FIGURE 4–24 Diffuse metastatic disease mimicking osteopoikilosis. *(A, B)* A CT scan through the pelvis and hips shows diffuse sclerotic foci consistent with metastatic disease. One examiner felt that this might represent the sclerotic foci of osteopoikilosis, however, which is a benign familial process. *(C)* An anteroposterior view of the pelvis shows a similar appearance; however, a destructive lytic lesion is seen in the right proximal femur, which makes metastatic disease more likely. This patient had metastatic prostate carcinoma. Compare this with *D* in a patient with known osteopoikilosis, and it is easy to see how the two entities can be confused. Clinical history is vital in the distinction.

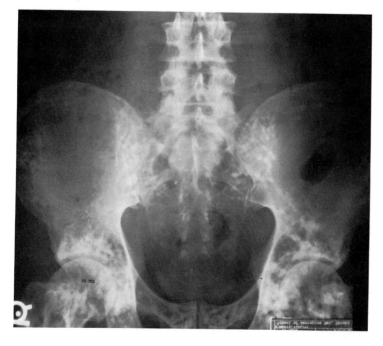

FIGURE 4–25 Osteopoikilosis. A more typical example of osteopoikilosis is shown in this example, in which the sclerotic foci are predominantly around the joints rather than diffusely spread throughout the bones.

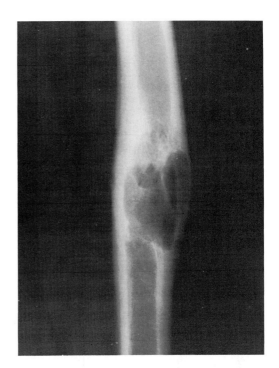

FIGURE 4–26 Nonossifying fibroma. A well-defined, slightly expansile lytic lesion is seen in a long bone, which is characteristic for a nonossifying fibroma. Unfortunately a biopsy of the lesion was performed, and the diagnosis was surgically confirmed.

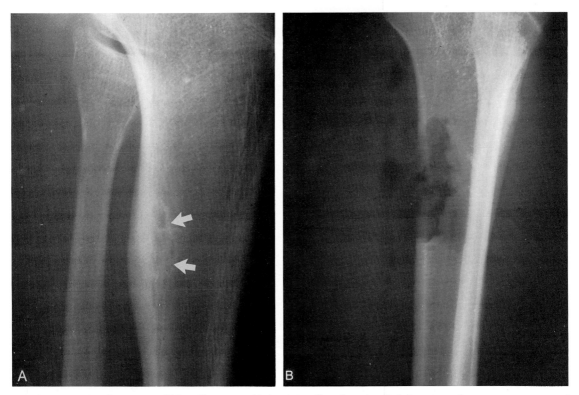

FIGURE 4–27 Healing nonossifying fibroma. *(A)* A minimally sclerotic, slightly expansile process is seen in the posterior proximal tibia (arrows). This was felt by the surgeons to represent a focus of infection or an osteoid osteoma even though the patient was asymptomatic. This is a characteristic appearance for a disappearing or healing nonossifying fibroma. The postsurgical appearance, which went on to a pathologic fracture, is shown in *B.* Surgery confirmed a nonossifying fibroma.

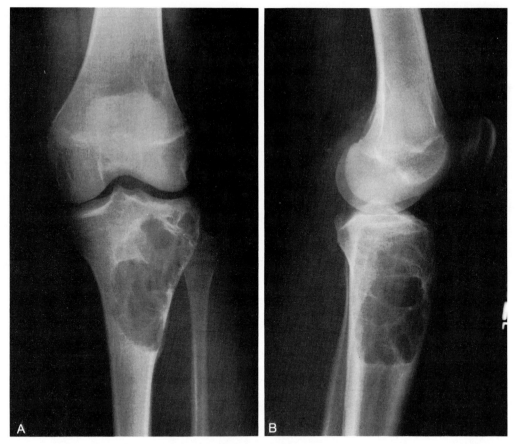

FIGURE 4–28 Nonossifying fibroma. *(A* and *B)* This well-defined, minimally expansile lytic lesion of the proximal tibia is characteristic for a nonossifying fibroma. It was felt by several radiologists to be a giant cell tumor; however, it has a sclerotic border and does not abut the tibial articular surface. Even though the patient was asymptomatic, a biopsy was performed and the diagnosis of a nonossifying fibroma was confirmed. (Case courtesy of Dr. Larry Yeager.)

(Fig. 4–28), and biopsy should be avoided. The asymptomatic nature is imperative to help distinguish them from most of the other lesions in the differential, and thereby preclude even giving a differential diagnosis. On occasion they are found to be multiple (Fig. 4–29), yet each lesion is so characteristic that they should be easily diagnosed.

Bone islands are not a radiographic dilemma when they are 1 cm or less. Occasionally, however, they grow to golf ball size and mimic sclerotic metastases (Fig. 4–30). They are always asymptomatic. Radiographically, two signs can be found to help distinguish giant bone islands from metastases: First, bone islands usually are oblong, with their long axis in the axis of stress on the bone (e.g., in a long bone they align themselves along the axis of the diaphysis); second, the margins of a bone island, if examined closely, will show bony trabeculae extending from the lesion into the normal bone in a spiculated

fashion.[10] (See Chapter 2.) This is characteristic of a bone island and helpful in differentiating it from more aggressive processes.

Unicameral bone cysts are often prophylactically packed so as to prevent fracture with subsequent deformity. When these cysts occur in the calcaneus, however, they should be left alone. They always occur in the anteroinferior portion of the calcaneus (Fig. 4–31), an area that does not receive undue stress. In fact, a pseudotumor of the calcaneus in the identical position is seen because of the absence of stress and resulting atrophy of bony trabeculae (Fig. 4–32). Calcaneal unicameral bone cysts are asymptomatic, only rarely fracture, and should not suffer the same fate as their counterparts in long bones.

Early in the course of its development a bone infarct can have a patchy or a mixed lytic-sclerotic pattern, or even resemble a permeative process (Figs. 4–33 and 4–34). In a patient with bone pain and a permeative bone lesion, many

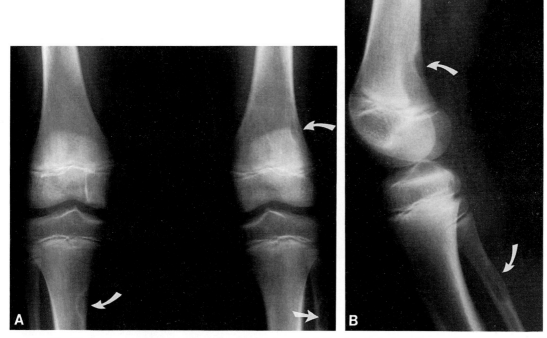

FIGURE 4–29 **Multiple nonossifying fibromas.** Multiple well-defined lytic lesions (arrows) are seen around the knees in this patient on the anteroposterior *(A)* and lateral *(B)* views, each of which is characteristic for a nonossifying fibroma.

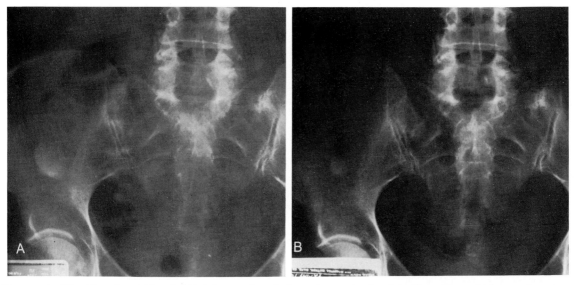

FIGURE 4–30 **Giant bone island.** *(A)* A large sclerotic focus is seen in the right iliac wing, which was thought to possibly represent an area of metastasis. *(B)* Old films from 5 years earlier were obtained, which showed a similar but much smaller process. This is characteristic for a growing bone island. Note in *A* how the lesion is somewhat spherical or oblong in the lines of trabecular stress, which is characteristic of a bone island.

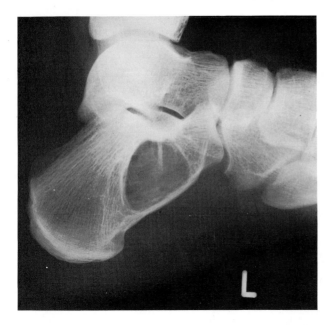

FIGURE 4–31 Unicameral bone cyst. A well-defined lytic lesion on the anteroinferior portion of the calcaneus, as in this example, is virtually pathognomonic for a unicameral bone cyst or simple bone cyst. Because this is an area of diminished stress it is thought not to be necessary to prophylactically curettage and pack this lesion in an effort to avoid a pathologic bone fracture, which is often done in the femur and humerus with unicameral bone cysts.

FIGURE 4–32 Pseudocyst of the calcaneus. An area of radiolucency is seen in the anteroinferior portion of the calcaneus that is similar to the example in Figure 4–31 but is not as well defined. This is a pseudocyst similar to the psuedocyst of the humerus that results from diminished stress through this region.

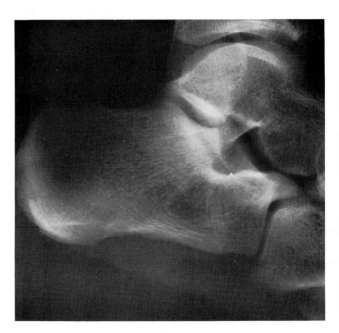

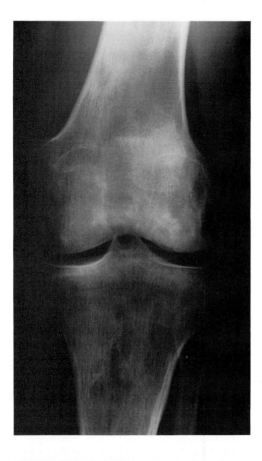

FIGURE 4–33 Early bone infarct. Patchy demineralization is seen in the distal femur and proximal tibia in this patient with systemic lupus erythematosus. The opposite leg was similarly involved. This is characteristic for early bone infarcts and should not be confused with infection or metastatic disease.

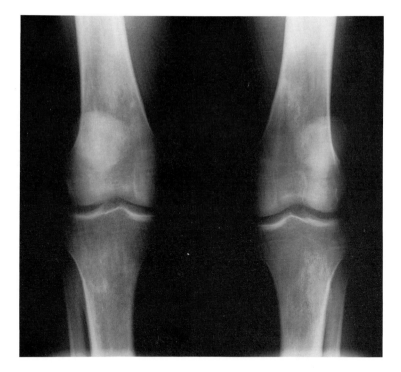

FIGURE 4–34 Bone infarct. A mixed lytic-sclerotic process is seen in the distal femurs and proximal tibias bilaterally in this patient with systemic lupus erythematosus. Because of pain in these regions a biopsy was performed, and bone infarct was confirmed. With this characteristic location and this appearance, even though suggestive of a more aggressive process, a biopsy of these lesions should not be performed.

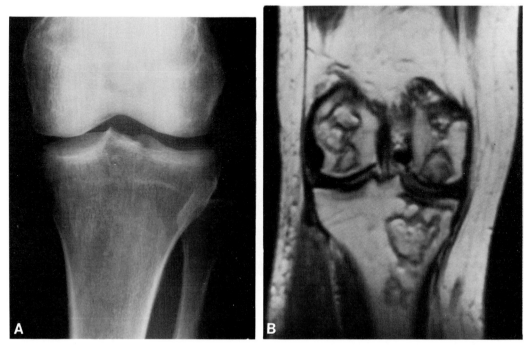

FIGURE 4–35 Bone infarct. (A) A plain film of the knee shows faint patchy sclerosis in the proximal tibia that was at first thought to be infection or malignancy. (B) MR imaging shows the characteristic serpiginous border seen with bone infarct. MR imaging can on occasion better characterize the ill-defined early bone infarct, as in this example.

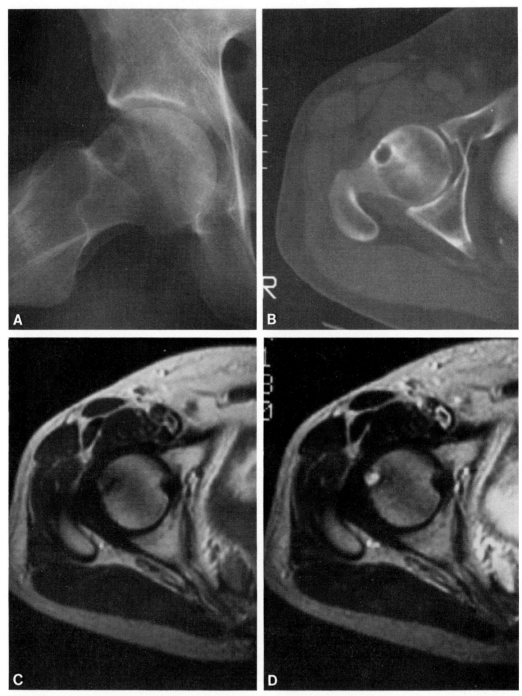

FIGURE 4–36 **Pitt's pit.** *(A)* A plain film of the right hip shows a well-defined lytic lesion in the lateral aspect of the femoral neck. It has a sclerotic border. This is a characteristic appearance of a synovial herniation pit, also called a Pitt's pit. *(B)* A CT scan through this lesion shows the typical subcortical location of a Pitt's pit. *(C)* A T1-weighted and *(D)* a T2-weighted MR image through the lesion show the low-signal T1 and high-signal T2 appearance, which is typical for a Pitt's pit.

aggressive disorders head the differential list and a biopsy soon ensues. If this process can be noted to be multiple and in the diametaphyseal region of a long bone, especially if the patient has an underlying disorder such as sickle cell anemia or systemic lupus erythematosus, areas of early bone infarction should be considered. In several instances the MR imaging appearance of an infarct has saved patients from biopsy when the plain films were equivocal (Fig. 4–35).[11]

A commonly encountered lytic lesion on the lateral aspect of the femoral neck was first described by Michael Pitt as a synovial herniation pit.[12] It has taken on the appropriate eponym of a "Pitt's pit." It is felt to be caused by surface erosion of the synovium and soft tissues around the hip, but its exact etiology is unknown. It has a characteristic plain film, CT, and MR appearance primarily because of its location and benign appearance (Fig. 4–36).

CONCLUSION

These are but a few of the many examples in skeletal radiology in which the well-trained radiologist can be of invaluable assistance to the clinician and the patient by helping to avert a needless biopsy. Dozens of other examples are nicely shown in normal variant textbooks, which are widely available. Because of the potential harm in performing a needless biopsy, these examples are stressed. When these lesions are encountered by the radiologist, a differential diagnosis should not be offered, as it will merely lead the surgeon to a biopsy in an attempt to reach a diagnosis. A biopsy in many of these entities not only is unnecessary, but also can be misleading.

REFERENCES

1. Barnes G, Gwinn J: Distal irregularities of the femur simulating malignancy. AJR 1974;122:180.
2. Resnick D, Niwayama G, Coutts RD: Subchondral cysts (geodes) in arthritic disorders: Pathologic and radiographic appearance of the hip joint. AJR 1977;128:799.
3. Martel W, Seeger FJ, Wicks JD, et al: Traumatic lesions of the discovertebral junction in the lumbar spine. AJR 1976;127:457.
4. Lipson S: Discogenic vertebral sclerosis with calcified disc. New Engl J Med 1991;325:794–799.
5. Helms C, Richmond B, Sims R: Pseudodislocation of the shoulder: A sign of an occult fracture. Emer Med 1986;18:237–241.
6. Goergen TG, Resnick D, Greenway G, et al: Dorsal defect of the patella (DDP): A characteristic radiographic lesion. Radiology 1979;130:333.
7. Helms C: Pseudocyst of the humerus. AJR 1979;131:287–292.
8. Minderhoud JM, Braakman R, Penning L: Os odontoideum: Clinical, radiological and therapeutic aspects. J Neurol Sci 1969;8:521.
9. Holt RG, Helms CA, Munk PL, Gillespy T III: Hypertrophy of C-1 anterior arch: Useful sign to distinguish os odontoideum from acute dens fracture. Radiology 1989;173:207–209.
10. Onitsuka H: Roentgenologic aspects of bone islands. Radiology 1977;124:607.
11. Munk PL, Helms CA, Holt RG: Immature bone infarcts: Findings on plain radiographs and MR scans. AJR 1989;152(3):547–549.
12. Pitt M, Graham A, Shipman J, Birkby W: Herniation pit of the femoral neck. AJR 1982;138:1115–1121.

Chapter

5

Trauma

Radiology of trauma to the skeletal system is such a large topic that entire volumes have been devoted to it. Lee Rogers has written the definitive work in his excellent book entitled *Radiology of Skeletal Trauma,*[1] and Jack and William Harris' outstanding book, *Radiology of Emergency Medicine,*[2] is a must read for anyone dealing with a large emergency department population. The leading orthopedic treatise on fractures is Rockwood and Green's multivolume text.[3] The following is merely an overview of selected cases that residents and medical students should be exposed to that can be studied in greater detail by referring to the texts mentioned above.

Before starting with specific examples the uninitiated or neophyte radiologist should keep a few key points in mind concerning radiology of trauma. First, have a high index of suspicion. Every radiologist in the world has missed fractures on radiographs because they were not sufficiently attuned to the fact that a fracture might be present. Oftentimes the history is either nonexistent or misleading, and the anatomic area of concern is therefore overlooked. When in doubt examine the patient! Orthopedic surgeons seldom miss seeing fractures on radiographs because they have examined the patient, they know where the patient hurts, and they have a high index of suspicion. Second, always get two radiographs at 90 degrees to each other in every trauma case. A high percentage of fractures are seen only on one view (the anteroposterior [AP] or the lateral) and will therefore be missed unless two views are routinely obtained. Third, once a fracture is identified don't forget to look at the rest of the film. About 10 per cent of all cases have a second

finding that often is as significant as, or even more significant than, the initial finding. Many fractures have associated dislocation, foreign bodies, or additional fractures, so be sure to examine the entire film.

SPINE

Examination of the Cervical Spine

The cervical spine (C-spine) is one of the most commonly radiographed parts of the body in a busy emergency department and can present the most difficulty in interpretation. Usually a cross-table lateral of the C-spine is obtained first, so as not to unduly move the patient who might have a cervical fracture. If the lateral C-spine appears normal, the remainder of the C-spine series, which may include flexion and extension views (if the patient can cooperate), is obtained.

What do you look for on the lateral C-spine? First, make certain that all seven cervical vertebral bodies can be visualized. A large number of fractures are missed because the shoulders obscure the lower C-spine levels (Fig. 5–1). If the entire C-spine is not visualized, repeat the film with the shoulders lowered.

Next, evaluate five parallel (more or less) lines for step-offs or discontinuity as follows (Fig. 5–2):

Line number 1 is in the prevertebral soft tissue. It extends down the posterior aspect of the airway; it should be several millimeters from the first three or four vertebral bodies and then move further away at the laryngeal cartilage; it should be less than one vertebral body width from the

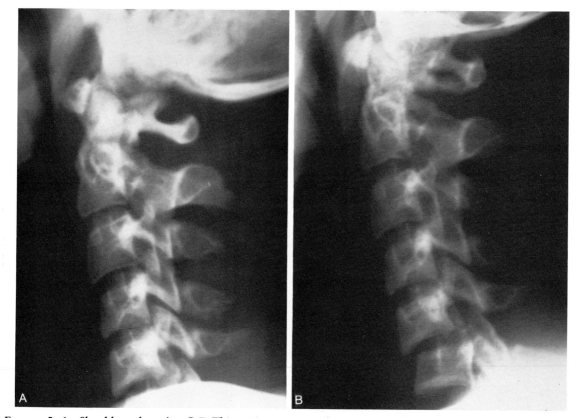

FIGURE 5–1 Shoulders obscuring C-7. This patient came to the emergency department after being injured as a result of diving into a shallow swimming pool. He had neck pain but no neurologic deficits. The initial radiograph obtained of the C-spine *(A)* was interpreted as being within normal limits. However, because of high-riding shoulders only five cervical vertebrae are visible. A repeat examination *(B)* with the shoulders lowered reveals a dislocation of C-5 on C-6. To visualize C-7 the shoulders were lowered even further. The C-7 vertebral body must be visualized on every lateral C-spine examination in a trauma setting.

anterior vertebral bodies from C-3 or C-4 to C-7; and it should be smooth in its contour.

Line 2 follows the anterior vertebral bodies and should be smooth and uninterrupted. Anterior osteophytes can encroach on this line and extend beyond it, and should therefore be ignored in drawing this line. Interruption of the anterior vertebral body line is a sign of a serious injury (Fig. 5–1B).

Line 3 is similar to the anterior vertebral body line (line 2) except that it connects the posterior vertebral bodies. Like line 2, it should be smooth and uninterrupted; any disruption signifies a serious injury.

Line 4, called the spinolaminal line, connects the posterior junction of the lamina with the spinous processes. The spinal cord lies between lines 3 and 4; therefore, any offset of either of these lines could mean that a bony structure is impinging on the cord. Severe neurologic deficits can result from very little force against the cord, and any bony structure lying on the cord must be recognized as soon as possible.

Line 5 is not really a line so much as a collection of points—the tips of the spinous processes. The spinous processes are quite variable in size and appearance, although C-7 usually has the largest. A fracture of one of the spinous processes, by itself, is not a serious injury, but it occasionally heralds other, more serious injuries. Also, who wants to miss a fractured spinous process, however innocuous, and then have the patient (after visiting another doctor) proclaim that you didn't see her "broken neck" on the radiograph?

After visually inspecting these five lines on the lateral C-spine, then inspect the C1-2 area a little more closely. Make certain that the anterior arch of C-1 is no greater than 2.5 mm from the dens (Fig. 5–3). Any greater separation than this (except in children, in whom up to 5.0 mm is normal) is suspicious for disruption of the transverse ligament between C-1 and C-2 (Fig. 5–4).

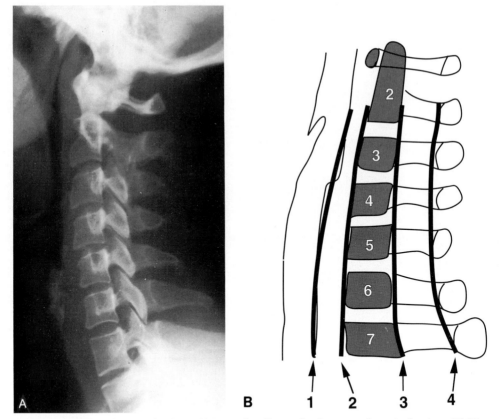

FIGURE 5–2   Normal lateral cervical spine. *(A)* Lateral radiograph of a normal cervical spine. *(B)* Diagrammatic representation of a lateral C-spine showing four parallel lines that should be observed in every lateral C-spine examination. Line 1 is the soft tissue line that is closely applied to the posterior border of the airway through the first four or five vertebral body segments and then widens around the laryngeal cartilage and runs parallel to the remainder of the cervical vertebrae. Line 2 demarcates the anterior border of the cervical vertebral bodies. Line 3 is the posterior border of the cervical vertebral bodies. Line 4, called the spinolaminal line, is drawn by connecting the junction of the lamina at the spinal process. It represents the posterior extent of the central canal, which contains the spinal cord itself. These lines should generally be smooth and parallel, with no abrupt step-offs.

The disc spaces are examined next to see that there is no inordinate widening or narrowing, either of which could indicate an acute traumatic injury. If a disc space is narrowed, it will usually be secondary to degenerative disease. Make certain that associated osteophytosis and sclerosis are present, however, before assuming the narrowing is due to degenerative disease.

An examination of the lateral C-spine as described above can be done in less than 1 minute. If this view is normal, then the remainder of the examination can be completed, including flexion and extension views. It is imperative that the patient initiate the flexion and extension without help from the technician or anyone else. A patient, if conscious and semialert, will not injure himself with voluntary flexion and extension and

will have muscle guarding, preventing motion, if an injury is present. Even gentle pressure to aid in flexion or extension can cause severe injury if a fracture or dislocation is present.

I would like to stress the importance of learning to look at lateral spine films with anterior facing either right or left. Many radiologists can only interpret images facing one way and become almost unable to function if the films are not placed on the viewbox in their preferred orientation. This is fine if they can control the film; however, in meetings where slides are shown, in books and journals, and on boards, they cannot turn the film to their liking. Get used to viewing lateral spine films (lateral chest films, too) in either anterior left or right orientation, or you will find yourself disadvantaged in many situations.

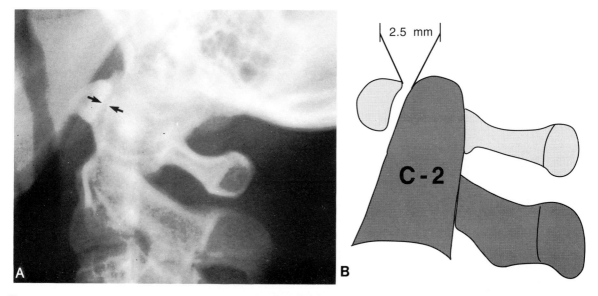

FIGURE 5–3   Normal C1-2. A lateral radiograph *(A)* and drawing *(B)* of the upper cervical spine, showing the normal distance of the anterior arch of C-1 to be less than 2.5 mm from the odontoid process of C-2 (arrows).

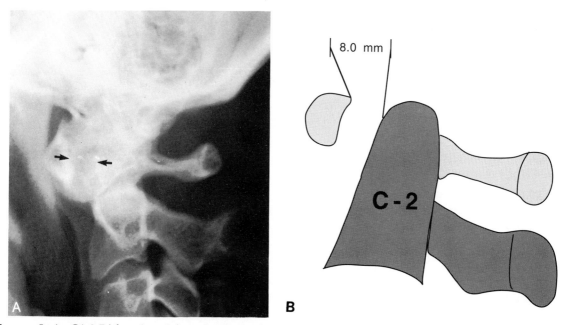

FIGURE 5–4   C1-2 Dislocation. A lateral radiograph *(A)* and drawing *(B)* of the upper cervical spine in a patient with trauma to the neck, which shows that the anterior arch of C-1 is 8 mm anterior to the odontoid process of C-2 (arrows). This is diagnostic of a dislocation of C-1 on C-2 and indicates rupture of the transverse ligaments, which normally hold these vertebral segments together.

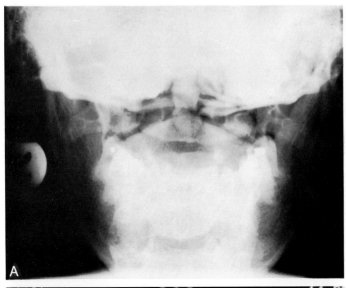

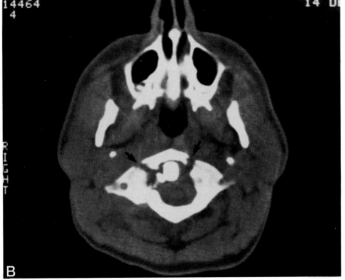

FIGURE 5–5 Jefferson's fracture. An AP open-mouth odontoid view *(A)* is suspicious for the lateral masses of C-1 being laterally displaced. However, because of overlying structures, this displacement is difficult to appreciate. Therefore, a CT examination *(B)* was obtained, which shows multiple fracture sites in the C-1 ring (arrows). This is called a Jefferson's fracture. CT is routinely used in spinal trauma because of the obvious shortcomings of plain films.

Examples of Fractures, Dislocations, and Other Abnormalities

A blow to the top of the head, such as when an object falls directly on the apex of the skull, can cause the lateral masses of C-1 to slide apart, splitting the bony ring of C-1. This is called a *Jefferson's fracture* (Fig. 5–5). It nicely illustrates how a bony ring will not break in just one place, but must break in several places. This rule is seldom violated. All of the vertebral rings, when fractured, must fracture in two or more places. The bony rings of the pelvis behave the same way. If you see only one fracture on the radiograph, you're certainly missing at least one more. Computed tomography (CT) is excellent at demonstrating the complete bony ring of C-1 and shows

the fractures, as well as any associated soft tissue mass, much better than plain films. In diagnosing a Jefferson's fracture on plain film the lateral masses of C-1 must extend beyond the margins of the C-2 body (Fig. 5–5A). Just seeing asymmetry of the spaces on either side of the dens is not enough to make the diagnosis, as these spaces can be normally asymmetric with rotation or with rotatory fixation of the atlantoaxial joint.

What is *rotatory fixation of the atlantoaxial joint?* This is a somewhat controversial, little understood process in which the atlantoaxial joint becomes fixed and the C-1 and C-2 bodies move en masse instead of rotating on each other. This condition is easily diagnosed with open-mouth odontoid views. In the normal odontoid view the spaces lateral to the dens (odontoid) are equal.

With rotation of the head to the left the space on the left widens, and with rotation to the right the space on the right widens. With rotatory fixation, one of the spaces is wider than the other and stays wider even with rotation of the head to the opposite side (Fig. 5–6). By itself, this is a relatively innocuous malady that is usually treated with a soft cervical collar and/or gentle traction. It is, however, occasionally associated with disruption of the transverse ligaments at C1-2 and is then a serious problem. Rotatory fixation usually presents spontaneously or after very mild trauma, such as that caused by sleeping in an unusual position.

Another relatively innocuous injury is a fracture of the C-6 or C-7 spinous process, called a *clay-shoveler's fracture*. Supposedly workers shoveling sticky clay in Australia (I've also read England and North Carolina—this is a vital distinction, and some future researcher can perhaps

straighten out this confusion) would toss the shovelfuls of clay over their shoulders; once in a while the clay would stick to the shovel, causing the ligaments attached to the spinous processes (supraspinous ligaments) to undergo a tremendous force, pulling on the spinous process and avulsing it. This fracture can occur at any of the lower cervical spinous processes (Fig. 5–7).

A *hangman's fracture* is an unstable, serious fracture of the upper cervical spine that is caused by hyperextension and distraction (such as hitting one's head on a dashboard). This is a fracture of the posterior elements of C-2 and, usually, displacement of the C-2 body anterior to C-3 (Fig. 5–8). Patients with this type of fracture actually do better than one might think. They often escape neurologic impairment because of the fractured posterior elements of C-2, which, in effect, cause a decompression and take pressure off the injured area. This is a simplistic explanation for a com-

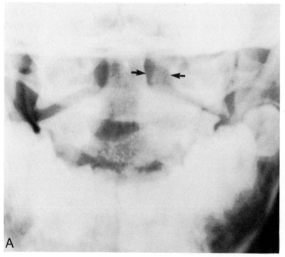

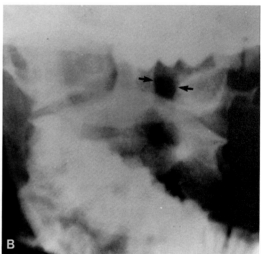

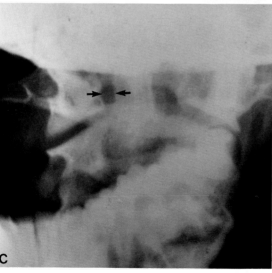

FIGURE 5–6 **Rotatory fixation of the atlantoaxial joint.** This patient came to the emergency department with pain and decreased motion in the cervical spine. An AP open-mouth odontoid view *(A)* shows that the space on the left side of the odontoid between the odontoid and the lateral mass of C-1 (arrows) is wider than the corresponding space on the right side. This is often due to rotation. Therefore, open-mouth odontoid views with right and left obliquities were obtained. Rotation of the patient's head to the left *(B)* causes the space on the left side of the odontoid process (arrows) to be wider than that on the right, which is appropriate. However, when the patient turns to the right *(C)* the space on the right (arrows) does not get wider than the space on the left. This is diagnostic of rotatory fixation of the atlantoaxial joint.

plex entity, but it seems to be a reasonable answer to why these patients often fare well.

Severe flexion of the cervical spine can cause a disruption of the posterior ligaments and anterior compression of a vertebral body. This is called a *flexion "teardrop" fracture* (Fig. 5–9). A teardrop fracture is usually associated with spinal cord injury, often from the posterior portion of the vertebral body being displaced into the central canal.

If severe enough, and if associated with some rotation, the apophyseal joint ligaments will rupture, and the facet joints dislocate and then override. This can result in locking of the facets in an overriding position, which in effect causes some stabilization to protect against further injury. This condition is called *unilateral locked facets* (Figs. 5–10 and 5–11), but occasionally it occurs bilaterally. When unilateral, the more inferior vertebral body is usually rotated, giving it a shorter AP length on a lateral film, which is a clue to the diagnosis (Fig. 5–11).

A "seat belt injury" is seen secondary to hyperflexion at the waist (as occurs in a car accident while the person is restrained by a lap belt). This causes distraction of the posterior elements and ligaments and anterior compression of the vertebral body. It usually involves the L-1 or L-2 level. Several variations of this injury can occur: A fracture of the posterior body is called a *Smith's fracture* and a fracture through the spinous process is called a *Chance fracture*. Horizontal fractures of the pedicles, laminae, and transverse processes can also occur (Fig. 5–12).

A somewhat controversial spinal abnormality that may or may not be caused by trauma is spondylolysis. *Spondylolysis* is a break or defect in the pars interarticularis portion of the lamina (Fig. 5–13). On oblique views the posterior elements form the figure of a Scottie dog, with the

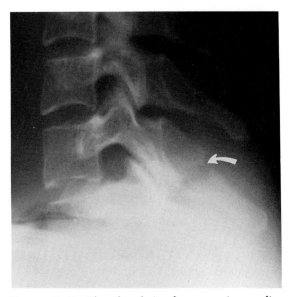

FIGURE 5–7 Clay-shoveler's fracture. A nondisplaced fracture of the C-7 spinous process (arrow) is noted, which is diagnostic of a clay-shoveler's fracture.

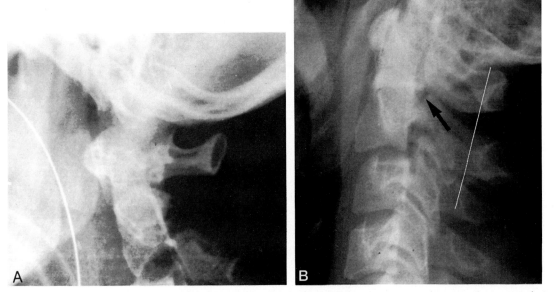

FIGURE 5–8 Hangman's fracture. *(A)* A lateral film of a patient with a hangman's fracture shows an obvious example of the posterior elements of the C-2 vertebral body fractured and displaced inferiorly. *(B)* The film of another patient shows a subtle fracture through the posterior elements of C-2 (arrow). A line drawn through the spinolaminal lines of the posterior elements shows the C-2 spinolaminal line to be offset in this example.

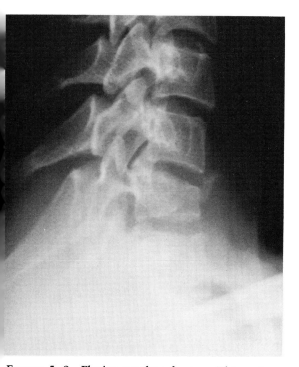

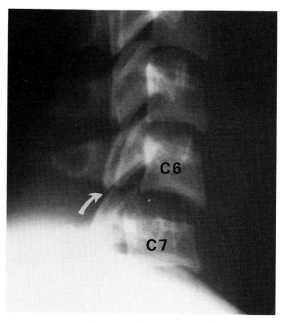

FIGURE 5–9 Flexion teardrop fracture. This patient suffered hyperflexion in a car accident and came to the emergency department with severe neurologic deficits. A lateral radiograph of the lower cervical spine shows wedging anteriorly of the C-7 vertebral body with some displacement of the posterior vertebral line of C-7 into the central canal. A small avulsion fracture off the anterior body is also noted.

FIGURE 5–10 Unilateral locked facets. The C6-7 disc space is abnormally widened, and the C-7 vertebral body is posteriorly located in relation to C-6. Also note the C-7 facets, which are dislocated and locked on the C-6 facets (arrow). When the facets are perched in this manner, the condition is termed locked facets, which in this example is unilateral.

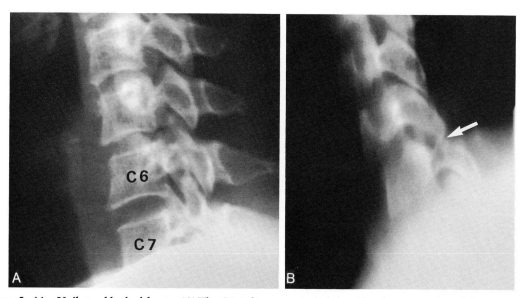

FIGURE 5–11 Unilateral locked facets. *(A)* The C6-7 disc space is slightly wider than normal, and the C-7 vertebral body is narrower in this view than the C-6 vertebral body, owing to abnormal rotation. The facets of C-7 are not well identified, but in the tomogram *(B)* they are shown to be overriding and locked (arrow).

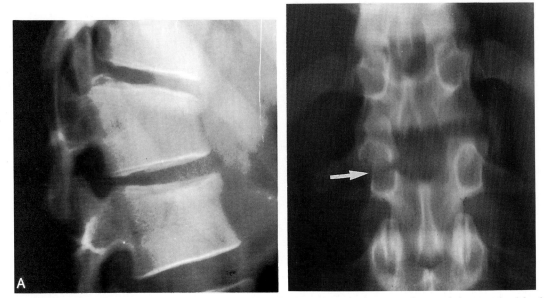

FIGURE 5–12   **Seat belt fracture.** Hyperflexion at the waist can cause anterior wedging of the vertebral body in the lower thoracic or upper lumbar region as shown in *A*. By itself, that is somewhat innocuous; however, *B* shows a horizontal fracture through the right transverse process and pedicle (arrow) resulting from extreme traction during the flexion injury. When fracture of the posterior elements occurs, this injury is considered to be unstable and potentially debilitating. Any anterior wedging injury to a vertebral body should have the posterior elements of that level closely inspected for interpedicular space widening.

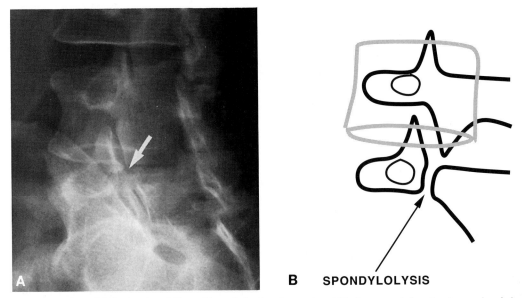

B   SPONDYLOLYSIS

FIGURE 5–13   **Spondylolysis.** An oblique film of the lumbar spine *(A)* shows a defect in the neck of the Scottie dog at L-5 (arrow), which is diagnostic of a spondylolysis. The drawing *(B)* shows the findings more clearly.

transverse process being the nose, the pedicle forming the eye, the inferior articular facet being the front leg, the superior articular facet representing the ear, and the pars interarticularis (which means the portion of the lamina that lies between the facets) equaling the dog's neck. If a spondylolysis is present, the pars interarticularis, or the neck of the dog, will have a defect or break. It often looks as if the Scottie dog has a collar around its neck. Although often difficult to visualize with MR, spondylolysis should be easily seen on CT (see Chapter 11). The cause of a spondylolysis is said by some investigators to be congenital and by others to be posttraumatic. Many believe that this is a stress-related injury from infancy that develops when toddlers try to walk and repeatedly fall on their buttocks, sending stress to their lower lumbar spine. The significance of spondylolysis is just as controversial as its cause. More and more clinicians are coming to the viewpoint that a spondylolysis is an incidental finding with no clinical significance in most cases. Certainly some patients have pain related to a spondylolysis and get relief after surgical stabilization, but such cases are less common.

If a spondylolysis is bilateral and the vertebral body in the more cephalad position slips forward on the more caudal body, spondylolisthesis is said to be present (Fig. 5–14). *Spondylolisthesis* may or may not be symptomatic and by itself has no clinical significance. If severe, it can cause neuroforaminal stenosis and can impinge on the nerve roots in the central spinal canal. If it is symptomatic, it can be surgically stabilized.

HAND AND WRIST

Several seemingly innocuous fractures in the hand require surgical fixation rather than just casting and, therefore, should be recognized by the radiologist as serious injuries. One such fracture is a fracture at the base of the thumb into the carpometacarpal joint, or a *Bennett's fracture* (Fig. 5–15). Because of the insertion of the strong thumb adductors at the base of the thumb it is almost impossible to keep the metacarpal from sliding off its proper alignment. It almost always requires internal fixation. The radiologist occasionally has to remind a nonorthopedic practitioner of this, as well as closely examine the alignment of a Bennett's fracture in plaster that has not been internally fixed with pins.

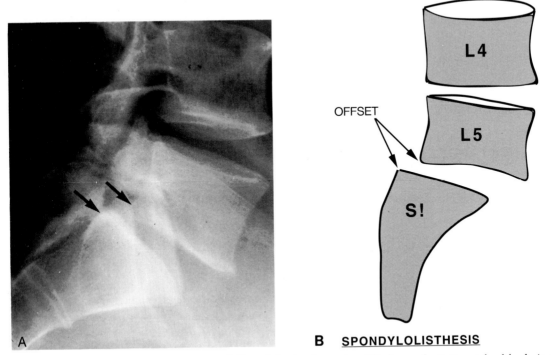

B **SPONDYLOLISTHESIS**

FIGURE 5–14 **Spondylolisthesis.** A lateral film of the lumbar spine *(A)* shows the L-5 vertebral body is slightly anteriorly offset on the S-1 body as noted by the posterior margins (arrows). The drawing *(B)* shows the findings more clearly. Because the offset is less than 25 per cent as measured by the length of the S-1 end-plate, it is termed a grade 1 spondylolisthesis. A grade 2 offset is more than 25 per cent but less than 50 per cent of the length of the S-1 end-plate.

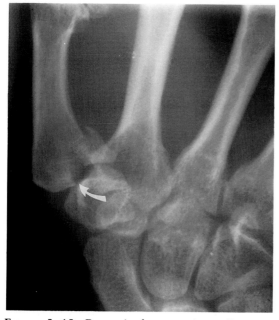

FIGURE 5–15 **Bennett's fracture.** A small corner fracture of the base of the thumb is noted that, at first glance, appears minor; however, it involves the articular surface of the base of the thumb (arrow), which makes this a serious injury that almost always requires internal fixation.

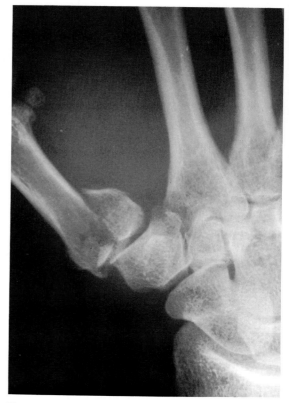

FIGURE 5–16 **Rolando's fracture.** A comminuted fracture of the base of the thumb that extends into the articular surface is a more serious type of Bennett's fracture and has been termed a Rolando's fracture.

A comminuted fracture of the base of the thumb that extends into the joint has been termed a *Rolando's fracture* (Fig. 5–16), and a fracture of the base of the thumb that does not involve the joint has been called a pseudo-Bennett's fracture.

A *mallet finger* or *baseball finger* is an avulsion injury at the base of the distal phalanx (Fig. 5–17) where the extensor digitorum tendon inserts. With the extensor tendon inoperative, the distal phalanx flexes without opposition. If not properly treated, this can result in a flexion deformity and inability to extend the distal phalanx.

Another innocent-appearing fracture that often requires internal fixation is an avulsion on the ulnar aspect of the first metacarpophalangeal joint (Fig. 5–18), which is where the ulnar collateral ligament of the thumb inserts. If the ulnar collateral ligament is torn, the function of the thumb can be impaired; therefore, this fracture can have a serious result if not properly treated. This injury is called a *gamekeeper's thumb* because of the propensity of old English game wardens to acquire it from breaking rabbits' necks between their thumbs and forefingers. A more current scenario is falling on a ski pole and having the pole jam into the webbing between the thumb and index finger. Kayakers occasionally suffer a gamekeeper's thumb when their paddles hit a rock. This avulsion injury usually requires pinning to securely fix the ligament.

A fall on the outstretched arm can result in any number of wrist fractures and dislocations. One serious such injury is the *lunate/perilunate dislocation*. This dislocation occurs when the ligaments between the capitate and the lunate are disrupted, allowing the capitate to dislocate from the cup-shaped articulation of the lunate. This is best seen on the lateral view. Ordinarily, on the lateral view, the capitate should be seen seated in the cup-shaped lunate (Figs. 5–19 and 5–20A). In a *dorsal perilunate dislocation* (occasionally the capitate dislocates volarly, but this is uncommon) the capitate and all of its surrounding bones, including the metacarpals, come to lie dorsal to a line drawn up through the radius and the lunate (Figs. 5–20B and 5–21). If the capitate then pushes the lunate volarly and tips it over, the line drawn up through the radius shows the lunate volarly displaced, and the line goes through the capitate. This has been termed a *lunate dislocation* (Figs. 5–20C and 5–22). The normal, perilunate, and lunate dislocations are

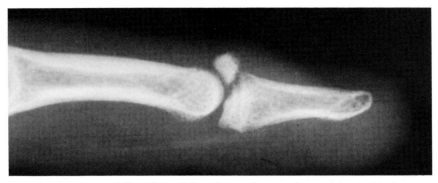

FIGURE 5–17   Mallet finger. A small avulsion injury is noted at the base of the distal phalanx, which is where the extensor digitorum tendon inserts. This injury is termed a mallet finger or baseball finger. It is often caused by a baseball striking the distal phalanx, causing the avulsion. (Case courtesy of Dr. Hideyo Minagi.)

FIGURE 5–18   Gamekeeper's thumb. A small avulsion injury on the ulnar aspect of the first metacarpophalangeal joint (arrow) is diagnostic of a gamekeeper's thumb. This is the insertion site for the ulnar collateral ligament, and usually requires internal fixation.

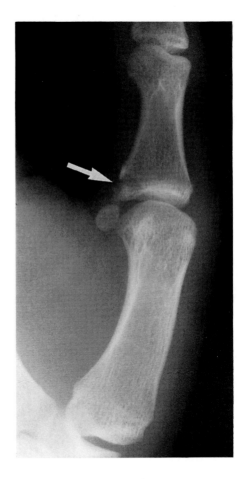

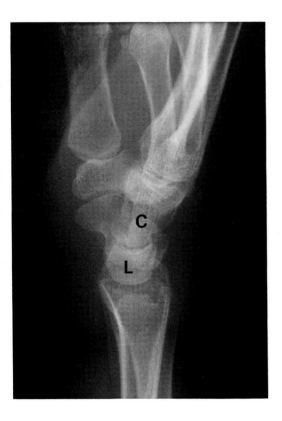

FIGURE 5–19   Normal lateral radiograph of the wrist. The normal lateral view should show the lunate (L) seated in the distal radius and the capitate (C) in turn seated in the lunate. A line drawn through the radius should connect all three structures. Compare this radiograph with the drawing in Figure 5–20A.

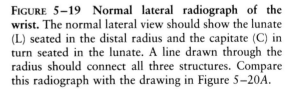

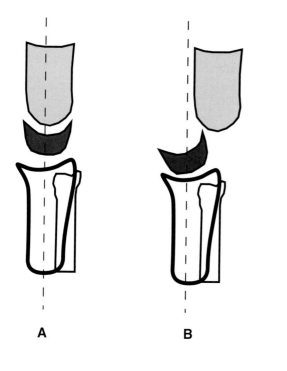
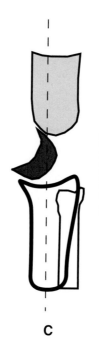

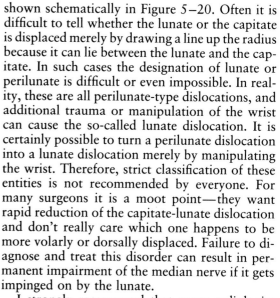

FIGURE 5–20 Schematic depiction of normal lateral wrist *(A)*, perilunate dislocation *(B)*, and lunate dislocation *(C)*. (The light shaded bone is the capitate; the dark shaded bone is the lunate. Ventral is to the left.)

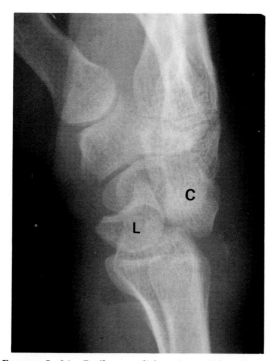

FIGURE 5–21 **Perilunate dislocation.** Although the lunate (L) is normal in relation to the distal radius, the capitate (C) and the remainder of the wrist are dorsally displaced in relation to the lunate. Compare this radiograph with the drawing in Figure 5–20B.

shown schematically in Figure 5–20. Often it is difficult to tell whether the lunate or the capitate is displaced merely by drawing a line up the radius because it can lie between the lunate and the capitate. In such cases the designation of lunate or perilunate is difficult or even impossible. In reality, these are all perilunate-type dislocations, and additional trauma or manipulation of the wrist can cause the so-called lunate dislocation. It is certainly possible to turn a perilunate dislocation into a lunate dislocation merely by manipulating the wrist. Therefore, strict classification of these entities is not recommended by everyone. For many surgeons it is a moot point—they want rapid reduction of the capitate-lunate dislocation and don't really care which one happens to be more volarly or dorsally displaced. Failure to diagnose and treat this disorder can result in permanent impairment of the median nerve if it gets impinged on by the lunate.

I strongly recommend that every radiologist get in the habit of looking at the alignment of the lunate and the capitate on every lateral wrist film. There's not a whole lot else to look for on the lateral view anyway. I see a missed perilunate dislocation every few years, which usually ends up in litigation.

A lunate or perilunate dislocation can be diagnosed on an AP view of the wrist by noting a triangular or pie-shaped lunate (Fig. 5–22B). Ordinarily the lunate has a rhomboid shape on the AP view, with the upper and lower borders parallel.

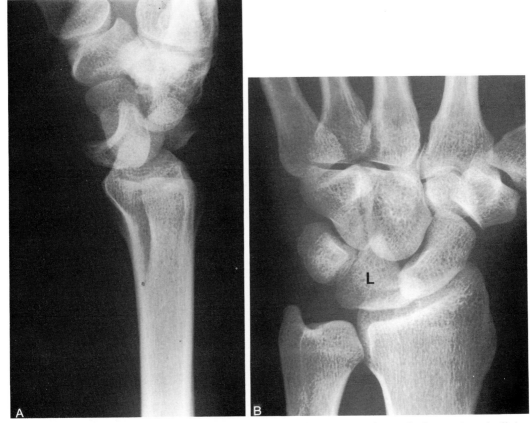

FIGURE 5–22 **Lunate dislocation.** This lateral radiograph of the wrist *(A)* shows the lunate tipped off the distal radius, whereas the capitate seems to be normally aligned in relation to the radius yet is dislocated from the lunate. Compare this with the drawing in Figure 5–20C. The AP view *(B)* shows a pie-shaped lunate rather than a lunate with a more rhomboid shape. A pie-shaped lunate (L) is diagnostic of a perilunate or lunate dislocation.

Several fractures are known to be associated with a perilunate dislocation, the most common of which is a transscaphoid fracture. The capitate, radial styloid, and triquetrum are also known to frequently fracture when a perilunate dislocation occurs. Often, the fractures are identified and treated, while the dislocation is overlooked.

One of the most difficult wrist fractures to radiologically identify is a *fracture of the hook of the hamate*. A special view, the carpal tunnel view, should be obtained when trying to see the hook of the hamate. This view is obtained with the wrist (palm down) flat on a radiograph plate and the fingers and palm pulled dorsally. The x-ray beam is angled about 45 degrees, parallel to the palm, so the carpal tunnel is in profile. The hook of the hamate is seen as a bony protuberance off the hamate on the ulnar aspect of the carpal tunnel. A fractured hook of the hamate is often well seen with the carpal tunnel view (Fig. 5–23) but can occasionally be difficult to pick up. A CT scan will often show an obvious fracture that the plain film does not (Fig. 5–24) and

should be considered in any possible carpal fracture when plain films are not diagnostic.

A fracture of the hook of the hamate most commonly occurs from a fall on the outstretched hand. A clinical setting that has gained attention in radiology and sports medicine circles is that of a professional athlete who participates in an activity in which the butt of a club, bat, or racket is held in the palm. Overswinging can result in the butt of the club levering off the hook of the hamate. This has been seen in professional baseball players, tennis players, and golfers. Why professionals? Amateurs usually are not strong enough to exert enough force to lever the hook off and, if they do, will usually terminate that activity, allowing healing. Professionals, however, continue their participation, which can lead to a nonunion of the fracture.

Another wrist injury that is seen after a fall onto the outstretched hand is *rotatory subluxation of the navicular*. This results from rupture of the scapholunate ligaments, which allows the scaphoid (navicular) to rotate dorsally. On an AP

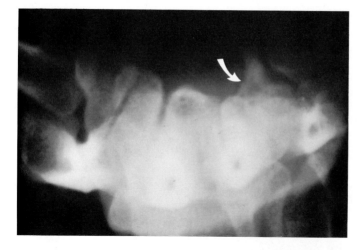

FIGURE 5–23   Fracture of the hook of the hamate. The hook of the hamate is seen on a carpal tunnel view in this patient, as well as an area of sclerosis with a faint cortical break (arrow). This represents a fracture at the base of the hook of the hamate.

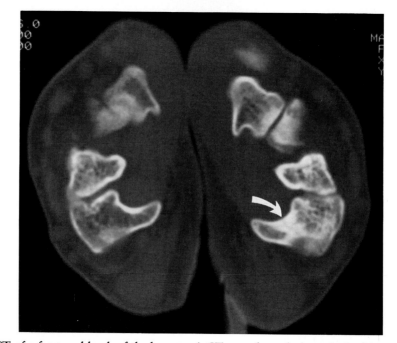

FIGURE 5–24   CT of a fractured hook of the hamate. A CT scan through the wrist in this patient shows a faint lucency surrounded by sclerosis in the left hook of the hamate (arrow), which represents a fracture with moderate reactive sclerosis. This could not be seen in the plain films, even in retrospect.

wrist radiograph a space is seen between the navicular and the lunate (Fig. 5–25) when ordinarily they are closely opposed. This space has been called the "Terry-Thomas" sign, after the famous British actor with a gap between his two front teeth. I prefer to call it the "David Letterman" sign.

A *fracture of the navicular* is a potentially serious injury because of the high rate of avascular necrosis that occurs with this injury. When avascular necrosis occurs, usually surgical intervention and bone grafting are required in order to obtain healing. This fracture can be difficult to

detect initially; therefore, whenever a fracture of the navicular is clinically suspect (trauma with pain over the snuffbox of the wrist) the wrist should be casted and repeat radiographs obtained in 1 week. Often the fracture is then visualized owing to the disuse osteoporosis and hyperemia around the fracture site. Thus, in the acute setting, a negative film does not exclude a fractured navicular. If avascular necrosis develops, it is the proximal fragment that undergoes aseptic necrosis because the blood supply to the navicular begins distally and runs proximally. A fracture with disruption of the blood supply thus leaves the

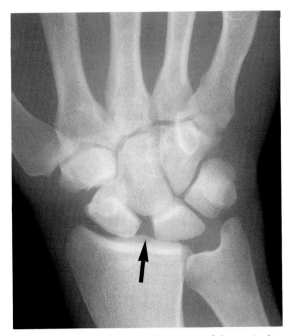

FIGURE 5–25 Rotatory subluxation of the navicular.
An AP view of the wrist shows a gap or space between the navicular and the lunate (arrow). This is abnormal and represents the "Terry-Thomas" sign, which means that the ligaments between the lunate and the scaphoid are ruptured. This is diagnostic of a rotatory subluxation of the navicular.

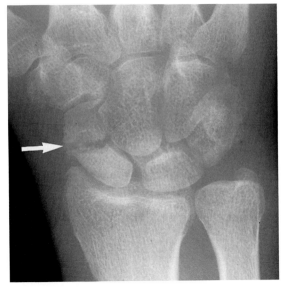

FIGURE 5–26 Avascular necrosis of the navicular.
An AP view of the wrist shows a fracture through the waist of the navicular (arrow). The proximal half of the navicular is slightly sclerotic in relation to the remainder of the carpal bones, which indicates avascular necrosis of the proximal half.

proximal pole without a vascular supply; hence it dies. Avascular necrosis is diagnosed by noting increased density of the proximal pole of the navicular as compared with the remainder of the carpal bones (Fig. 5–26).

Avascular necrosis can occur in other carpal bones, most commonly the lunate. This is called *Kienböck's malacia* and is most often caused by trauma, although some investigators claim it is idiopathic. The disease is diagnosed by noting increased density of the lunate bone, which may or may not go on to collapse and fragment (Fig. 5–27). It often requires surgical bone grafting and occasionally removal, or proximal carpal row fusion. Kienböck's malacia is said to have an increased incidence in patients who have shortening of the ulna in relation to the radius—called negative ulnar variance. Positive ulnar variance (the ulna is longer than the radius) is associated with an increased incidence of triangular fibrocartilage tears.

An avulsion fracture that is frequently seen is a *triquetral fracture*. The fracture is best seen on the lateral film, which shows a small chip of bone on the dorsum of the wrist (Fig. 5–28). This is virtually pathognomonic of avulsion off the triquetrum.

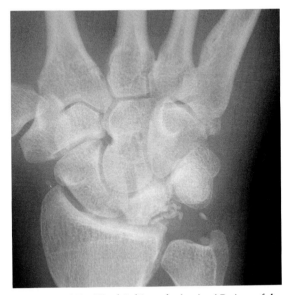

FIGURE 5–27 Kienböck's malacia. An AP view of the wrist reveals the lunate to be sclerotic and abnormal in shape. The lunate has collapsed owing to aseptic necrosis. This is known as Kienböck's malacia. Note that the ulna is shorter than the radius—negative ulnar variance—which is said to be related to an increased incidence of Kienböck's malacia.

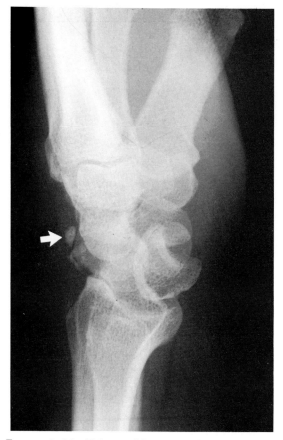

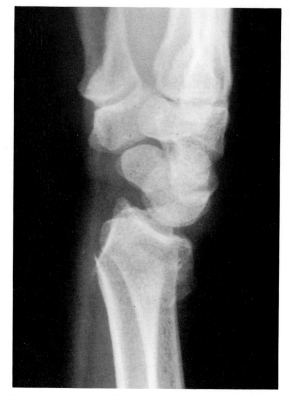

FIGURE 5—29 Colles' fracture. A fracture of the distal radius with dorsal angulation is noted, which has been termed a Colles' fracture (volar is to the left).

FIGURE 5—28 Triquetral fracture and perilunate dislocation. A perilunate or lunate dislocation is present (it is difficult to classify exactly which has occurred, since both the lunate and the capitate are out of their normal positions). Compare this radiograph with the drawing in Figure 5–20A. A small avulsion is seen on the dorsum of the wrist (arrow), which is virtually diagnostic of an avulsion off the triquetrum. It is often associated with a lunate or perilunate dislocation.

ARM

One of the most common fractures of the forearm is a fracture of the distal radius and ulna after a fall on the outstretched arm. This results in dorsal angulation of the distal forearm and wrist and is called a *Colles' fracture* (Fig. 5–29). When the fracture angulates volarly it is called a *Smith's fracture* (Fig. 5–30). A Smith's fracture is a much less common occurrence than a Colles' fracture. Sometimes the radius and ulna suffer a traumatic insult, and the force on the bones causes bending instead of a frank fracture. This has been termed *plastic bowing deformity of the forearm* (Fig. 5–31) and is often treated by breaking the bones (under anesthesia, of course) and resetting them. Left untreated, a plastic bowing deformity can result in reduced supination and pronation.

The forearm is a two-bone system that has some of the same properties as a bony ring. For example, a solid ring cannot break in only a single place; it must break in at least two points (try to break a pretzel—not a soft New York pretzel—in only one place). Likewise, the rings in the spine or pelvis always break in at least two places. In the forearm a fracture of one bone should be accompanied by a fracture of the other. If the second fracture is not present, a dislocation of the nonfractured bone usually occurs. The most common example of this is a fracture of the ulna with a dislocation of the proximal radius (Fig. 5–32). This is called a *Monteggia's fracture*. (It has also been termed a "nightstick injury" from the policeman hitting someone with a nightstick: the person being hit instinctively raises an arm for protection and the nightstick falls on the ulna, fracturing it and dislocating the radial head.) The dislocated radial head can be missed clinically and go on to aseptic necrosis with subsequent elbow dysfunction. Therefore, any time the forearm is fractured the elbow must be examined to exclude a dislocation.

A fracture of the radius with dislocation of the distal ulna is called a *Galleazzi's fracture* (Fig. 5–33). This is much less common than a Mon-

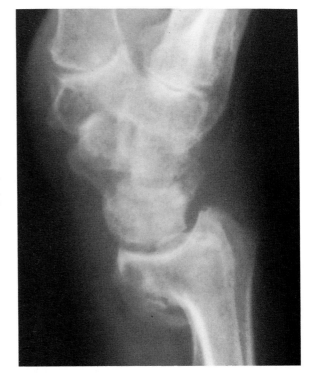

FIGURE 5–30 **Smith's fracture.** A fracture of the distal radius with volar angulation such as this is called a Smith's fracture. This injury is much less common than the Colles' fracture shown in Figure 5–29 (volar is to the left).

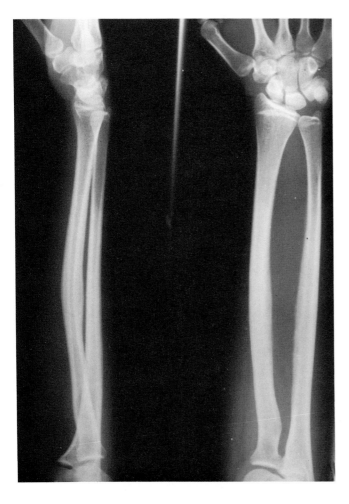

FIGURE 5–31 **Plastic bowing deformity of the forearm.** These AP and lateral views of a child's forearm show the radius to be abnormally bowed. This condition has been termed a plastic bowing deformity of the forearm and occurs only in children.

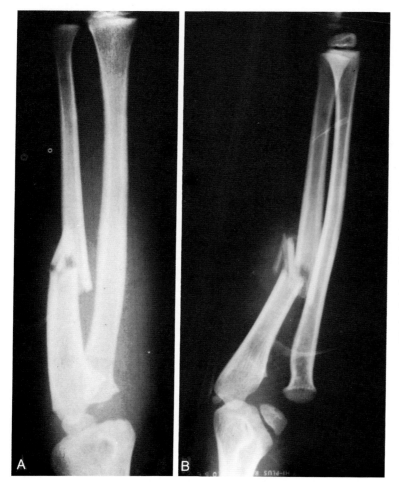

FIGURE 5–32 Monteggia's fracture. A blow to the forearm, such as with a policeman's nightstick, can result in a fracture of the ulna. Although the head of the radius appears normally placed on the AP view *(A)*, the lateral examination *(B)* reveals the head of the radius to be displaced. Failure to recognize this abnormality can result in death of the radial head with subsequent elbow dysfunction. This illustrates the importance of always obtaining two views of a bone in an injury.

teggia's fracture, and because the deformity of the dislocated ulna is usually obvious, it is rarely missed clinically.

A helpful indicator of a fracture about the elbow is a displaced posterior fat pad. Ordinarily the posterior fat pad is not visible on a lateral view of the elbow because it is tucked away in the olecranon fossa of the distal humerus. When the joint becomes distended with blood secondary to a fracture, the posterior fat pad is displaced out of the olecranon fossa and is visible on the lateral view (Fig. 5–34). Therefore, in the setting of trauma a visible posterior fat pad indicates a fracture. In an adult (epiphyses closed) the fracture site is almost always the radial head (Fig. 5–34B). In a child (epiphyses open) it is usually indicative of a supracondylar fracture (Fig. 5–35). Often the fracture itself is not visualized, and heroic steps are taken by clinicians and radiologists alike to demonstrate the fracture. These steps include oblique views, special radial head views, tomograms, and even CT scans and MR imaging. These are costly and unnecessary attempts to document pathology that will be treated identically whether or not it is radiographically recorded. So long as there is no obvious deformity or loose body it does not matter if the fracture is definitely identified or not in a patient with a posttraumatic painful elbow and a visible posterior fat pad.

Couldn't an infection cause a joint effusion and a displaced posterior fat pad? Of course, but the clinical setting would not be to rule out a fracture. In fact, any elbow effusion will cause a posterior fat pad to be visible.

The anterior fat pad also gets displaced with a joint effusion. Ordinarily it is visible as a small triangle just anterior to the distal humeral diaphysis on a lateral film (Fig. 5–36). With an effusion it gets displaced superiorly and outward from the humerus and has been called a "sail" sign because it resembles a spinnaker sail (Figs. 5–34 and 5–35). I have seen only one example of a displaced anterior fat pad without a visible posterior fat pad and that was in a patient with a prior elbow fracture who probably scarred down the joint posteriorly, preventing it from distending enough to push the fat pad out of the fossa.

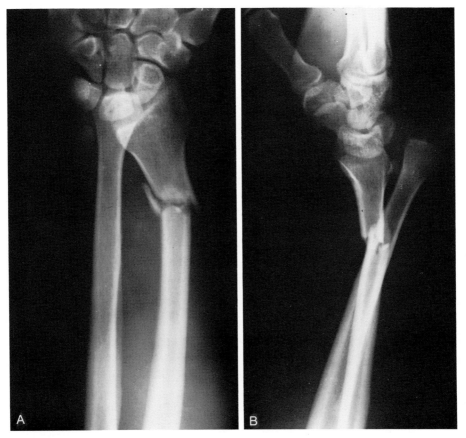

FIGURE 5–33 Galleazzi's fracture. A fracture of the distal radius in this patient is seen on the AP view *(A)* without a definite fracture of the ulna. The lateral view *(B)* shows an obvious dislocation of the distal ulna, which would almost certainly not be missed clinically. This has been termed a Galleazzi's fracture and is much less common than a Monteggia's fracture.

Therefore, I usually don't care what the anterior fat pad looks like and find it easier to concentrate on the presence or absence of the posterior fat pad. Keep things as simple as possible. Why be concerned over the appearance of two fat pads when one will do quite nicely?

Shoulder dislocations are generally easily diagnosed, both clinically and radiographically. The most common shoulder dislocation is the anterior dislocation. It is at least ten times more common than the posterior dislocation. For all practical purposes, these are the only two types of shoulder dislocations to be concerned about.

An anterior dislocation occurs when the arm is forcibly externally rotated and abducted. This is commonly seen when football players "arm tackle," when kayakers "brace" with the paddle above their heads and allow their arms to get too far posterior, when skiers plant their uphill pole and get it stuck, and as a result of similar athletic positions. Radiographically, the diagnosis is easily made on an AP shoulder film: the humeral

head is seen to lie inferiorly and medial to the glenoid (Fig. 5–37). The humeral head often impacts against the inferior lip of the glenoid, causing an indentation on the posterosuperior portion of the humeral head called a *Hill-Sachs deformity.* A Hill-Sachs deformity is said to indicate a greater likelihood of recurrent dislocation, and some surgeons use it as an indicator to surgically intervene so as to prevent a recurrence. A bony irregularity or fragment off the inferior glenoid, which occurs from the same mechanism as does the Hill-Sachs deformity, is called a *Bankhart deformity.* This deformity is not nearly so common as the Hill-Sachs.

A posterior dislocation can be a difficult diagnosis to make, both clinically and radiographically. An AP view may look normal, or nearly so. On the AP view of a normal shoulder the humeral head should slightly overlap the glenoid (Fig. 5–38), forming a "crescent sign." In a patient with a posterior dislocation this crescent of bony overlap is often absent and a small space is

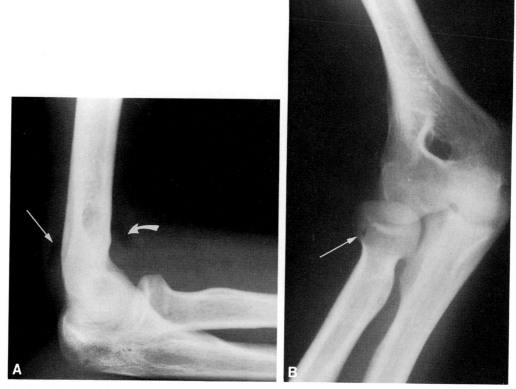

FIGURE 5–34 Displaced fat pads about the elbow. On the lateral view of the elbow in this patient *(A)* the posterior fat pad is visible (arrow) and the anterior fat pad is elevated and anteriorly displaced (curved arrow). These findings indicate a fracture about the elbow, which in an adult should be in the radial head. An oblique view in this patient *(B)* shows the fracture of the radial head (arrow). Even without definitely seeing the fracture on the radiographs it should be surmised to be present when the posterior fat pad is visualized in the setting of trauma. The elevated and displaced anterior fat pad has been termed a "sail" sign because it resembles a spinnaker sail.

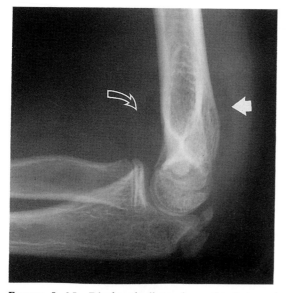

FIGURE 5–35 Displaced elbow fat pads. A lateral view of the elbow in this patient shows a posterior fat pad (arrow) and a "sail" sign anteriorly (curved arrow). This is indicative of a fracture about the elbow, which in a child (the epiphyses are open) usually means a supracondylar fracture.

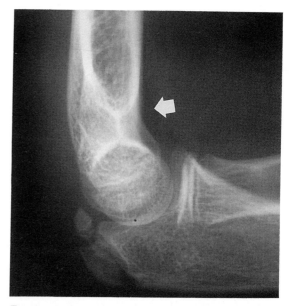

FIGURE 5–36 Normal anterior fat pad of the elbow. Note the lucency just anterior to the humerus of this normal elbow (arrow), and compare this with the "sail" sign of the anterior fat pads in Figures 5–34 and 5–35.

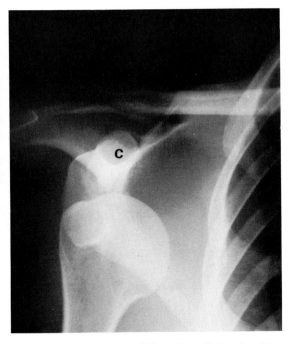

FIGURE 5–37 **Anterior dislocation of the shoulder.** An AP view of the right shoulder shows the humeral head to lie medial to the glenoid and inferior to the coracoid process (C). This is diagnostic of an anterior dislocation of the shoulder.

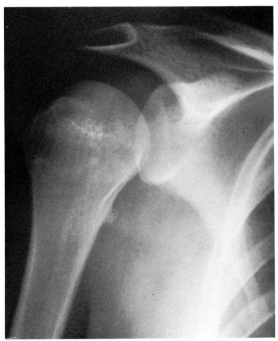

FIGURE 5–38 **Normal AP view of the shoulder.** Note on this example of a normal shoulder that the humeral head slightly overlaps the glenoid. This has been termed the "crescent sign."

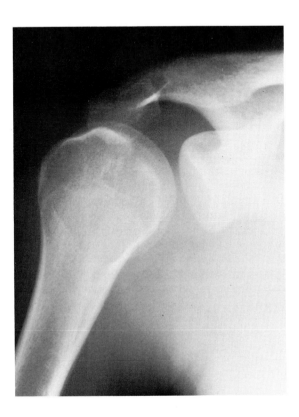

FIGURE 5–39 **Posterior dislocation of the shoulder.** Note that the humeral head in this patient is slightly displaced from the glenoid on the AP view. This is termed absence of the "crescent sign" and is often seen with a posterior dislocation. Compare this with Figure 5–38.

seen between the glenoid and the humeral head (Fig. 5–39).

The best way to unequivocally diagnose a dislocated shoulder is to obtain a transscapular view. An axillary view will show basically the same thing but requires the patient to move his arm and shoulder, which can be painful and can even re-dislocate the shoulder if it has spontaneously reduced itself. The transscapular view is obtained by angling the x-ray beam across the shoulder in the same plane as the blade of the scapula. This gives an *en face* view of the glenoid, and the humeral head can easily be related to it as either normal, anterior (Fig. 5–40), or pos-

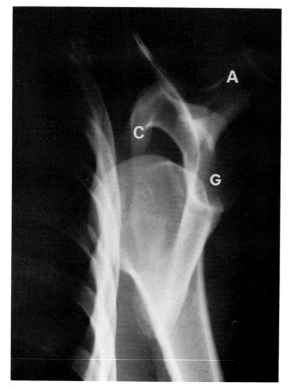

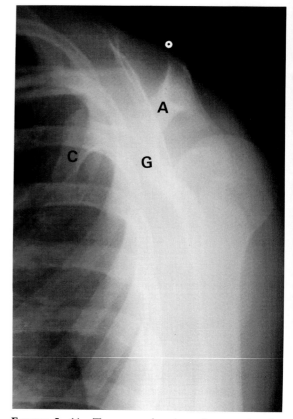

FIGURE 5–40   Transscapular view of an anterior dislocation. This transscapular view of the shoulder is obtained by aiming the x-ray beam parallel to the shoulder blade. The coracoid process (C) can be seen anteriorly, and the spine of the acromion (A) can be seen posteriorly. Both of these structures extend inwardly and meet at the glenoid (G). In this example the humeral head is seen to lie outside of the glenoid in an anterior direction.

FIGURE 5–41   Transscapular view of a posterior dislocation. The transscapular view in this patient is more difficult to appreciate; however, the coracoid process (C) and the acromion (A) can still be identified, and the position of the glenoid (G) can be extrapolated. The humeral head is seen to lie posterior to where the glenoid lies.

terior (Fig. 5–41). Because of overlapping ribs and clavicles the exact anatomy is often difficult to discern on the transscapular view. To find the glenoid one has to find the coracoid, the spine of the acromion, and the blade of the scapula. These three structures all lead to the glenoid and form a "Y" around it. All one has to do to find the center of the glenoid is to find two of those bony landmarks—usually the coracoid and the blade of the scapula. The humeral head can then be found and its position determined.

I was recently involved in a court case where an ER doc and a radiologist both missed a posterior dislocation in a patient who fell and had shoulder pain. The patient had the diagnosis made 2 weeks later and needed surgery—he was left with some permanent shoulder disability. The radiologist's lawyer argued that a community hospital radiologist should not be expected to diagnose such a rare disorder, even though the

"University radiologist" (me) said it should be routinely identified. You certainly cannot expect to pass boards if you miss a posterior dislocation on your exam—this is bread and butter radiology.

An entity that can be mistaken for a dislocated shoulder is a traumatic hemarthrosis that displaces the humeral head inferolaterally on the AP film. Because the anterior dislocation displaces inferomedially it should not be confused with this. The posterior dislocation will easily be excluded by looking at a transscapular view. This is termed a pseudodislocation and is discussed more fully in Chapter 4.

If a fracture about the shoulder is suspected and the plain films are negative or equivocal, a CT scan should be performed. Any complex joint, such as the shoulder or hip, is best examined with CT scanning when the full extent of the fracture needs to be identified (Fig. 5–42).

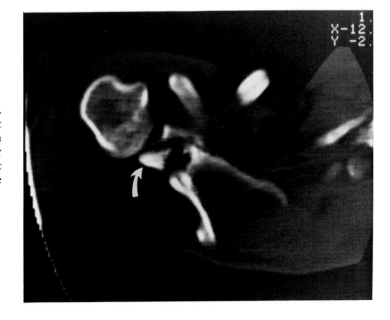

FIGURE 5–42   **Fracture of the glenoid.**
A CT scan of the shoulder in this patient
who had a fracture identified on a plain
film shows extension into the articular
portion with a possible loose fragment
(arrow). The plain film did not show the
fracture extending into the joint.

PELVIS

Fractures of the pelvis, and especially those
involving the acetabulum, can be difficult to evaluate completely with plain films alone. Because
plain films often do not show free fragments and
subtle fractures, CT scanning should be considered in almost all acetabular fractures (Fig.
5–43).

Sacral fractures are said to occur in half of the
cases that have pelvic fractures, yet radiologists
see a lot of pelvic fractures without seeing very
many sacral fractures. Why is this? Simple—we
miss a lot of sacral fractures. They can be difficult
to see on even the best of films because the sacrum
is often hidden by bowel gas. In looking for sacral
fractures one should examine the arcuate lines of
the sacrum bilaterally to see if they are intact.
Fractures often interrupt these lines and, because
of the side-to-side asymmetry, can be easily spot-
ted (Fig. 5–44).

Sacral stress fractures occur commonly in patients who are osteoporotic or who have undergone radiation therapy. These present as patchy
or linear sclerosis in the sacral ala that may or
may not show cortical disruption (Fig. 5–45).
They should be differentiated from metastatic
disease because of their characteristic location,
appearance, and history of prior radiation and
by the presence of a cortical break. These are
often bilateral and have a pathognomonic appearance on bone scan called a "Honda sign"
(Fig. 5–46). They also have a characteristic MR
appearance with geographic involvement of one
or both sacral alae with low signal on T1WI,
which may or may not have high signal on T2WI
(Fig. 5–47).

Avulsion injuries affect the pelvis quite often
and should be easily recognized by radiologists.
On occasion an avulsion can appear somewhat
"aggressive," and if it is not diagnosed radiographically, a biopsy might be performed. This
action can be calamitous, as avulsion injuries
have been known to mimic malignant lesions histologically, with a misdiagnosis leading to radical
treatment (Fig. 5–48). Therefore, when an avulsion injury is a consideration, it becomes a "don't
touch" lesion (see Chapter 4). Common sites for
pelvic avulsion include the ischium, the superior
and inferior anterior iliac spines (Fig. 5–49), and
the iliac crest. Such injuries are fairly common in
long jumpers, sprinters, hurdlers, gymnasts, and
cheerleaders.

The symphysis pubis is another area in the
pelvis that can demonstrate radiologic findings as
a result of stress. In ultramarathoners, marathon
cross-country skiers, and soccer players the
symphysis occasionally undergoes degenerative
changes (Figs. 5–50 and 5–51). The hallmarks
of degenerative disease (osteoarthritis) are sclerosis, joint space narrowing, and osteophytosis.
In certain joints, however, erosions occur as a
result of degenerative joint disease. These joints
include the temporomandibular joint (TMJ), the
acromioclavicular (AC) joint, and the sacroiliac
(SI) joint. These are easy to remember because
they are the "letter joints"—the TMJ, the AC,
and the SI. The symphysis pubis also behaves in
this manner. Ordinarily when erosions are a fea-

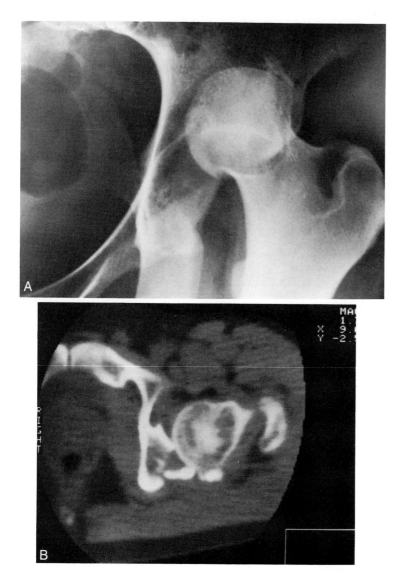

FIGURE 5–43 **Dislocation of the hip.** *(A)* An AP plain film of the left hip shows dislocation of the femoral head, which lies superior to the acetabulum. Fractures are easily identified on the CT scan *(B)*. A cortical break through the articular surface of the posterior acetabulum, as well as the dislocation, is identified.

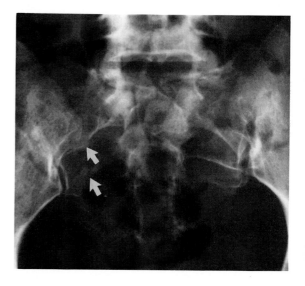

FIGURE 5–44 **Fracture of the sacrum.** An AP view of the sacrum in this patient shows normal arcuate lines on the left side of the sacrum that are interrupted on the right side (arrows). Interruption of these lines indicates a fracture through this portion of the sacrum.

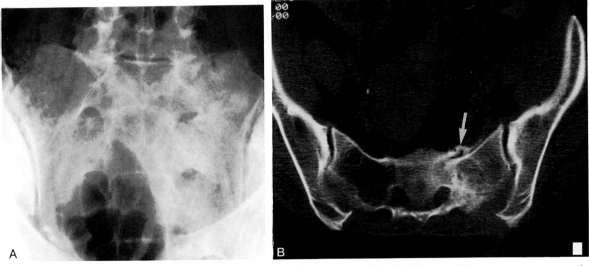

A   B

FIGURE 5–45   **Stress fracture of the sacrum.** *(A)* Faint sclerosis is noted in the left part of the sacrum as compared with the right in this patient complaining of pelvic pain. A radionuclide bone scan showed increased isotope uptake on the left half of the sacrum, and metastatic disease was postulated. A CT scan through this region *(B)* demonstrates a cortical disruption (arrow) indicative of a fracture. This is a characteristic plain film and CT appearance of a stress fracture of the sacrum.

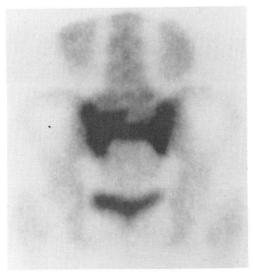

FIGURE 5–46   **"Honda Sign."** A radionuclide bone scan in a patient with bilateral sacral insufficiency (or stress) fractures shows increased uptake in the sacrum corresponding to an "H," which has been termed a "Honda sign." This finding is virtually pathognomonic for sacral stress fractures.

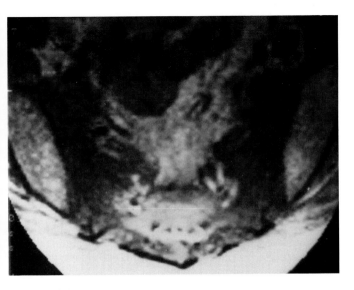

FIGURE 5–47   **MR imaging of sacral insufficiency fracture.** A T1-weighted coronal MR image through the sacrum in the patient with the bone scan shown in Figure 5–46 reveals areas of low signal corresponding to the edema and reactive bone around the sacral stress fractures. Much of the area of low signal will get increased in signal on a T2-weighted sequence. Why get an MR image if the bone scan is pathognomonic? A good question. The MR image is certainly not necessary if the bone scan had been performed already, and the bone scan would not be needed if the MR image were the first study.

103

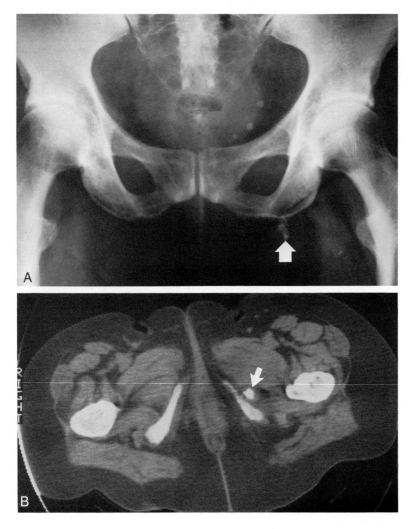

FIGURE 5–48 Avulsion off the ischium. (A) An AP view of the pelvis shows calcification extending off the left ischium (arrow) in a patient complaining of pain at this site. Note the irregular cortical surface, suggesting periostitis. The CT scan shows dense calcification adjacent to the ischium (arrow). These findings are characteristic for an ischial avulsion, and a biopsy should not be done.

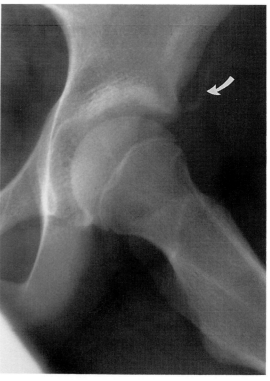

FIGURE 5–49 Avulsion from anterior inferior iliac spine. A plain film of the pelvis shows a calcific density near the anterior inferior iliac spine (arrow), which is typical for an avulsion of the rectus femoris muscle.

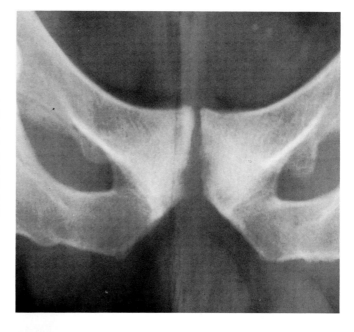

FIGURE 5–50 **Osteoarthritis of the symphysis pubis.** Sclerosis with erosion is noted at the symphysis in this ultramarathoner complaining of severe pubic pain. This is characteristic of degenerative disease or osteoarthritis at this site in an overuse setting, such as in an ultramarathoner. Erosions are ordinarily not seen in degenerative disease except in certain joints, such as the symphysis pubis, the SI joints, and the AC joints.

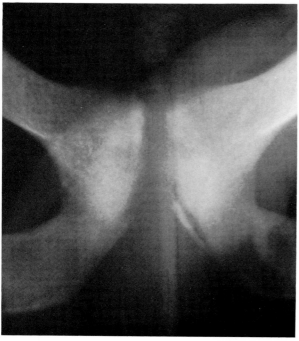

FIGURE 5–51 **Osteoarthritis of the symphysis pubis.** This is another example of sclerosis and erosive changes at the symphysis pubis in an ultramarathoner.

ture of an articular process, osteoarthritis (degenerative joint disease) is not in the differential diagnosis. It should be if the TMJ, the AC joint, the SI joint, or the symphysis is involved, however.

When the sacroiliac joints are involved with degenerative joint disease, the condition can closely resemble an HLA-B27 spondyloarthropathy (Fig. 5–52) and lead to erroneous diagnosis and treatment. Large osteophytes can develop across the SI joints and mimic sclerosis (Fig. 5–53) or even a tumor (Fig. 5–54).

LEG

Overt fractures in the femur and lower leg are, for the most part, straightforward and deserve no special radiologic treatment for fear of missing subtle abnormalities. Stress fractures, however, need to be considered in anyone with hip or leg pain, as overlooking the diagnosis can lead to catastrophe. The most serious stress fracture—and fortunately one of the rarest—is the femoral neck stress fracture. It has been divided into three types by orthopedic surgeons: type 1, sclerosis without a fracture line evident (Fig. 5–55); type

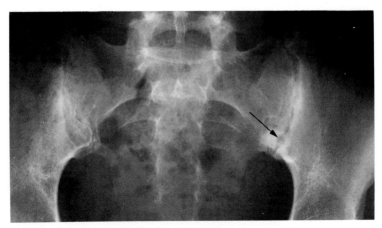

FIGURE 5–52 Osteoarthritis of the sacroiliac joint. Sclerosis and erosions (arrow) are seen in the left SI joint in this young, professional dancer. Although this finding has the appearance of an inflammatory arthritis, it is also seen in degenerative disease or osteoarthritis secondary to overuse.

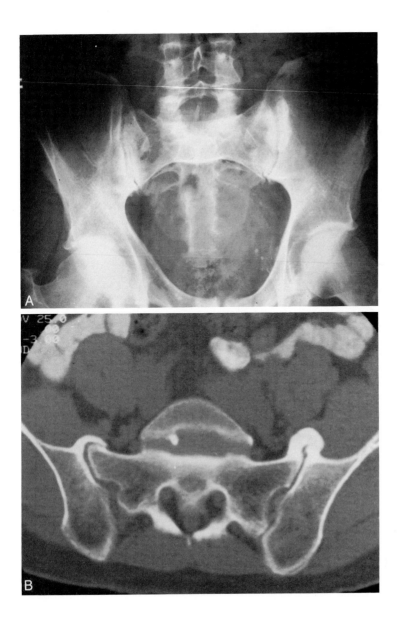

FIGURE 5–53 Sacroiliac osteophytes. An AP view of the pelvis *(A)* in this marathoner shows dense sclerosis over both SI joints. A CT scan through this area *(B)* demonstrates dense, bridging osteophytes characteristic of degenerative disease.

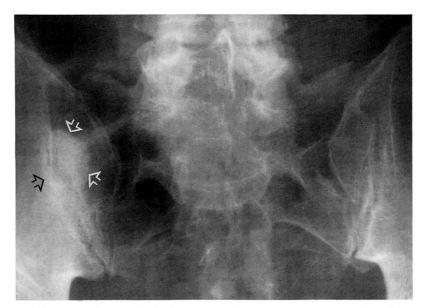

FIGURE 5–54   **Sacroiliac osteophytosis.** A focal area of sclerosis is seen overlying the right SI joint (arrows) in this elderly patient. A metastatic process was a diagnostic consideration. This is characteristic, however, of a sacroiliac osteophyte seen in degenerative disease of the SI joints. (Case courtesy of Dr. G. El-Khoury.)

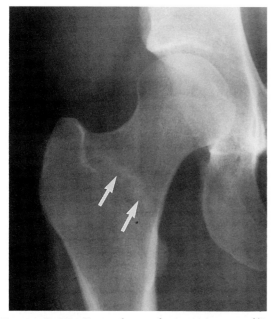

FIGURE 5–55   **Femoral stress fracture.** An area of linear sclerosis (arrows) is seen at the base of the femoral neck in a neophyte runner with hip pain. This finding is diagnostic of a stress fracture of the femur. (Case courtesy of Dr. David Simms.)

2, a lucent fracture line without displacement (Fig. 5–56); type 3, a displaced fracture is evident. The prognosis is best for a type 1 and worst for a type 3 fracture. Many surgeons believe that type 2 and type 3 fractures require internal fixation, whereas a type 1 fracture requires total bed rest for at least 3 to 4 weeks. Many type 1 fractures progress to complete fractures with displacement (type 3) with continued weight bearing; therefore, these are considered very serious lesions.

Stress fractures also occur in the distal diaphysis of the femur and in the proximal, middle, and distal thirds of the tibia. All of these stress fractures need to be treated with the utmost caution, since complete fractures are not uncommon with continued stress (Figs. 5–57 and 5–58). Sclerosis in a weight-bearing bone that has a horizontal or oblique linear pattern should be considered a stress fracture until proved otherwise. Occasionally a stress fracture will appear somewhat aggressive, with aggressive periostitis and no definite linearity to the sclerosis (Fig. 5–59). If the fracture is mistaken for a tumor and a biopsy is performed, it can be confused with a malignancy, with subsequent radical therapy. Therefore, in such cases a biopsy should not be done under any circumstances. If the clinical presentation is unusual for a stress fracture and the plain films are not diagnostic, take additional films 1 or 2 weeks later. Sometimes CT and MR imaging will better delineate the lesion and may show normal soft tissues. Stress fractures can be difficult to diagnose radiologically early on but should be straightforward after several weeks. A history of repetitive stress is not always obtained, so the diagnosis should not depend solely on the history.

An unusual stress fracture that for unknown reasons is seen almost exclusively in females is a

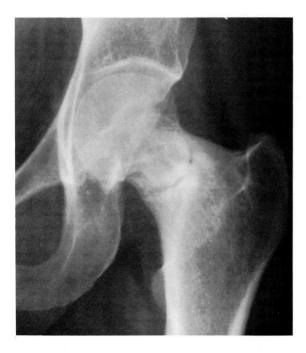

FIGURE 5–56 Stress fracture of the femoral neck. A linear lucency with surrounding sclerosis is seen in the femoral neck in this jogger with hip pain. This is a severe femoral neck stress fracture.

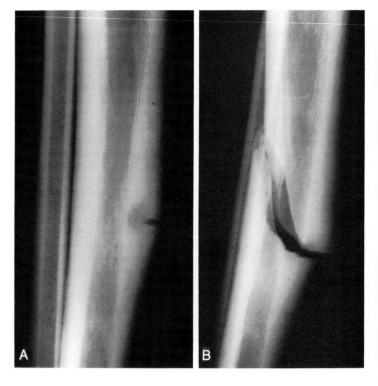

FIGURE 5–57 Stress fracture with completion. *(A)* A linear lucency is seen in the anterior cortex of the tibia in this runner, which is diagnostic for a stress fracture. *(B)* This radiograph shows the result of continued exercise. The stress fracture went on to a complete fracture, which illustrates why any stress fracture of a long bone should be protected.

fibular stress fracture (Fig. 5–60). The fibula is ordinarily not thought of as a weight-bearing bone, but in certain people it must serve as such.

One final stress fracture that deserves mention because it is frequently misdiagnosed clinically and overlooked radiographically is the calcaneal stress fracture (Fig. 5–61). It is often misdiagnosed clinically as a "heel spur" or plantar

fasciitis and can be a subtle radiographic finding. MR imaging can be helpful in cases in which plain films are negative (Fig. 5–62).

Overt fractures in the lower extremity are uncommonly missed on radiographs; however, a few exceptions should be noted. Hip fractures in the elderly population can be difficult to detect (Fig. 5–63), and a high index of suspicion should

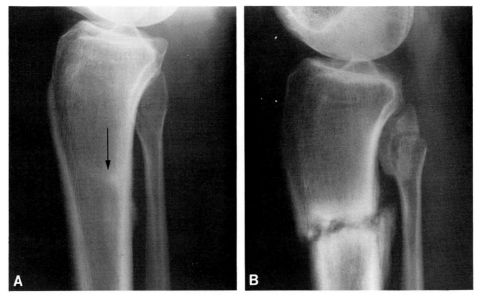

FIGURE 5–58 **Stress fracture with completion.** *(A)* A faint linear sclerotic area (arrow) is seen, which is characteristic for a stress fracture of the proximal tibia. *(B)* This radiograph shows the result of continued exercise in this patient: a complete fracture of the tibia and of the proximal fibula.

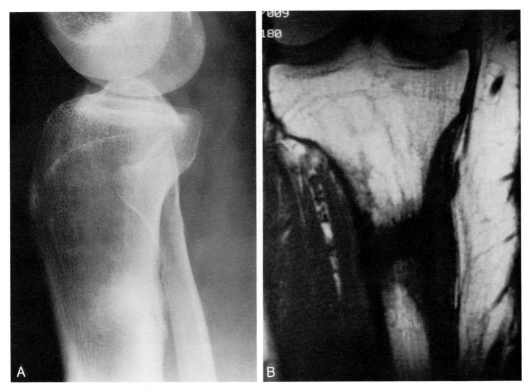

FIGURE 5–59 **Stress fracture of the tibia.** *(A)* An irregular focus of sclerosis is seen in the posterior proximal tibia with adjacent periostitis. There was concern that this might represent a primary bone tumor, and the surgeons recommended a biopsy. An MR imaging scan was performed *(B)*, however, showing a linear low-signal area running obliquely across the tibia, which is characteristic of a stress fracture. No significant soft tissue mass was found. The patient's recent history included an increase in his jogging, and a stress fracture was diagnosed based on these images.

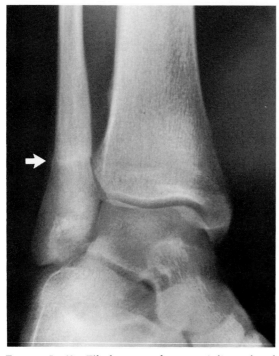

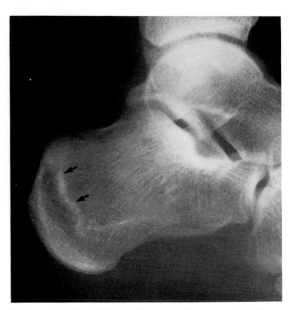

FIGURE 5–60 Fibular stress fracture. A linear band of sclerosis with adjacent periostitis (arrow) is seen in the distal fibula in this young woman jogger. This is diagnostic for a stress fracture of the fibula.

FIGURE 5–61 Calcaneal stress fracture. A linear band of sclerosis is seen in the posterior calcaneus (arrows), which is diagnostic for a stress fracture of the calcaneus.

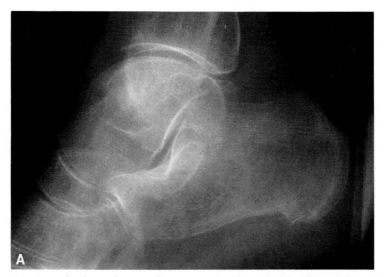

FIGURE 5–62 MR imaging of calcaneal stress fracture. *(A)* A lateral plain film of the calcaneus of an elderly woman with heel pain and a history of lung carcinoma shows only osteoporosis. *(B)* A radionuclide bone scan reveals diffuse increased uptake throughout the calcaneus. The question of whether to treat the calcaneus with radiation for metastatic lung carcinoma or to do a biopsy first was a dilemma. *(C)* An MR imaging scan was obtained to get a better idea of where the met might be. This sagittal T1-weighted image shows a linear low-signal area (arrow) which is characteristic for a stress fracture. Obviously, no biopsy or radiation was necessary.

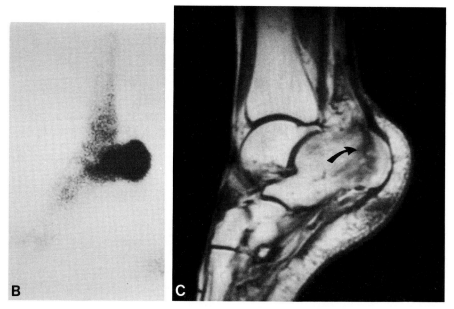

FIGURE 5–62 *Continued*   For legend see opposite page.

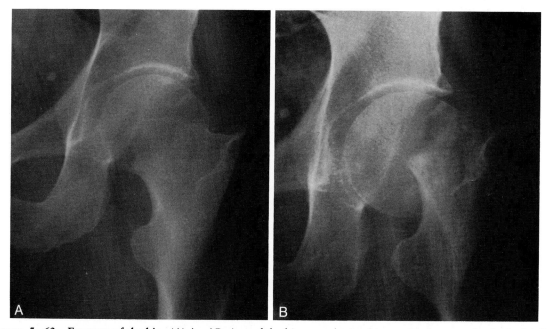

FIGURE 5–63   **Fracture of the hip.** *(A)* An AP view of the hip was obtained in an elderly man after he had fallen. It was interpreted as normal, and the patient was dismissed from the emergency department. Two weeks later the patient returned to the emergency department because he was unable to walk. Another radiograph was obtained *(B)*, and this shows a complete fracture through the femoral neck. In retrospect the fracture can be faintly seen in *A* and should have been picked up initially. Fractures of the hip in the elderly can be difficult to see and should be diligently searched for with additional views when the clinical setting is appropriate.

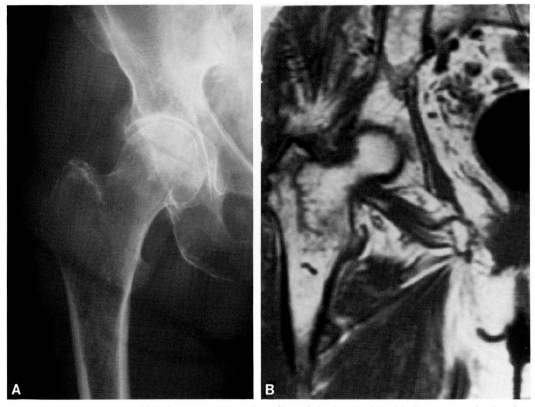

FIGURE 5–64 MR imaging of hip fracture. *(A)* A plain film of the hip in this elderly patient who has hip pain following a fall does not show a fracture. *(B)* A T1-weighted MR image shows linear low signal in the intertrochanteric region, which is typical for a hip fracture.

be maintained. A negative plain film in an elderly patient with hip pain after trauma (even relatively mild trauma) does not exclude a femoral neck fracture. Additional examinations, such as tomograms, CT, or MR imaging, should be considered before ruling out a fracture. MR imaging has proved to be very useful in diagnosing hip fractures when plain films are negative (Fig. 5–64) and, even though expensive, can actually reduce the overall costs by ensuring that no fractures are missed.

Another fracture that can be difficult to exclude on routine plain films is a tibial plateau fracture (Fig. 5–65). Many emergency rooms routinely take a cross-table lateral view of the knee to look for a fat/fluid level in the suprapatellar recess. This finding indicates that a fracture has occurred and allowed fatty marrow to enter the joint; it has a high correlation with a tibial plateau fracture. In the appropriate clinical setting tomograms, CT, or MR imaging may be necessary to make the diagnosis.

A serious fracture in the foot that can be missed radiographically when little or no displacement occurs is the so-called Lisfranc's fracture (Fig. 5–66). It is named after a famous surgeon in Napoleon's army who would do forefoot amputations in patients with gangrenous toes after frostbite. The Lisfranc's fracture is a fracture-dislocation of the tarsometatarsals. If the dislocation is minimal, it can be easily overlooked. A key to normal alignment is that the medial border of the second metatarsal should always line up with the medial border of the second cuneiform, and the medial border of the fourth metatarsal should line up with the medial border of the cuboid. If they do not, a Lisfranc's fracture-dislocation should be suspected. This fracture is seen most commonly as a result of catching the forefoot in something such as a hole in the ground, or in a horseback rider falling and hanging by the forefoot in the stirrups. It is not uncommonly seen as a neurotrophic or Charcot's joint in diabetics.

A fracture of the calcaneus can be difficult to appreciate on routine radiographs. Boehler's angle is a normal anatomic landmark that should be looked for in every foot film when trauma has

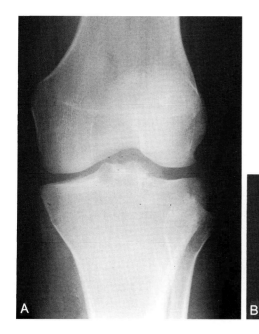

FIGURE 5–65 **Tibial plateau fracture.** *(A)* An AP view of the knee shows no obvious abnormalities at first glance. However, a CT scan with reformations of the knee *(B)* demonstrates a plateau fracture of the lateral tibia. Note the rounded sclerosis, which in retrospect can be barely appreciated in *A*. *(C)* A T1 coronal MR image shows a tibial plateau fracture that was barely discernable on plain films. MR is an excellent imaging choice for subtle fractures. Tibial plateau fractures are probably the most commonly missed fractures about the knee.

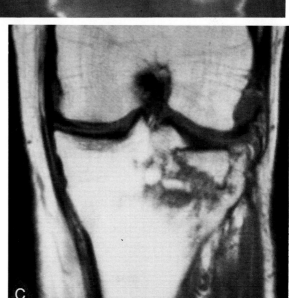

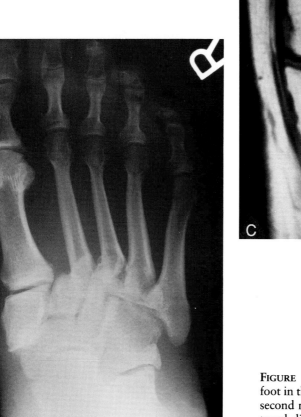

FIGURE 5–66 **Lisfranc's fracture.** An AP view of the foot in this patient shows a space between the first and second metatarsals with the base of the second metatarsal displaced off the second cuneiform. This is indicative of a Lisfranc's fracture-dislocation.

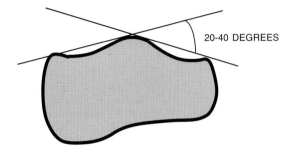

FIGURE 5–67 Boehler's angle in a normal calcaneus. This drawing shows the normal calcaneus with a line across the anterior process extending to the apex of the calcaneus, intersecting with a line from the posterior portion of the calcaneus to the apex. This is termed Boehler's angle, and when it becomes flattened or less than 20 degrees, a calcaneal fracture should be diagnosed.

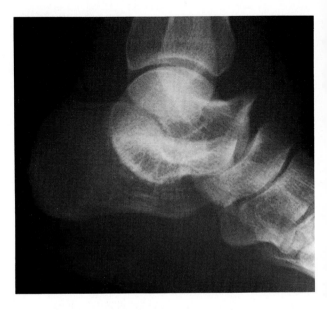

FIGURE 5–68 Calcaneal fracture. Boehler's angle in this calcaneus is less than 20 degrees, which is indicative of a fracture of the calcaneus.

occurred (Fig. 5–67). If the angle is narrower than 20 degrees, a compression of the calcaneus is indicated, such as is seen with jumping injuries (Fig. 5–68). This fracture has been termed a "lover's fracture," for the propensity of lovers to jump out of windows when discovered in compromising surroundings by apparently larger or armed jealous suitors.

CONCLUSION

This fairly simplified overview of some commonly overlooked fractures and dislocations should in no way be interpreted as a substitute for the more complete texts listed in the bibliography. For most residents and medical students it can serve as a starting point, however, and perhaps stimulate reading in more depth on some of the topics.

REFERENCES

1. Rogers LF: Radiology of Skeletal Trauma. New York, ed 2. Churchill Livingstone, 1993.
2. Harris JH Jr, Harris WH: The Radiology of Emergency Medicine, ed 3. Baltimore, Williams & Wilkins, 1993.
3. Rockwood CA Jr, Green DP: Fractures in Adults, ed 3. Philadelphia, JB Lippincott Co, 1993.

Chapter

6

Arthritis

The radiologic study of arthritis can be extremely difficult for the inexperienced because of the wide variety of patterns of disease, which produces a tremendous amount of overlap among the various diseases. What at first seems to be simple characterization of disease entities is found by the more experienced observer to be broad generalizations that may or may not fit into any one category of disease.

This chapter gives an overview of radiologic evaluation of arthritis with the caveat that it is, by necessity, a simplified version and in no way complete. If one is interested in greater detail or more accuracy, I would urge reading either Debbie Forrester's excellent monograph[1] on the subject or Anne Brower's superb book.[2] The definitive work on this subject is Don Resnick's six-volume tome,[3] but you can't read even the arthritis portion during a 4-year residency—it's best used as a reference.

The majority of arthritides are most easily examined and categorized by looking at their effect on the hands. Forrester recommends a search pattern that she calls the ABC'S, with the "A" indicating alignment, "B" standing for bone mineralization, "C" standing for cartilage and including a search for erosions, and the "S" standing for soft tissues. I would add to this search pattern by making it the ABCD'S, with the "D" indicating distribution of the pathology. Although this is implied in Forrester's search pattern, I feel that it cannot be overemphasized.

In general, if the distribution of the arthropathy can be determined, the differential diagnosis becomes very short (Table 6–1). Although on paper this sounds quite nice, it can on occasion be difficult to accurately determine the distribution of the arthropathy. The distribution of the arthropathy is difficult to determine when it is not clearly distal or proximal but is more general, such as occurs with gout, multicentric reticulohistiocytosis (MRH), and sarcoid. It can also be difficult to accurately determine the distribution when advanced disease is present, such as occurs with severe rheumatoid arthritis. With severe rheumatoid arthritis the proximal nature of the pathology is not so apparent because of involvement with the metacarpophalangeal joints and even the phalangeal joints. In a similar manner, when psoriatic disease, Reiter's syndrome, or osteoarthritis are severely advanced, they can involve the more proximal portion of the hand and wrist, although this is unusual.

Side-to-side symmetry of the arthropathy is occasionally helpful in selecting a differential diagnosis (Table 6–2). Primary osteoarthritis, rheumatoid arthritis, and MRH are classically described as bilaterally symmetric. Exceptions occur quite frequently, however, so that bilateral symmetry in these disorders is probably only on the order of 80 to 90 per cent. Rheumatoid arthritis is a common offender of the bilateral symmetry rule, and one should not be surprised if rheumatoid arthritis is seen to be asymmetric in up to 20 to 25 per cent of cases.

Involvement of joints other than the hand and wrist is not a common feature with most of the arthritides. In general, when a large joint such as the shoulder, hip, or knee is involved with arthritis only a few entities need to be considered (Table 6–3). Although it must be emphasized that almost any arthritis can affect almost any

TABLE 6–1 Arthropathy Distribution in Hands and Wrists

Distal	Proximal
Psoriasis	Rheumatoid arthritis
Reiter's syndrome	Calcium pyrophosphate dihydrate crystal deposition disease (CPPD)
Osteoarthritis	

TABLE 6–2 Bilateral Symmetry of Arthropathy

Primary osteoarthritis
Rheumatoid arthritis
Multicentric reticulohistiocytosis

TABLE 6–3 Large Joint Involvement

Osteoarthritis (degenerative joint disease)	Ankylosing spondylitis
Rheumatoid arthritis	Pigmented villonodular synovitis
Calcium pyrophosphate dihydrate crystal deposition disease (CPPD)	Synovial osteochondromatosis
	Infection

TABLE 6–4 Sacroiliac Joint Involvement

Anklosing spondylitis	Osteoarthritis (degenerative joint disease)
Inflammatory bowel disease	Infection
Psoriasis	Gout
Reiter's syndrome	Hyperparathyroidism

TABLE 6–5 Normal Mineralization

Osteoarthritis (degenerative joint disease)	Gout
Calcium pyrophosphate dihydrate crystal deposition disease (CPPD)	Multicentric reticulohistiocytosis
	Pigmented villonodular synovitis
	Synovial osteochondromatosis

joint, the diseases listed in Table 6–3 probably will account for 90 per cent or more of the large joint arthropathies.

Involvement of certain joints can often give a clue as to the underlying disease process. For example, if the sacroiliac (SI) joints are involved, the differential diagnosis is as listed in Table 6–4. Again, almost any arthritis can affect any joint, but if the SI joint is involved, using Table 6–4 for the differential diagnosis will give a 95 per cent or better chance of having the right answer.

Demineralization will occur around any joint that has pain, swelling, and hyperemia. Almost any of the arthritides can cause this to occur, yet there are a few entities that tend not to be associated with demineralization (Table 6–5). Normal mineralization in the presence of an arthritis only indicates that there is no underlying hyperemia and probably no associated pain or at least long-standing pain at the time the x-ray was obtained. Normal mineralization often indicates an old, burned-out arthritis that was at one time painful and probably associated with demineralization. Nevertheless, when normal mineralization is noted around a joint that is abnormal, the entities in Table 6–5 should be strongly considered.

The above-mentioned differential diagnoses are to be considered generalizations and are, for the most part (except when mentioned), probably not more than 75 to 85 per cent accurate. They are a nice starting point, however, for developing the differential diagnosis. I cannot overemphasize that the exceptions are exceedingly common. There are probably more missed diagnoses in the field of arthritis than in almost any other area of radiology. The remainder of this chapter gives a brief overview of arthritides with which most radiologists should be familiar. Rather than provide an in-depth description of each process—which can be obtained in any of the major radiology texts—I give salient discriminating points that might make it easier to differentiate one process from another.

OSTEOARTHRITIS

The most common arthritis seen by radiologists is osteoarthritis, or degenerative joint disease (DJD). It is felt to be caused by trauma—either overt or as an accumulation of microtrauma over the years. The hallmarks of DJD are joint space

TABLE 6–6 Hallmarks of Degenerative Joint Disease

Sclerosis
Osteophytes
Joint space narrowing

narrowing, sclerosis, and osteophytosis (Table 6–6) (Fig. 6–1). If all three of these findings are not present on the radiograph, another diagnosis should be considered.

Joint space narrowing is the least specific finding of the three, yet it is virtually always present in DJD. Unfortunately it is also seen in almost every other joint abnormality, so by itself it means little.

Sclerosis should be present in varying amounts in all cases of DJD unless severe osteoporosis is present. Osteoporosis causes the sclerosis to be diminished. For instance, in long-standing rheumatoid arthritis where the cartilage has been destroyed, DJD often occurs with little sclerosis. Osteophytosis will be diminished in the setting of osteoporosis also. Otherwise, sclerosis and osteophytosis should be prominent in DJD.

The only disorder that will cause osteophytes without sclerosis or joint space narrowing is diffuse idiopathic skeletal hyperostosis (DISH). This common bone-forming disorder at first glance resembles DJD except there is no joint space (or disc space in the spine) narrowing and there is no sclerosis (Fig. 6–2). DISH is not felt to be caused by trauma or stress, as is DJD, and is not painful or disabling, as DJD can be. Millions of dollars per year are awarded to government employees on retirement for "disability" payments for supposed DJD acquired on their jobs when in fact they have DISH and are misdiagnosed. It is hoped that such errors will be rectified in the future as more radiologists become informed of the difference between DJD and DISH.

Osteoarthritis is divided into two types: primary and secondary. Secondary osteoarthritis is what radiologists refer to when speaking of DJD. It is, as mentioned, secondary to trauma of some sort. It can occur in any joint in the body but is particularly common in the knees, hips, and spine.

Primary osteoarthritis is a familial arthritis that affects middle-aged females almost exclusively, and is seen only in the hands. It affects the distal interphalangeal (DIP) joints, the proximal interphalangeal (PIP) joints, and the base of the thumb in a bilaterally symmetric fashion (Fig. 6–3). If the arthritis is not bilaterally symmetric, the diagnosis of primary osteoarthritis should be questioned (Fig. 6–4).

A type of primary osteoarthritis that can be very painful and debilitating is erosive osteoarthritis. It has the identical distribution as mentioned for primary osteoarthritis but is associated

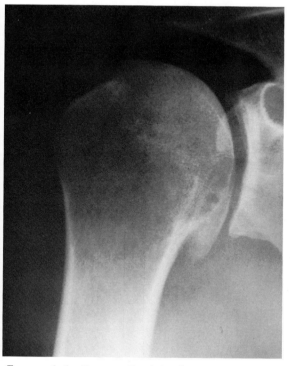

FIGURE 6–1 Degenerative joint disease of the shoulder. This former professional baseball pitcher with long-standing shoulder pain has joint space narrowing, subchondral sclerosis, and osteophytosis, which are hallmarks of degenerative joint disease (DJD).

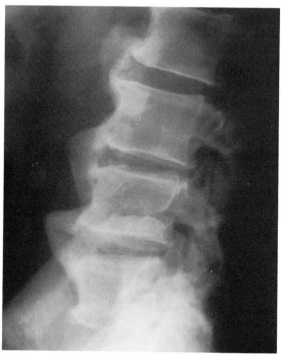

FIGURE 6–2 Diffuse idiopathic skeletal hyperostosis. A lateral of the lumbar spine shows extensive osteophytosis without significant disc space narrowing or sclerosis. This is a classic picture for diffuse idiopathic skeletal hyperostosis (DISH).

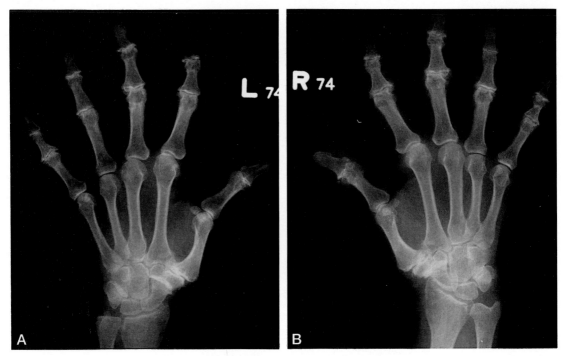

FIGURE 6–3 Primary osteoarthritis. A radiograph of the hands in a patient with primary osteoarthritis shows classic findings of osteophytosis, joint space narrowing, and sclerosis at the distal interphalangeal joints, the proximal interphalangeal joints, and the base of the thumb. This was bilaterally symmetric in this patient, which is seen by comparing the left hand *(A)* with the right hand *(B)*. This is typical for primary osteoarthritis.

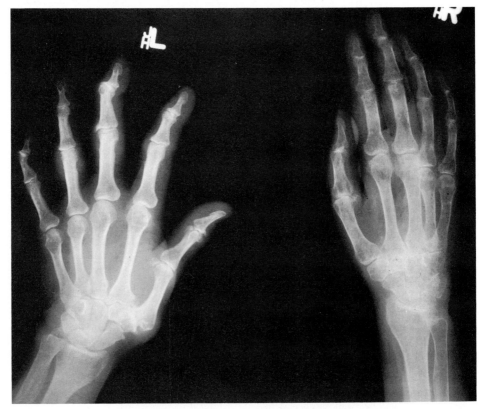

FIGURE 6–4 Lack of bilateral symmetry in primary osteoarthritis. This patient has classic radiographic findings of primary osteoarthritis in the left hand; however, the right hand shows only osteoporosis and soft tissue wasting without evidence of osteoarthritis. The reason for the lack of bilaterality is that this patient has long-standing right-sided paralysis, which has blocked the onset of the arthritic changes in the right hand.

with severe osteoporosis of the hands as well as erosions. It is somewhat uncommon, and radiologists generally see little of this disorder. Residents tend to mention erosive osteoarthritis in every example of joint erosions encountered whether it is in the hands, knees, hips, or wherever. This is totally inappropriate because erosive osteoarthritis only occurs in the hands, and there it has a characteristic distribution, which should make for an easy diagnosis.

There are a few exceptions to the classic triad of findings seen in DJD (sclerosis, narrowing, and osteophytes). Several joints also exhibit erosions as a manifestation of DJD. I call these joints the "letter joints" because they are all often called by their initials: the TMJ (temporomandibular joint), the AC (acromioclavicular) joint, and the SI (sacroiliac) joints; the symphysis pubis behaves similarly (Table 6–7). When erosions are seen in one of these joints DJD must be considered, or inappropriate treatment can be expected (Fig. 6–5).

Another process that can occasionally be seen in DJD is a subchondral cyst or geode (taken from the geologic term used when a volcanic rock has a gas pocket that leaves a large cavity in the rock). Geodes are cystic formations that occur around joints in a variety of disorders (Table 6–8). Presumably, one method by which they form is synovial fluid being forced into the subchondral bone, causing a cystic collection of joint fluid. They seldom cause problems by themselves but are often misdiagnosed as something more sinister (Fig. 6–6) (see Chapter 4).

RHEUMATOID ARTHRITIS

Rheumatoid arthritis is a connective tissue disorder of unknown cause that can affect any synovial-lined joint in the body. The radiographic hallmarks are soft tissue swelling, osteoporosis,

TABLE 6–7 Joints That Exhibit Erosions with Osteoarthritis

Temporomandibular (TMJ)	Acromioclavicular (AC)
Sacroiliac (SI)	Symphysis pubis

TABLE 6–8 Diseases That Cause Subchrondral Cysts (Geodes)

Rheumatoid arthritis	Calcium pyrophosphate dihydrate crystal deposition disease (CPPD)
Degenerative joint disease	Avascular necrosis

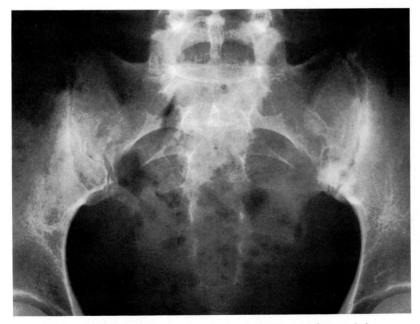

FIGURE 6–5 Osteoarthritis of the SI joint. A young woman, who is a professional dancer, complained of left-sided hip pain. This anteroposterior (AP) film of the pelvis demonstrated left SI joint sclerosis, joint irregularity, and erosions. A complete workup to rule out an HLA-B27 spondyloarthropathy was negative, and no laboratory or clinical evidence for infection was found. Her clinical history pointed to this process being completely occupation related, and an aspiration biopsy to rule out infection was therefore not performed. This is not an unusual appearance for DJD of the SI joints.

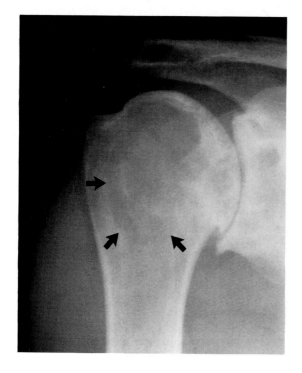

FIGURE 6–6 Subchondral cyst or geode of the shoulder. This patient has marked DJD of the shoulder with joint space narrowing, sclerosis, and osteophytosis. A large lytic process (arrows) seen in the humeral head is a subchondral cyst or geode, which often occurs in association with DJD. Because of the DJD in the shoulder, a biopsy to rule out a more sinister lesion in the humeral head should be avoided.

joint space narrowing, and marginal erosions (Table 6–9). In the hands it is classically a proximal process that is bilaterally symmetrical (Fig. 6–7). There are so many exceptions to these

TABLE 6–9 Hallmarks of Rheumatoid Arthritis

Proximal and bilaterally symmetric (hands)	Osteoporosis
	Joint space narrowing
Soft tissue swelling	Marginal erosions

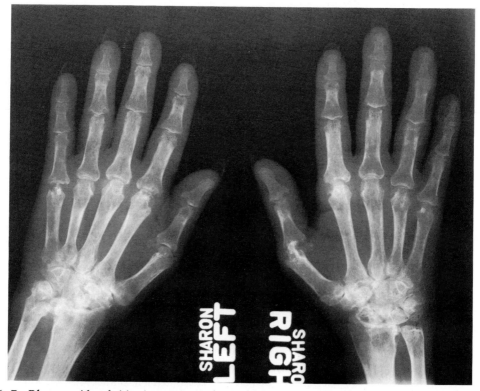

FIGURE 6–7 Rheumatoid arthritis. An erosive arthritis that primarily affects the carpal bones and the metacarpophalangeal joints is seen that has osteoporosis and soft tissue swelling (note the soft tissue over the ulnar styloid processes). It is a bilaterally symmetrical process in this patient, which is classic.

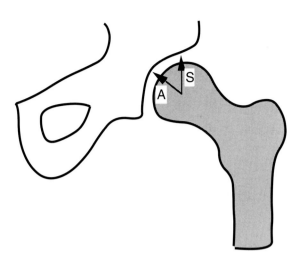

FIGURE 6–8 Routes of migration of the femoral head. Osteoarthritis of the hip tends to cause superior (S) migration of the femoral head in relation to the acetabulum, whereas rheumatoid arthritis tends to cause axial (A) migration of the femoral head in relation to the acetabulum.

rules, however, that I have come to regard them as no better than 80 per cent accurate. Rheumatoid arthritis has a large variety of appearances and can be difficult to diagnose with any degree of assurance from its radiographic appearance alone.

Rheumatoid arthritis in large joints is fairly characteristic in that it causes a lot of joint space narrowing and is associated with marked osteoporosis. Erosions may or may not be present and tend to be marginal, that is, away from the weight-bearing portion of the joint. In the hip the femoral head tends to migrate axially, whereas in osteoarthritis it tends to migrate superolaterally (Figs. 6–8 and 6–9). In the shoulder the humeral head tends to be "high-riding" (Fig. 6–10). Other things to think of when confronted with a high-riding shoulder are a torn rotator cuff and calcium pyrophosphate dihydrate crystal deposition disease (CPPD) (Table 6–10).

TABLE 6–10 Diseases That Cause a High-riding Shoulder

Calcium pyrophosphate dihydrate crystal deposition disease (CPPD)	Rheumatoid arthritis
	Torn rotator cuff

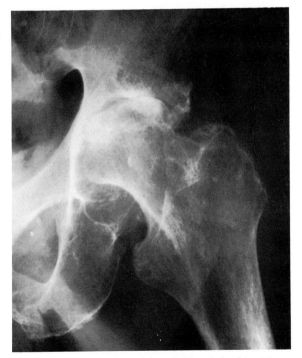

FIGURE 6–9 Rheumatoid arthritis of the hip. Note the severe joint space narrowing in this patient with rheumatoid arthritis. The femoral head has migrated in an axial direction with fairly concentric joint space narrowing. Minimal secondary degenerative changes have occurred, as noted by the sclerosis in the superior portion of the joint; however, these have been diminished somewhat by the osteoporosis that usually accompanies rheumatoid arthritis.

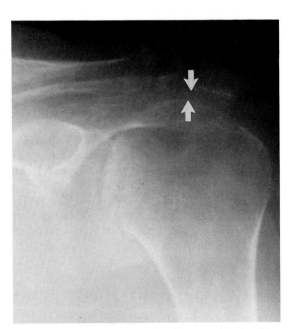

FIGURE 6–10 Rheumatoid arthritis in the shoulder. An AP view of the shoulder in this patient with rheumatoid arthritis shows that the distance between the acromion and the humeral head is diminished (arrows). Ordinarily this space is about one fingerbreadth in width to allow the rotator cuff to move freely. This is a common finding in rheumatoid arthritis as well as in CPPD or with a torn rotator cuff.

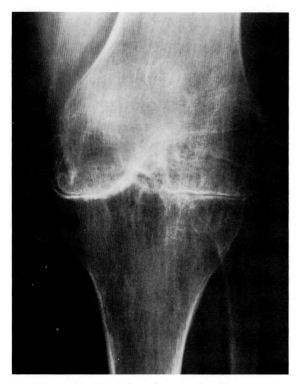

FIGURE 6–11 Secondary degenerative disease in the knee in a patient with rheumatoid arthritis. This patient has a history of long-standing rheumatoid arthritis. An AP view of the knee shows severe osteoporosis and joint space narrowing. Secondary DJD is occurring as evidenced by the sclerosis and osteophytosis; however, these findings are out of proportion to the severe joint space narrowing. When DJD narrows a joint to this extent, the osteophytosis and sclerosis are invariably much more pronounced.

When rheumatoid arthritis is long-standing, it is not unusual for secondary DJD to superimpose itself on the findings one would expect with rheumatoid. This picture of DJD differs somewhat from that usually seen in that the sclerosis and osteophytes are considerably diminished in severity as compared with the joint space narrowing (Fig. 6–11).

HLA-B27
SPONDYLOARTHROPATHIES

A group of diseases that was formerly called "rheumatoid variants" is now known as the "seronegative HLA-B27 positive spondyloarthropathies." What was wrong with "rheumatoid variants"? It was short and concise. It has been replaced with a polysyllabic mouthful that is perhaps more descriptively correct, but so what? That is the problem with most academicians— make it sound more erudite and maybe everyone will think we're smarter than we really are. They

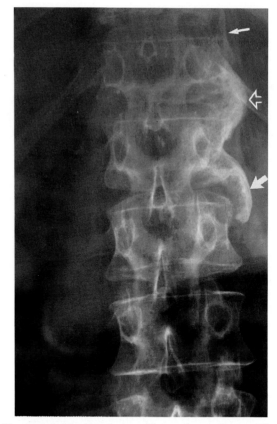

FIGURE 6–12 Psoriasis with syndesmophytes. The large paravertebral ossification on the left side of the T12-L1 disc space (open arrow) is difficult to differentiate between an osteophyte and a syndesmophyte. Either could have this appearance. However, the paravertebral ossification at the left L1-2 disc space (solid arrow) definitely has a vertical rather than a horizontal orientation, as does the faint ossification seen at the T11-12 disc space (small arrow). These definitely represent syndesmophytes. Therefore, it makes sense to logically assume that the ossification at the T12-L1 disc space is almost certainly a syndesmophyte as well. This patient has large nonmarginal asymmetric syndesmophytes, which are typical of psoriatic arthritis or Reiter's syndrome. This patient indeed has psoriasis.

shouldn't be so insecure. I liked "rheumatoid variants."

These disorders are all linked to the HLA-B27 histocompatibility antigen. Included in this group of diseases are ankylosing spondylitis, inflammatory bowel disease, psoriatic arthritis, and Reiter's syndrome. They are characterized by bony ankylosis, proliferative new-bone formation, and predominantly axial (spinal) involvement.

One of the more characteristic findings is that of syndesmophytes in the spine. A syndesmophyte is a paravertebral ossification that resembles an osteophyte except that it runs vertically, whereas an osteophyte has its orientation in a horizontal axis. Sometimes deciding whether a particular paravertebral ossification is an osteophyte or a syndesmophyte is difficult based on its orientation alone (Fig. 6–12). Bridging osteophytes and large syndesmophytes can have a similar appearance, with both having an orientation halfway between vertical and horizontal. How should one evaluate those examples? Easy—ignore them. Look at the other vertebral bodies and use the ossifications on them to determine whether you are dealing with osteophytes or syndesmophytes. If no other level is involved, you might just have to make the diagnosis based on something else. In other words, sometimes you just will not be able to tell one from the other.

Syndesmophytes are classified as to whether they are marginal and symmetric or nonmarginal and asymmetric. A marginal syndesmophyte has its origin at the edge or margin of a vertebral body and extends to the margin of the adjacent vertebral body. Marginal syndesmophytes are invariably bilaterally symmetric as viewed on an anteroposterior (AP) spine film. Ankylosing spondylitis classically has marginal, symmetric syndesmophytes (Fig. 6–13). Inflammatory bowel disease has an identical appearance when the spine is involved.

Nonmarginal, asymmetric syndesmophytes are generally large and bulky. They emanate from the vertebral body away from the end-plate or margin and are unilateral or asymmetric as viewed on an AP spine film (Figs. 6–12 and 6–14). Psoriatic arthritis and Reiter's syndrome classically have this type of syndesmophyte.

Involvement of the SI joints is common in the HLA-B27 spondyloarthropathies. The patterns of involvement, like the patterns of involvement of the spine, are somewhat typical for each disorder. Ankylosing spondylitis and inflammatory bowel disease typically cause bilaterally symmetric SI joint disease that is initially erosive and progresses to sclerosis and fusion (Figs. 6–15 and 6–16). It is extremely unusual to have asymmetric or unilateral SI joint disease in these two disorders. Another entity that can have bilateral SI joint erosions is hyperparathyroidism. Subperiosteal resorption along the SI joints mimics erosive changes. This is more commonly seen in children.

Reiter's syndrome and psoriatic arthritis can exhibit unilateral or bilateral SI joint involvement. It is said that it is bilateral about 50 per cent of the time. It is often asymmetric when it

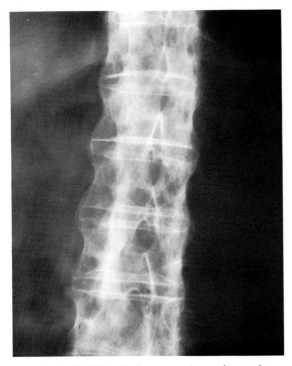

FIGURE 6–13 Marginal symmetric syndesmophytes in a patient with ankylosing spondylitis. Bilateral marginal syndesmophytes are seen bridging the disc spaces throughout the lumbar spine in this patient. This is a "bamboo spine" and is classic for ankylosing spondylitis or inflammatory bowel disease.

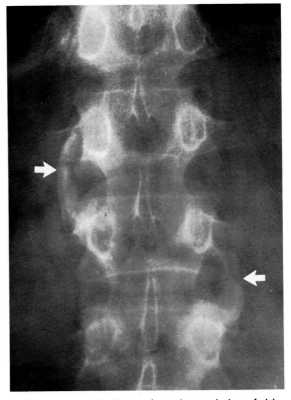

FIGURE 6–14 Syndesmophytes in psoriatic arthritis. Large, bulky, nonmarginal asymmetric syndesmophytes (arrows) are seen in this patient with psoriatic arthritis.

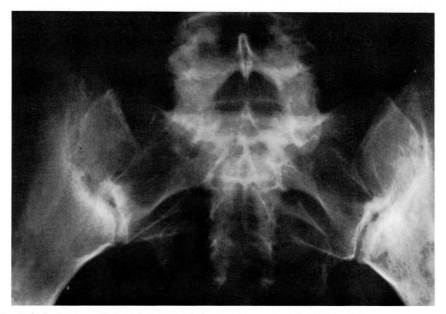

FIGURE 6–15 Ankylosing spondylitis. Bilateral, symmetric SI joint sclerosis and erosions are seen in this patient with ankylosing spondylitis. Inflammatory bowel disease could have an identical appearance. Although this is classic for these two disorders, it would not be that unusual for psoriatic disease or Reiter's syndrome to have this appearance. Hyperparathyroidism can also have this appearance. It would be unlikely for infection or DJD to be bilateral in this fashion.

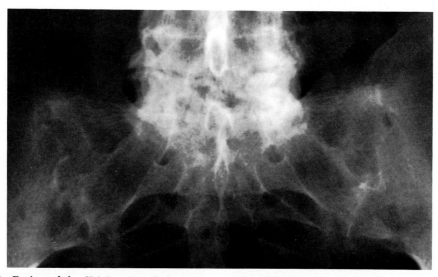

FIGURE 6–16 Fusion of the SI joints in ankylosing spondylitis. Bilateral complete fusion of the SI joints in this patient with ankylosing spondylitis makes the SI joints totally indistinguishable. Inflammatory bowel disease could have a similar appearance. I have not seen other disease processes affect the SI joints to this extent, with the exception of long-standing paralysis.

is bilateral, but exact symmetry can be difficult to assess. Therefore, when it is definitely bilateral and not clearly asymmetric, I consider the SI joints to be in the bilateral symmetric category. This means that if I have a case with bilateral, symmetric SI joint disease, it could be caused by any of the four HLA-B27 spondyloarthropathies. If I have a case with unilateral (or clearly asym-

metric) SI joint involvement, I can confidently exclude ankylosing spondylitis and inflammatory bowel disease; I would consider Reiter's syndrome and psoriatic disease. In this example I would have to also consider infection and DJD (don't forget that DJD can cause erosions in the SI joints) (Figs. 6–5 and 6–17) and in older patients gout. Computed tomography (CT) is very

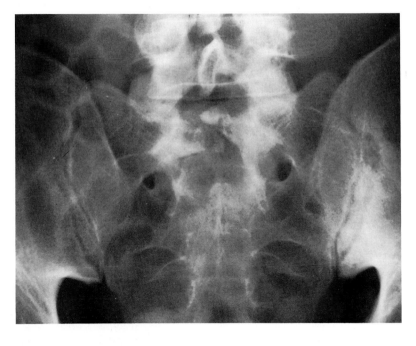

FIGURE 6–17 Psoriasis with SI joint disease. Unilateral SI sclerosis and erosions are seen in this patient with psoriasis. Ankylosing spondylitis and inflammatory bowel disease virtually never have this appearance.

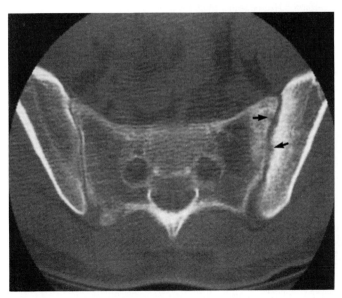

FIGURE 6–18 CT of the SI joints in psoriasis. A CT scan through the SI joints in this patient with psoriasis shows unilateral SI joint sclerosis and erosions (arrows) typical for psoriasis or Reiter's syndrome.

helpful in examining the SI joints and is considered by many to be the diagnostic procedure of choice because of the unobstructed view of the entire joint (Fig. 6–18).

That is, in a nutshell, my approach to the SI joints (Table 6–4). Other considerations in the differential are too uncommon for me to worry about for the most part, and you shouldn't either.

Large joint involvement with the HLA-B27 spondyloarthropathies is uncommon (except for ankylosing spondylitis) but occurs often enough to warrant learning about. In general, the arthropathy will resemble rheumatoid arthritis with the typical features thereof (Fig. 6–19). The hips

are involved in up to 50 per cent of the patients with ankylosing spondylitis.

Small joint involvement, specifically the hands and feet, is not commonly seen in ankylosing spondylitis and inflammatory bowel disease and tends to resemble rheumatoid arthritis. Psoriasis causes a distinctive arthropathy that is characterized by its distal predominance, proliferative erosions, soft tissue swelling, and periostitis. The erosions are different from the clean-cut, sharply marginated erosions seen in all other erosive arthritides in that they have fuzzy margins with wisps of periostitis emanating from them (Fig. 6–20A). The severe forms are often associated

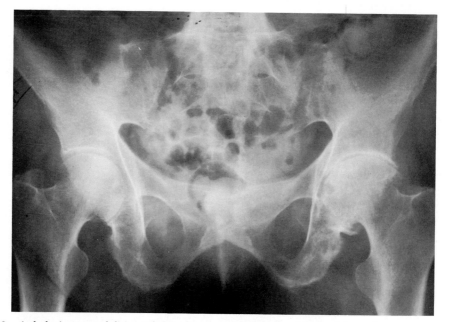

FIGURE 6–19 **Ankylosing spondylitis with hip disease.** An AP view of the pelvis in this patient with ankylosing spondylitis shows bilateral complete fusion of the SI joints. Concentric left hip joint narrowing is present with axial migration of the femoral head. The hip changes would be typical findings in rheumatoid arthritis or, as in this example, ankylosing spondylitis. Note the secondary DJD changes in the hip as well.

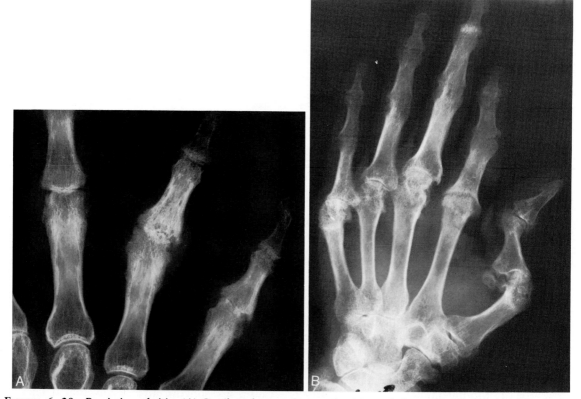

FIGURE 6–20 **Psoriatic arthritis.** *(A)* Cartilage loss at the proximal interphalangeal joints of the third, fourth, and fifth digits in this hand is apparent, with erosions noted most prominently in the third digit. These erosions are not sharply demarcated but are covered with fluffy new bone, which are termed proliferative erosions. Note also the periostitis along the shafts of each of the proximal phalanges. *(B)* Advanced psoriatic arthritis. Fusion or ankylosis is apparent across the proximal interphalangeal joints of the second through the fifth digits. Several of the distal interphalangeal joints are also ankylosed. Severe joint space narrowing at the metacarpophalangeal joints is noted. This distal arthritis is typical for psoriatic arthritis in advanced stages.

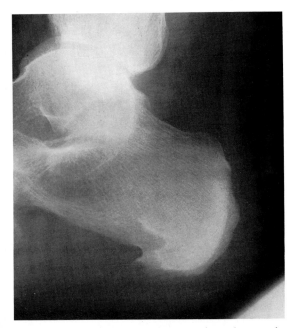

FIGURE 6–21 Reiter's syndrome. A lateral view of a calcaneus in a patient with Reiter's syndrome shows poorly defined new bone on the inferior margin of the calcaneus with a calcaneal spur that is also poorly defined. This is typical of psoriatic arthritis or Reiter's syndrome as opposed to the well-formed calcaneal spur in DJD.

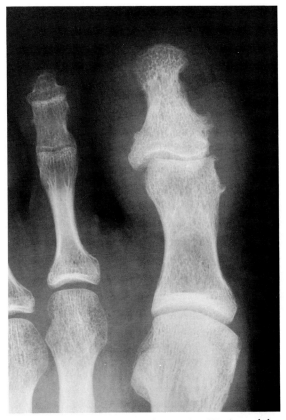

FIGURE 6–22 Reiter's syndrome. An AP view of the great toe in a patient with Reiter's syndrome shows fluffy periostitis in the erosions adjacent to the interphalangeal joint of the great toe. Marked soft tissue swelling is also present throughout the great toe. These changes are typical in appearance and location for Reiter's syndrome or psoriasis.

with bony ankylosis across joints (Fig. 6–20*B*) and mutilans deformities. A fairly common finding is a calcaneal heel spur that has fuzzy margins as opposed to the well-corticated heel spur seen in DJD or after trauma (Fig. 6–21).

Reiter's syndrome causes changes that are identical in every respect with those of psoriasis with the exception that the hands are not as commonly involved (Fig. 6–22). Therefore, I recommend storing the findings for psoriasis and Reiter's syndrome on a single neuron and saving the other for a phone number or something else.

CRYSTAL-INDUCED ARTHRITIS

The crystal-induced arthritides include gout and pseudogout (CPPD). Ochronosis and a few other arcane crystal deposition diseases are so rare that they don't deserve mention except to say that you will probably never see an example outside of a textbook or teaching file.

Gout

Gout is a metabolic disorder that results in hyperuricemia and leads to monosodium urate crystals being deposited in various sites in the body, especially joint cartilage. The actual causes

of the hyperuricemia are myriad, including inherited, and are not germane to this discussion.

The arthropathy caused by gout is very characteristic radiographically, yet it is seldom seen anymore. Why is that? Because it takes 4 to 6 years for gout to cause radiographically evident disease, and almost all patients are successfully treated long before the destructive arthropathy occurs.

The classic radiographic findings are well-defined erosions, often with sclerotic borders or overhanging edges; soft tissue nodules that calcify in the presence of renal failure; and a random distribution in the hands without marked osteoporosis (Fig. 6–23). I know of no other disorder that typically has erosions with sclerotic margins; therefore, this is a very specific finding for gout. It typically affects the metatarsophalangeal joint of the great toe (called podagra) (Fig. 6–24). In advanced stages it can be very deforming (Fig. 6–25). Patients with gout often have chondrocalcinosis because they have an increased chance

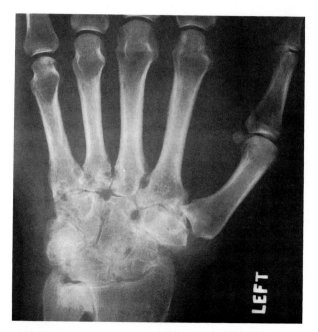

FIGURE 6–23 **Gout.** Sharply marginated erosions, some with a sclerotic margin, are noted throughout the carpus and proximal metacarpals. These erosions are classic in gout. Note the absence of marked demineralization.

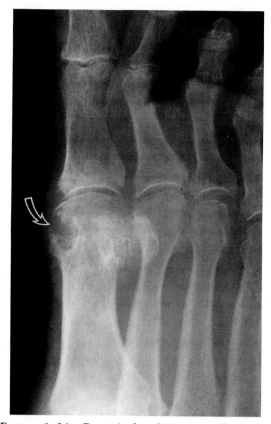

FIGURE 6–24 **Gout.** A sharply marginated erosion with an overhanging edge (arrow) is seen in the metatarsophalangeal joint in the great toe in this patient with gout. This appearance and location are classic for gout, whereas psoriasis and Reiter's syndrome usually involve the interphalangeal joint and do not have erosions that are this sharply marginated.

of having pseudogout (CPPD). Up to 40 per cent of the patients with gout concomitantly have CPPD.

It is worth repeating that patients must have clinically evident gout for years before changes will be apparent on a radiograph, and it is getting to be rare to find such a case. Also, even though erosions with overhanging edges can occur with gout, they can occur in other disorders as well and are by no means pathognomonic.

Pseudogout

CPPD crystal deposition disease causes much confusion among radiologists as well as other specialists. It is actually quite simple if you don't read all the conflicting literature. First, what do you call it? Is it pseudogout or CPPD? Who cares? Call it either, or both, or Fred. Many academicians say that it should be called pseudogout only when symptoms are present. Do we call lung cancer something else if the patient is asymptomatic? Of course not. For all practical purposes the terms pseudogout and CPPD are synonymous, and argument over the issue is academic balderdash.

CPPD has a classic triad: pain, cartilage calcification, and joint destruction. The patient may have any combination of one or more of this triad at any one time. Each of these signs and symptoms will be dealt with individually in some detail, but note that two of the three are radiographic findings. This disorder is best diagnosed radiographically.

The pain of CPPD is nonspecific. It can mimic that of gout (hence the term pseudogout) or infection or just about any arthritis. It typically is

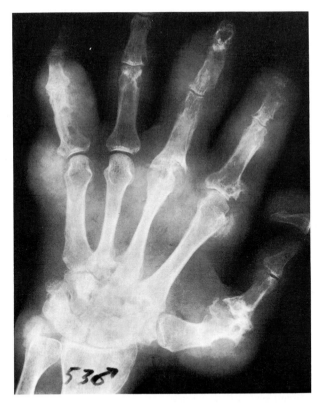

FIGURE 6–25 **Advanced gout.** Marked diffuse and focal soft-tissue swelling is present throughout the hand and wrist in this patient with long-standing gout. Destructive, large, well-marginated erosions, some with overhanging edges, are noted near multiple joints. The focal areas of soft tissue swelling are called tophi, some of which are calcified. These calcify only with coexistent renal disease.

intermittent over many years until DJD occurs and becomes the main cause of pain.

Cartilage calcification, known as chondrocalcinosis, can occur in any joint but tends to affect a few select sites in the overwhelming majority of patients. These are the medial and lateral compartments of the knee (Fig. 6–26), the triangular fibrocartilage of the wrist (Fig. 6–27), and the symphysis pubis. Chondrocalcinosis in these areas is virtually diagnostic of CPPD. When CPPD crystals occur in the soft tissues, such as in the rotator cuff of the shoulder, a radiograph cannot differentiate between CPPD and calcium hydroxyapatite, which occurs in calcific tendinitis. Some refer to the deposition of calcium hydroxyapatite (CHA) crystals in soft tissues as HAD— HydroxyApatite Deposition. It is by far the most commonly seen source of soft tissue calcification. HAD does not occur in the joint cartilage except in extremely rare cases; therefore, all chondrocalcinosis can be considered CPPD. This, for some reason, is confounding to many people. Many established academicians have a hard time accepting the fact that if chondrocalcinosis is present CPPD crystals are the only possible culprit. Monosodium urate crystals in gout are not radiographically visible. CHA does not occur in cartilage. In fact, no other radiographically visible crystal in cartilage has been described. It couldn't

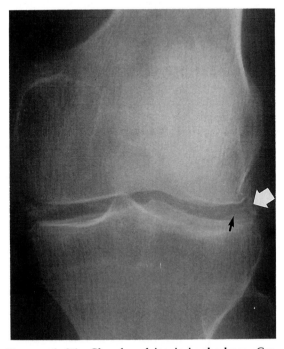

FIGURE 6–26 **Chondrocalcinosis in the knee.** Cartilage calcification, known as chondrocalcinosis, is seen in the fibrocartilage (large arrow) and in the hyaline articular cartilage (small arrow) in this patient with CPPD.

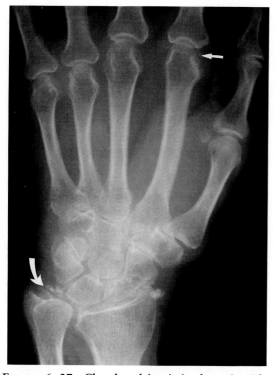

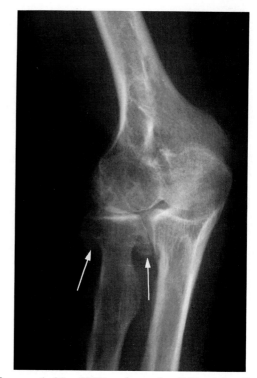

FIGURE 6–27 Chondrocalcinosis in the wrist. This patient with CPPD exhibits chondrocalcinosis in the triangular fibrocartilage of the wrist (curved arrow). A small amount of chondrocalcinosis is also seen in the second metacarpophalangeal joint (small arrow). Triangular fibrocartilage calcification is one of the more common locations for chondrocalcinosis to occur.

FIGURE 6–28 CPPD arthropathy. DJD of the elbow is seen in this patient with CPPD. Note the joint space narrowing with minimal sclerosis and the large osteophytes (arrows). Osteophytes of this nature are termed "drooping" osteophytes and are often seen in CPPD. The elbow is an unusual place for DJD to occur except in the setting of CPPD or trauma.

be simpler: chondrocalcinosis equals CPPD. So what's the fuss all about? Beats me.

The joint destruction or arthropathy of CPPD is virtually indistinguishable from that of DJD. In fact, it is DJD. It's caused by CPPD crystals eroding the cartilage. There are a few features of DJD caused by CPPD that will help to distinguish it from DJD caused by trauma or overuse. The main difference is one of location. CPPD has a proclivity for the shoulder, the elbow (Fig. 6–28), the radiocarpal joint in the wrist (Fig. 6–29), and the patellofemoral joint of the knee. These areas are not normally involved by DJD from wear and tear (such as the DIP joints of the hand, the hip, and the medial compartment of the knee). When DJD is seen in the joints that CPPD tends to involve, a search for chondrocalcinosis should be made. If necessary, a joint aspiration for CPPD crystals may be necessary to confirm the diagnosis.

Occasionally the arthropathy of CPPD accelerates, and severe destruction occurs to such an extent that a neuropathic or Charcot's joint is mimicked on the radiograph (Fig. 6–30). This has been termed a pseudo-Charcot's joint. It is not a true Charcot's joint because of the presence of sensation.

Three diseases have a high degree of association with CPPD. These are primary hyperparathyroidism, gout, and hemochromatosis. This is not a differential diagnosis for chondrocalcinosis. These diseases tend to occur at the same time that CPPD occurs. If the patient has one of these three disorders, he is more likely to have CPPD than is a normal person. There is probably no good reason to work up every patient with chondrocalcinosis for one of the three associated diseases, since they are so uncommon and CPPD is extremely common. Several texts list many other disorders that are supposedly associated with CPPD, such as acromegaly, diabetes, Wilson's disease, and hypophosphatasia, but the recent work in this field does not support this.

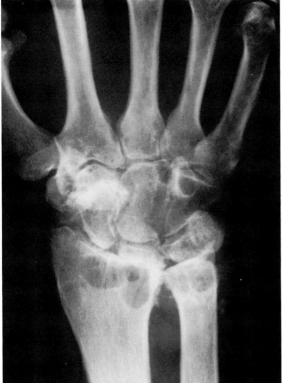

FIGURE 6–29 CPPD arthropathy. Marked DJD at the radiocarpal joint is seen in this patient with CPPD. Severe joint space narrowing and sclerosis with large subchondral cysts or geodes are hallmarks of DJD. This is an unusual location for DJD except in the setting of CPPD.

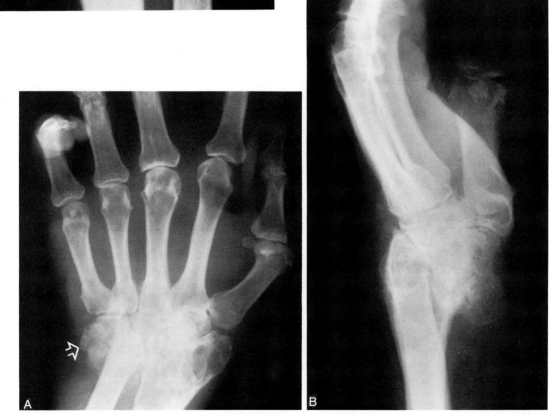

FIGURE 6–30 Pseudo-Charcot's joint in CPPD. This patient with CPPD shows severe joint destruction in the carpus primarily at the radiocarpal joint. Large subchondral cysts or geodes are noted (A). Heterotopic new bone or joint debris is also seen (arrow). (B) Dislocation of the radiocarpal joint is seen, with the entire carpus lying volarly in relation to the radius. The findings of severe joint destruction, heterotopic new bone, and dislocation are classic for a Charcot's joint. This patient, however, had sensation in this joint; therefore, it is not a true Charcot's or neuropathic joint but a pseudo-Charcot's joint, which is occasionally seen in CPPD.

COLLAGEN-VASCULAR DISEASES

Scleroderma, systemic lupus erythematosus (SLE), dermatomyositis, and mixed connective tissue disease are all grouped together as collagen-vascular diseases. The striking abnormalities in the hands in each of these disorders are osteoporosis and soft tissue wasting. SLE characteristically has severe ulnar deviation of the phalanges (Fig. 6–31). Erosions are generally not present in these diseases. Soft tissue calcifications are typically present in scleroderma (Fig. 6–32) and dermatomyositis. Mixed connective tissue disease is an overlap of scleroderma, SLE, polymyositis, and rheumatoid arthritis. Obviously it has a myriad of radiographic findings.

SARCOID

Sarcoidosis causes deposition of granulation tissue in the body, primarily in the lungs but also in the bones. In the skeletal system it has a predilection for the hands, where it causes lytic destructive lesions in the cortex. These often have a lace-like appearance (Fig. 6–33). Sarcoid can also affect the joints in the hand, causing DJD-like changes.

HEMOCHROMATOSIS

Twenty to 50 per cent of patients with hemochromatosis have a characteristic arthropathy in the hands that should suggest the diagnosis. Hemochromatosis is a disease of excess iron that gets deposited in tissues throughout the body, leading to fibrosis and eventual organ failure. The characteristic arthropathy classically involves the second through fourth metacarpophalangeal joints. The radiographic changes are essentially those of DJD (joint space narrowing, sclerosis, and osteophytes) (Fig. 6–34). Up to 50 per cent of the patients with hemochromatosis also have CPPD; therefore, when looking at the hands a search should be made for triangular fibrocartilage chondrocalcinosis. Another finding that is often seen in hemochromatosis is called "squaring" of the metacarpal heads. They appear enlarged and block-like as a result of the large osteophytes commonly seen in this disorder. In fact the osteophytes are often called "drooping" because of the unusual way they hang off the joint margin.

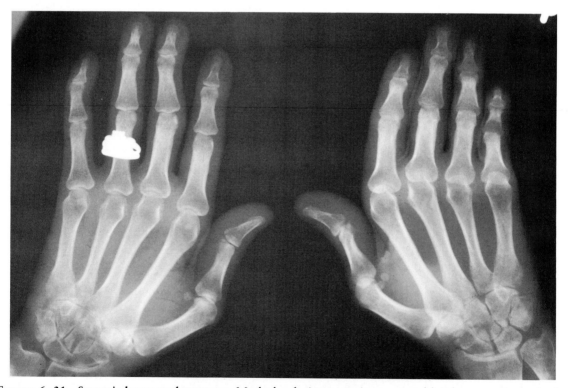

FIGURE 6–31 **Systemic lupus erythematosus.** Marked soft tissue wasting, as noted by the concavity in the hypothenar eminence, occurs with ulnar deviation of the phalanges and is seen primarily in the right hand in this patient. These are hallmarks of SLE.

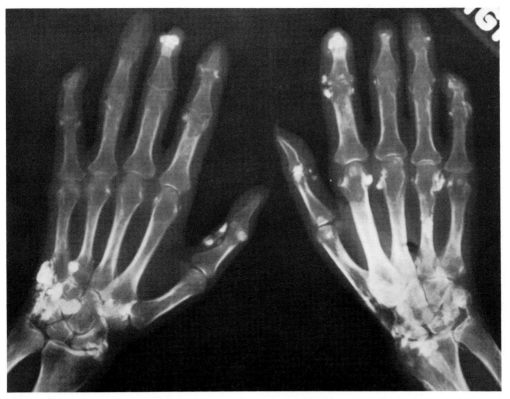

FIGURE 6–32 Scleroderma. Diffuse subcutaneous soft tissue calcification is seen throughout the hands and wrist in this patient with scleroderma. Soft tissue wasting and osteoporosis are also present as well as bone loss in multiple distal phalanges secondary to the vascular abnormalities often present in this disease.

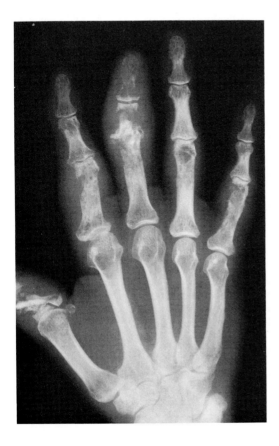

FIGURE 6–33 Sarcoid. An AP view of the hand in this patient with sarcoid demonstrates classic changes of bony involvement with this granulomatous process. Note the lace-like pattern of destruction seen most prominently in the proximal phalanges and the distal third phalanx. Soft tissue swelling and some areas of severe bony dissolution are also noted, which occur in more advanced patterns of sarcoid. These changes are typically limited to the hands but can rarely occur in other parts of the skeleton.

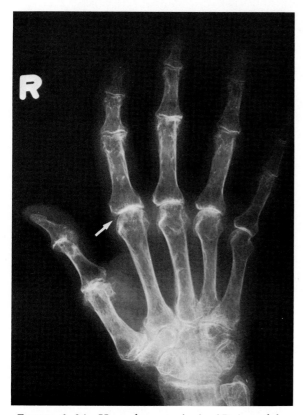

FIGURE 6–34 **Hemochromatosis.** An AP view of the hand in this patient with hemochromatosis shows severe joint space narrowing throughout the hand, which is most marked at the metacarpophalangeal joints. Associated sclerosis at the metacarpophalangeal joints with large osteophytes seen off the metacarpal heads suggests DJD. These are unusual joints for DJD to occur in, yet this is the classic appearance of hemochromatosis. No chondrocalcinosis is seen in the triangular cartilage in this patient; however, a small amount of chondrocalcinosis can be seen at the second metacarpophalangeal joint (arrow). Fifty percent of patients with hemochromatosis also have CPPD.

MULTICENTRIC RETICULOHISTIOCYTOSIS

MRH is a very rare disorder that probably has no place in a fundamentals book such as this. However, I have probably seen more cases of this disorder in the past 10 years than I have seen of gout. This disorder was termed lipoid dermatoarthritis up until a few years ago. It is a disorder of cutaneous xanthomas that are associated with a mutilating arthritis of the hands, which is very characteristic. Multiple erosions, predominantly in the phalanges, are found that are strikingly bilaterally symmetric and not associated with osteoporosis (Figs. 6–35 and 6–36). Rheumatoid

arthritis usually comes to mind because of the erosions and bilateral symmetry; however, the distal distribution and lack of osteoporosis are against rheumatoid. MRH can proceed to an arthritis mutilans, or spontaneously arrest.

NEUROPATHIC OR CHARCOT'S JOINT

The radiographic findings for a Charcot's joint are characteristic and almost pathognomonic. A classic triad has been described that consists of joint destruction, dislocation, and heterotopic new bone (Fig. 6–37). Multiple other findings have been described that do not seem to be as useful as the classic triad.

Joint destruction is seen in every arthritis encountered and, therefore, seems very nonspecific; however, nothing causes as severe destruction in a joint as a Charcot's joint. Early in the development of a Charcot's joint the joint destruction may merely appear to be joint space narrowing. It is extremely difficult to make the diagnosis this early. In the spine, instead of joint space destruction, there is disc space destruction (Fig. 6–38).

Dislocation, like joint destruction, can be present in varying degrees. Early on the joint may have subluxation instead of dislocation.

Heterotopic new bone has also been termed "debris" and consists of soft tissue calcification or clumps of ossification adjacent to the joint. It, too, can be present in varying amounts.

The most commonly seen Charcot's joint today is in the foot of a diabetic. It typically affects the first and second tarsometatarsal joints in a fashion termed a Lisfranc's fracture (Fig. 6–39). Lisfranc was Napoleon's surgeon, and he gained fame for saving the lives of soldiers with gangrenous toes from frostbite by doing a forefoot amputation at the tarsometatarsal junction.

Tabes dorsalis from syphilis is seldom seen today. I have only encountered one case of a Charcot's joint in syphilis in the past 10 years, and I've been around some pretty raunchy residents. More commonly seen is a Charcot's joint in a patient with paralysis who continues to use the affected limb for support. A Charcot's joint that is also seen on occasion is the so-called pseudo-Charcot's joint in CPPD (Fig. 6–30).

The shoulder can become a Charcot's joint in patients with syringomyelia, which has a so-called "atrophic Charcot" appearance. This refers to its tendency to have no debris or heterotopic new bone, and the proximal humerus has a tapered appearance likened to a licked candy stick.

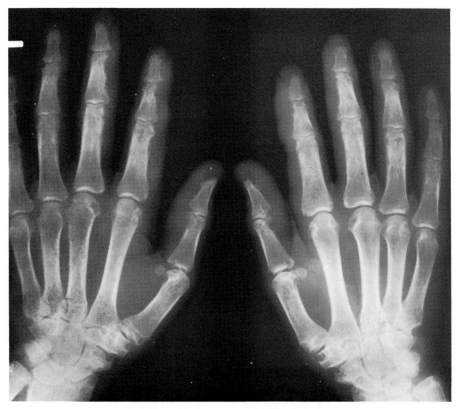

FIGURE 6–35 Multicentric reticulohistiocytosis. An AP view of the hand in this patient reveals multiple soft tissue nodules seen best in the second and third digits bilaterally with diffuse erosions that are sharply demarcated and strikingly bilaterally symmetric. There is little or no osteoporosis. These changes are classic for multicentric reticulohistiocytosis.

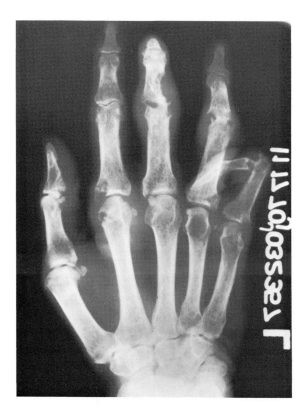

FIGURE 6–36 Multicentric reticulohistiocytosis. A markedly destructive erosive process that was bilaterally symmetric and associated with soft tissue nodules is seen, which is characteristic for multicentric reticulohistiocytosis. Note the sharply marginated erosions and the relative lack of osteoporosis.

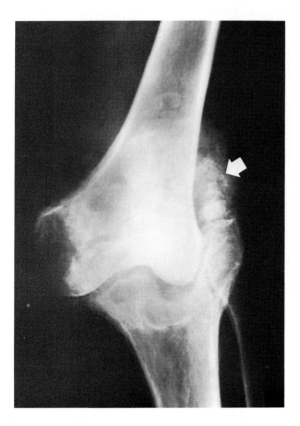

FIGURE 6–37 **Charcot's joint.** An AP view of the knee in this patient with tabes dorsalis shows the classic changes of a neuropathic or Charcot's joint. Note the severe joint destruction, the subluxation, and the heterotopic new bone (arrow).

←

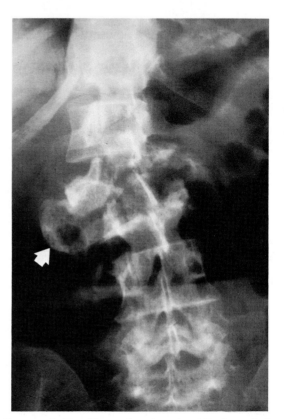

FIGURE 6–38 **Charcot's spine.** An AP view of the spine in this paraplegic shows severe destruction of the L-2 and L-3 vertebral bodies and the intervening disc space, heterotopic new bone (arrow), and malalignment or dislocation.

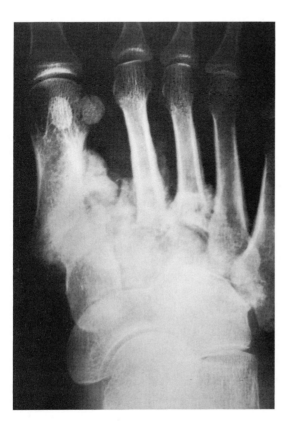

←

FIGURE 6–39 **Lisfranc Charcot's joint.** Dislocation of the second and third metatarsals along with joint destruction and large amounts of heterotopic new bone are present in the foot of this diabetic. These findings are classic for a Charcot's joint that has been termed a Lisfranc's fracture-dislocation. It is most commonly seen secondary to trauma rather than as a Charcot's joint but is the most common neuropathic joint seen today.

HEMOPHILIA, JUVENILE RHEUMATOID ARTHRITIS, AND PARALYSIS

Why would two clinically disparate entities like juvenile rheumatoid arthritis (JRA) and hemophilia be covered in the same section? Because this is a radiology book, and they are radiographically indistinguishable. As with several other processes covered in this book, you might as well store these two on a single neuron and save the other neuron for something important.

The classic findings for JRA and hemophilia are overgrowth of the ends of the bones (epiphyseal enlargement) associated with gracile diaphyses (Fig. 6–40). Joint destruction may or may not be present (Figs. 6–41 and 6–42). A finding that is purported to be classic for JRA and hemophilia is widening of the intercondylar notch of the knee. I find this sign variable and difficult to use. I have never seen it present when the other classic signs were not also present and obvious.

Another process that can mimic the findings in JRA and hemophilia is a joint that has undergone disuse from paralysis (Fig. 6–43). It has always been said that the reason the epiphyses are overgrown in JRA and hemophilia is because

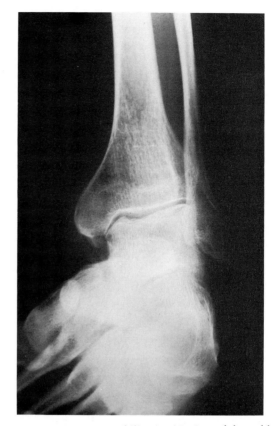

FIGURE 6–41 **Hemophilia.** An AP view of the ankle in this patient with hemophilia shows subtle changes of overgrowth of the distal tibia and fibula as compared with the diameter of the diaphyses. Some joint destruction of the tibiotalar joint is also noted.

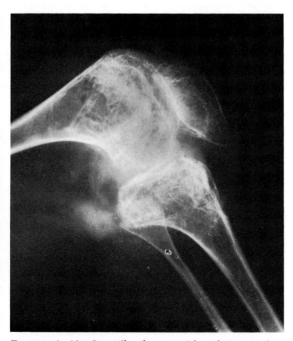

FIGURE 6–40 **Juvenile rheumatoid arthritis.** A lateral view of the knee in this patient with JRA shows the classic findings of overgrowth of the ends of the bones and associated gracile diaphyses. These changes can also be seen in hemophilia or paralysis patients.

of the hyperemia; however, a lot of other things cause hyperemia without affecting the size of the epiphyses. The thing that JRA, hemophilia, and paralysis have in common is disuse. I believe that this is what causes the overgrowth of the ends of the bones seen in all three disorders.

SYNOVIAL OSTEOCHONDROMATOSIS

Synovial osteochondromatosis, a relatively common disorder, is caused by a metaplasia of the synovium, resulting in the deposition of foci of cartilage in the joint. It is most commonly seen in the knee, hip, and elbow. Most of the time these cartilaginous deposits calcify and are readily seen on a radiograph (Figs. 6–44 and 6–45). Up to 30 per cent of the time the cartilaginous deposits do not calcify. In these cases all that is seen on the radiograph is a joint effusion unless erosions or joint destruction occur (Fig. 6–46).

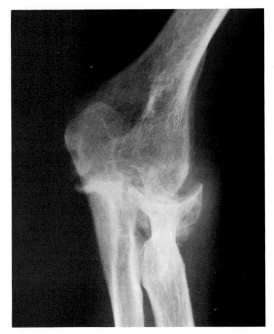

FIGURE 6–42 **Hemophilia.** An AP view of the elbow in this patient with hemophilia shows overgrowth of the ends of the bones, in particular the head of the radius, and marked joint destruction. JRA could certainly cause an appearance such as this.

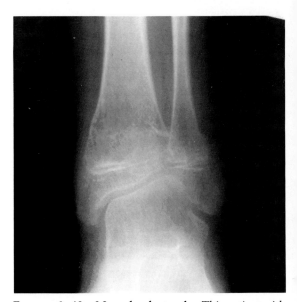

FIGURE 6–43 **Muscular dystrophy.** This patient with muscular dystrophy has changes similar to those of JRA and hemophilia, which consist of overgrowth of the ends of the bones and a tibio-talar slant. This appearance is frequently found in patients with paralysis.

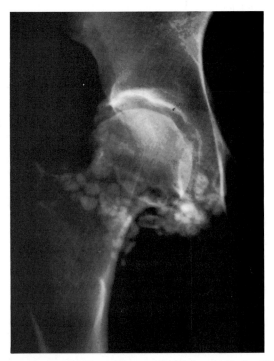

FIGURE 6–44 **Synovial osteochondromatosis.** An AP view of the hip in this patient with left hip pain shows multiple calcified loose bodies in the hip joint, which is virtually diagnostic of synovial osteochondromatosis.

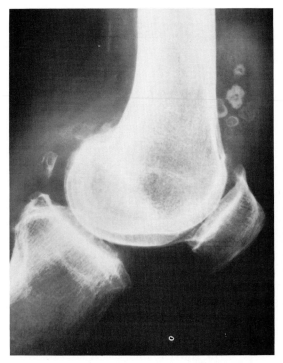

FIGURE 6–45 **Synovial osteochondromatosis.** Multiple calcified loose bodies are seen in the suprapatellar space of the knee in this patient, which is virtually diagnostic of synovial osteochondromatosis.

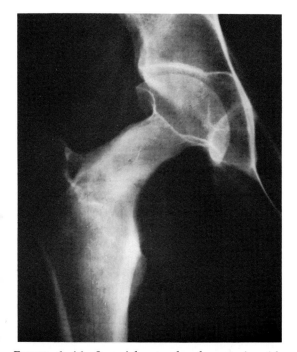

FIGURE 6–46 **Synovial osteochondromatosis without calcification.** An AP view of the hip in this patient shows the femoral neck to be virtually whittled down, with the femoral head undercut, giving an apple core appearance. This has occurred from the pressure erosion of multiple nonossified loose bodies in the joint. This is nonossified synovial osteochondromatosis, which is probably more properly termed synovial chondromatosis. It usually does not cause this degree of bony erosion and is indistinguishable from pigmented villonodular synovitis.

The calcifications begin in the synovium and then tend to shed into the joint, where they can cause symptoms of free fragments or "joint mice." They then embed into the synovium and tend not to be free in the joint after a while. It is usually necessary to perform a complete synovectomy to relieve the symptoms.

PIGMENTED VILLONODULAR SYNOVITIS

Pigmented villonodular synovitis (PVNS) is a chronic, inflammatory process of the synovium that causes synovial proliferation. A swollen joint with lobular masses of synovium occurs, which causes pain and joint destruction (Fig. 6–47). It seldom, if ever, calcifies. It has been termed giant cell tumor of tendon sheath and tendon sheath xanthoma when it occurs in a tendon sheath, which is not unusual. Overall, PVNS is rare, and most radiologists will encounter only a few cases in their careers. PVNS looks radiographically identical to noncalcified synovial osteochondro-

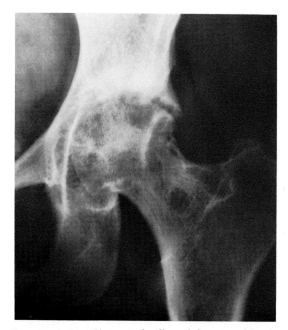

FIGURE 6–47 **Pigmented villonodular synovitis.** An AP view of the hip in this patient shows joint space destruction and bony erosions throughout the femoral head and neck. PVNS or synovial chondromatosis (nonossified) could have this appearance.

matosis, yet it is much less common. Therefore, whenever PVNS is a consideration, mention synovial osteochondromatosis (noncalcified).

SUDECK'S ATROPHY

Also known as shoulder-hand syndrome and reflex sympathetic dystrophy, Sudeck's atrophy is a poorly understood joint affliction that typically occurs after minor trauma to an extremity, resulting in pain, swelling, and dysfunction. Severe osteoporosis and swelling are seen radiographically (Fig. 6–48). The disorder typically affects the distal part of an extremity, such as a hand or foot, yet intermediate joints, such as the knee and hip, are thought by some to occasionally be involved. The pain usually subsides, but the osteoporosis may persist. The swelling, with time, will subside, and the skin may become atrophic. It is important for the radiologist to recognize the aggressive osteoporosis in this disorder so the treating physician can begin aggressive physical therapy.

JOINT EFFUSIONS

Radiology residents often go to great extremes to determine whether or not a joint—be it a knee, hip, shoulder, elbow, or whatever—has an effusion. There are some good signs of joint effu-

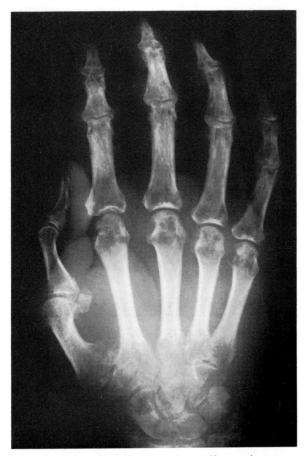

FIGURE 6–48 Sudeck's atrophy. Diffuse soft tissue swelling and marked osteoporosis that is so aggressive it has a spotty or permeative appearance around the joints is noted in this patient with severe hand pain and dysfunction after minor trauma. This is characteristic of Sudeck's atrophy.

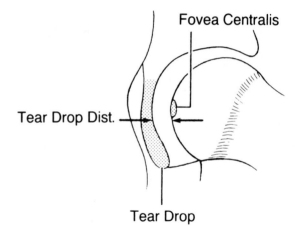

FIGURE 6–49 Drawing of the teardrop measurement. The teardrop measurement is the distance from the medialmost aspect of the femoral head to the nearest portion of the adjacent acetabulum (arrows). Widening of this distance as compared with the opposite hip is indicative of a joint effusion.

sions (which I will review), and there are some that are used that are invalid. The thing that amazes me is all the attention it gets because when all is said and done, in most cases, it doesn't make any difference whatsoever. With the exception of the elbow (see Chapter 5), and possibly the hip, treatment is never predicated on the radiographic finding of a joint effusion.

Most joint effusions are clinically obvious and do not require radiographic validation. As mentioned earlier, the elbow is an exception. In the setting of trauma to the elbow an effusion indicates a fracture. The radiographic signs of an elbow effusion are generally clearly seen and have proved to be valid. Clinical determination of an elbow effusion can be difficult; therefore, the radiologist can be very helpful in this area.

Clinical determination of a hip effusion is also difficult. The presence of a hip effusion can be valuable in certain clinical settings. For instance,

in a patient with pain in the hip and an effusion the joint should be aspirated to rule out an infection. If only pain were present, an aspiration would probably not be performed. The radiology literature mentions displacement of the fat stripes about the hip as being an indicator for an effusion, but this has been proved to be fallacious. The only fat pad around the hip that gets displaced with an effusion is the obturator internus, and it is seldom seen. The remainder of the fat pads are far removed from the joint capsule and are not directly influenced by the joint.

A radiographic sign in the hip that does work for indicating an effusion is called the teardrop sign. Leonard Swischuk first brought this sign to my attention by its application in pediatric patients. I have used it in adults as well with good results. The teardrop is an anatomic landmark at the medial aspect of the hip joint (Fig. 6–49) that is made up of several bony structures bounding the acetabulum medially. The teardrop measurement is the distance from the medialmost part of the femoral head to the medialmost extent of the acetabulum (which is the teardrop). This measurement—inappropriately called the teardrop measurement—should be equal in both hips. An effusion will push the femoral head laterally and give the affected side a wider teardrop distance (Fig. 6–50). The teardrop distance is a valid indicator of an effusion in children. It is valid in adults only when no long-standing joint abnormality, such as DJD or an old fracture, is present. A difference in the teardrop distance from one hip to the other of as little as 1 mm is significant in the appropriate clinical setting. It would be

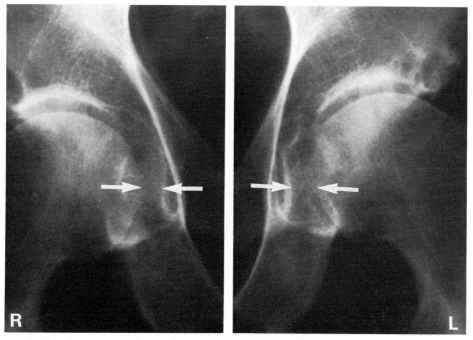

FIGURE 6–50 Widened teardrop. The teardrop distance in this patient on the left side (arrows) is slightly wider than that on the right side (arrows), which is indicative of a hip joint effusion. This patient had a hip joint infection on the left side.

FIGURE 6–51 Knee joint effusion. This patient has fat and fluid in his knee, with widely distended fat pads (arrows). The suprapatellar fat pad is bounded by a layer of fluid that has a fat-fluid level (small arrows). This film was taken with the beam directed laterally so as to demonstrate a fat-fluid level that might indicate a fracture. The anterior femoral fat pad can just barely be identified.

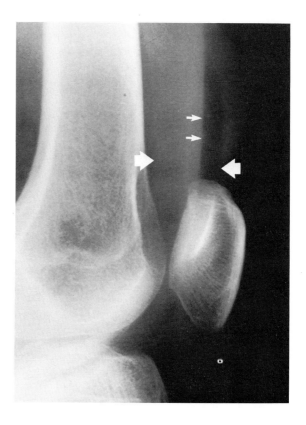

better to aspirate a few normal hips rather than risk missing a hip infection that might destroy the hip if diagnosed late.

The radiographic sign for a knee effusion that seems to be the most reliable is the measurement of the distance between the suprapatellar fat pad and the anterior femoral fat pad (Fig. 6–51). A distance between these two fat pads of more than 10 mm is definite evidence for an effusion. A distance of less than 5 mm is normal. A distance of 5 to 10 mm is no-man's-land. I usually call an effusion if the distance is greater than 5 mm, realizing that I'm probably overcalling a few. I am also aware that it doesn't make any difference if there is an effusion in the knee or not—the patient gets treated the same regardless. If it were vital to the patient, you could aspirate the joint or perform a magnetic resonance (MR) imaging study to find out. I should emphasize that we never do an MR exam just to see if there is fluid in the joint.

Shoulder effusions are difficult to detect unless they are massive enough to displace the humeral head inferiorly, as with a fracture and hemarthrosis (see Chapter 5). Fortunately, as with most other joints, treatment is not based on the presence or absence of an effusion, so it hardly matters. The same is true in the ankle, wrist, and smaller joints.

AVASCULAR NECROSIS

Avascular necrosis (AVN), or aseptic necrosis, can occur around almost any joint for a host of reasons, including steroids, trauma, various underlying disease states, and even idiopathically. It is often seen in renal transplant patients.

The hallmark of AVN is increased bone density at an otherwise normal joint. Increased density at a joint usually indicates DJD; however, if osteophytes and joint space narrowing are not present, another disorder should be considered.

The earliest sign of AVN is a joint effusion. This often is not radiographically visible or is so nonspecific as to not help with the diagnosis unless the clinical setting had already raised suspicion for AVN. The next sign for AVN is a patchy or mottled density (Fig. 6–52). In the knee this density increase can occur throughout an entire condyle, while in the hip it often involves the entire femoral head. Next, a subchondral lucency develops that forms a thin line along the articular surface (Fig. 6–53). This lucent line has been described as being an early indicator for AVN when in fact it is a late finding. Also, the lucent line stage is often not present in the evolution of AVN. Therefore, using the lucent line as one of the main criteria for AVN can lead to missing early findings or missing the diagnosis completely. I would estimate that I see a lucent line in only 20 per cent or fewer of the cases of AVN in our hospital.

The final sign in AVN is collapse of the articular surface and joint fragmentation (Fig. 6–54). I must stress that these changes all occur on only one side of a joint, which makes for an easy di-

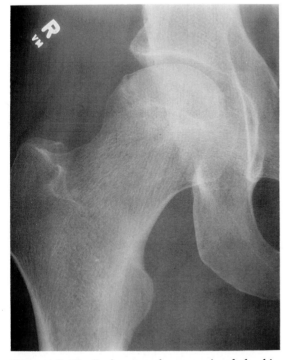

FIGURE 6–52 Early avascular necrosis of the hip. Patchy sclerosis is present throughout the femoral head in this patient with a renal transplant and avascular necrosis of the right hip. No subchondral lucency or articular surface irregularity in the weight-bearing region is yet present with the exception of a small cortical irregularity seen laterally.

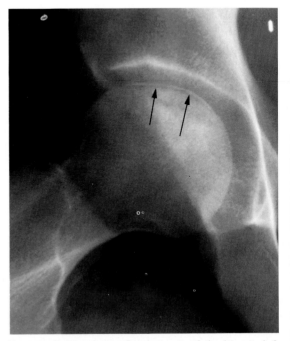

FIGURE 6–53 Avascular necrosis of the hip. A definite subchondral lucency (arrows) is seen in the weight-bearing portion of this hip with avascular necrosis. Patchy sclerosis throughout the femoral head is also noted.

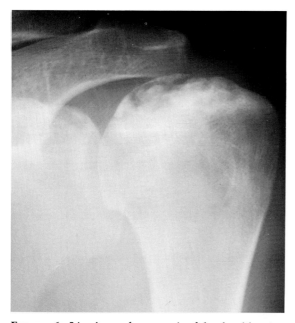

FIGURE 6–54 **Avascular necrosis of the shoulder.** Articular surface collapse is present in this shoulder with long-standing avascular necrosis. Dense bony sclerosis is also present.

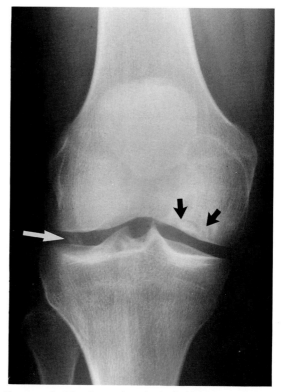

FIGURE 6–55 **Osteochondritis dissecans.** A small focal area of avascular necrosis in the medial condyle of the femur (arrows) is present, which is an area of osteochondritis dissecans. Part of the area of avascular necrosis has shed a bony fragment (large arrow) that is loose in the joint and known as a joint mouse.

agnosis, since almost everything else around joints involves both sides.

MR imaging plays a valuable role in the early diagnosis of AVN throughout the skeletal system but especially in the hip where it is more sensitive than even radionuclide scans. The use of MR imaging in AVN of the hip is discussed more fully in Chapter 13: MR Imaging: Miscellaneous Uses.

A form of AVN that is smaller and more focal than that just described is osteochondritis dissecans. It is thought to be due to trauma, although many believe that it is primarily idiopathic. It is most commonly found in the knee at the medial femoral condyle (Fig. 6–55) but also is seen frequently in the dome of the talus (Fig. 6–56) and occasionally in the capitellum (Fig. 6–57). Osteochondritis dissecans often leads to a small fragment of bone being sloughed off and becoming a free fragment in the joint—a "joint mouse" (Fig. 6–55).

→

FIGURE 6–56 **Osteochondritis dissecans of the talus.** A focal area of avascular necrosis in the talus as seen here (arrows) is called osteochondritis dissecans. The talus is the second most common site after the knee and, as in the knee, can cause a joint mouse or loose body in the joint.

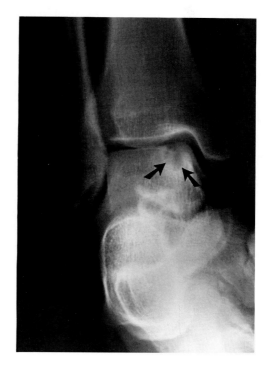

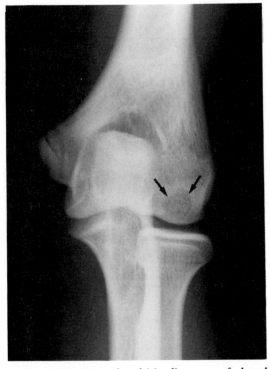

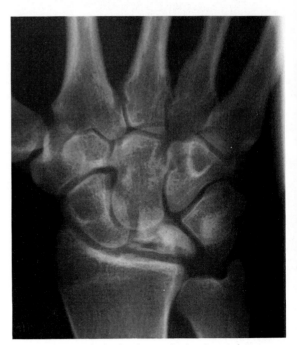

FIGURE 6–57 Osteochondritis dissecans of the elbow. The third most common site for osteochondritis dissecans is in the capitellum of the elbow. The faint lucency seen in this capitellum (arrows) was at first felt to be a chondroblastoma or an area of infection.

FIGURE 6–59 Kienböck's malacia. Avascular necrosis of the lunate, or Kienböck's malacia, is demonstrated in this patient. Note the increased density and partial fragmentation of the lunate.

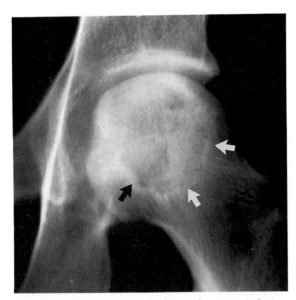

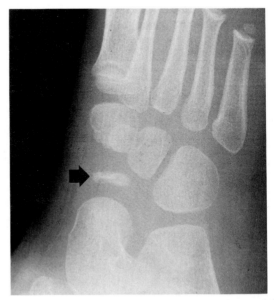

FIGURE 6–58 Geode in the hip. A large cystic lesion (arrows) is seen in this patient with avascular necrosis of the hip. Note the adjacent patchy sclerosis indicative of avascular necrosis. A subchondral cyst or geode should be considered any time a lytic lesion is found around a joint.

FIGURE 6–60 Köhler's bone disease. Flattening and sclerosis of the tarsal navicular (arrow) in children is thought by many to be avascular necrosis and is called Köhler's bone disease. Others have found this to be an asymptomatic normal variant and believe that it is an incidental finding.

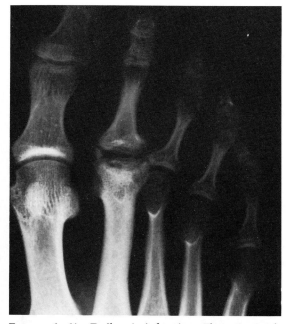

FIGURE 6–61 Freiberg's infraction. Flattening, collapse, and sclerosis of the second metatarsal head, as seen in this patient, is typical of avascular necrosis or Freiberg's infraction. It can also involve the third or fourth metatarsal heads. Note the compensatory hypertrophy of the cortex of the second metatarsal, which is invariably found with this disorder.

AVN is one of the disorders around joints in which subchondral cysts or "geodes" can occur. It is the only one of the four disorders (rheumatoid arthritis, DJD, and CPPD being the others) that can have an essentially normal joint and have a geode (Fig. 6–58). The other abnormalities will have joint space narrowing and/or osteophytes, osteoporosis, chondrocalcinosis, or other findings.

A host of names have been ascribed to epiphyseal AVN, usually with the eponym being the first person to describe the disorder. These are thought to be idiopathic for the most part but can also occur secondary to trauma. A few of the more common bones involved are the following: the carpal lunate—Kienböck's malacia (Fig. 6–59); the tarsal navicular—Köhler's bone disease (Fig. 6–60); the metatarsal heads—Freiberg's infraction (Fig. 6–61); the femoral head—Legg-Perthes; the ring apophyses of the spine—

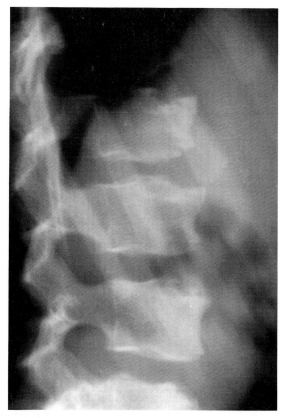

FIGURE 6–62 Scheuermann's disease. Avascular necrosis of the apophyseal rings of the vertebral bodies is called Scheuermann's disease. He originally described a painful kyphosis with multiple vertebral bodies involved. It is most commonly seen without kyphosis or pain and with only a few vertebral bodies involved.

Scheuermann's disease (Fig. 6–62); and the tibial tubercle—Osgood-Schlatter disease, also called surfer's knees.

REFERENCES

1. Forrester DM, Brown JC: The Radiology of Joint Disease, ed 3. Philadelphia, WB Saunders Co., 1987.
2. Brower AC: Arthritis in Black and White. Philadelphia, WB Saunders Co., 1988.
3. Resnick D: Diagnosis of Bone and Joint Disorders, ed 3. Philadelphia, WB Saunders Co., 1995.

Chapter

7

Metabolic Bone Disease

Most of the literature on metabolic bone disease is steeped in biochemistry, physiology, histology, internal medicine, and other arcane pursuits that can be quite confusing for a poor radiology resident who just wants a few pearls and illustrations. Frankly, it's a tough topic. I will, by necessity, keep it simple; but this is an important topic about which every radiologist should have at least a superficial fund of knowledge. I have excluded disorders such as pseudo- and pseudo-pseudo hypoparathyroidism that are unlikely to be seen and have tried to cover the more commonly seen disorders.

OSTEOPOROSIS

Osteoporosis is diminished bone quantity in which the bone is otherwise normal. This contrasts with osteomalacia, in which the bone quantity is normal but the bone itself is abnormal in that it is not normally mineralized. Osteomalacia results in excess nonmineralized osteoid. It is not possible in the vast majority of cases to distinguish between osteoporosis and osteomalacia on plain films.

The causes of osteoporosis are myriad, the most common of which is senile osteoporosis, or osteoporosis of aging. This is seen most commonly in postmenopausal females and is a major public health concern because of the increase of spinal and hip fractures in this patient population. Another name for this type of osteoporosis is primary osteoporosis.

Secondary osteoporosis implies that an underlying disorder, such as thyrotoxicosis or renal disease, has caused the osteoporosis. Only about 5 per cent of osteoporosis has an underlying cause. The differential diagnosis for secondary osteoporosis is quite long and probably should not be memorized, as one cannot even be sure if it is osteoporosis or osteomalacia based on the plain films. Therefore, the differential for presumed osteoporosis would have to include the causes of osteomalacia. The list gets too long to be of any real help to anyone.

The main radiographic finding in osteoporosis is thinning of the cortex. This is best demonstrated in the second metacarpal at the middiaphysis (Figs. 7–1 and 7–2). The normal metacarpal cortical thickening should be approximately one fourth to one third the thickness of the metacarpal (Fig. 7–3). In osteoporosis this cortical thickness is decreased. The metacarpal cortex (and all bony cortices, for that matter) decreases normally with age and is less for women than for men of the same age. Several tables have been published that give the normal metacarpal cortical measurement, with age and sex adjustments to allow determination of normal. Unfortunately these tables only determine the mineralization of the peripheral skeleton and do not seem to correlate to whether or not spinal or hip fractures will occur.

Measurement of the axial bone mineral content can be done by one of several methods that use computed tomography (CT) to assess the bone quantity in the spine. There is much debate over which method is superior and even whether or not knowing the bone mineral content is clinically helpful, since just knowing the age and sex of the patient is fairly accurate for predicting the bone mass quantity. Most agree that knowing the

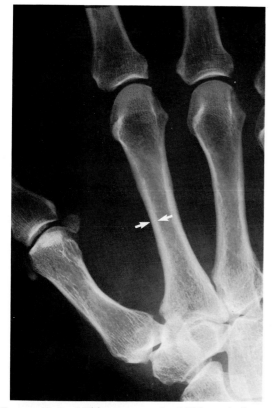

FIGURE 7–1 Mild osteoporosis. Mild cortical narrowing (arrows) at the mid-second metacarpal is noted in this patient with renal osteodystrophy. Note the calcification around the first metacarpophalangeal joint. Compare this cortical width with that of the normal width in Figure 7–3.

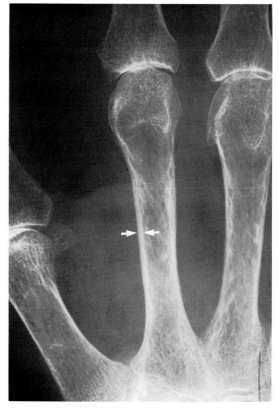

FIGURE 7–2 Marked osteoporosis. Marked cortical narrowing (arrows) of the mid-second metacarpal cortex is present in this patient with severe osteoporosis. Also note the intracortical tunneling, which occurs with more rapid forms of osteoporosis.

FIGURE 7–3 Normal mineralization. Note the cortical width (arrows) of the mid-second metacarpal in this patient with normal mineralization. The width of the cortex is easily greater than one third of the total width of the metacarpal.

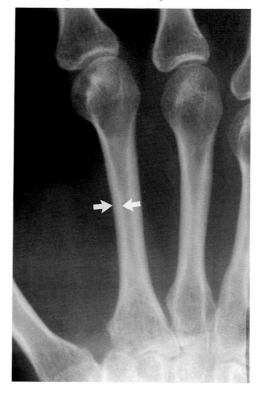

axial bone mineral measurement does not help to predict which patients are at risk for spinal and hip fractures.

Exercise and proper diet (whatever that is) seem to help delay the onset of primary osteoporosis as much as anything. Calcium additives have not been shown to reverse the process of primary osteoporosis. Estrogen therapy has been found to be beneficial in delaying primary osteoporosis but is controversial in regards to its side effects. If it is inevitable and cannot be treated in most cases, why go to a huge expense to diagnose it? That's one of the reasons this is a controversial topic.[1]

Because we cannot accurately give the causes of osteoporosis by looking at a radiograph and cannot even differentiate it from osteomalacia, it is a topic that is frustrating for many radiologists to deal with. Most of us would rather comment on something we can give a diagnosis on or at least a short differential. In general, when decreased bone mass is present on a radiograph the odds are that osteoporosis is present. However, because the disease process could just as easily be osteomalacia it is recommended that the term "osteopenia" be used. This is a generic term that includes both osteoporosis and osteomalacia. When used it also implies that the observer knows he cannot separate the two entities and is an educated person. It is radiographically correct but perhaps a bit pretentious.

A type of osteoporosis that can be seen in a patient of any age is disuse osteoporosis. It results from immobilization from any cause, most commonly after treatment of a fracture. The radiographic appearance of disuse osteoporosis is different from senile osteoporosis in that it occurs somewhat more rapidly and gives the bone a patchy or even a permeative appearance (Fig. 7–4). This is from the osteocytic resorption in the cortex, causing intracortical holes. If allowed to continue with disuse, the bone would resemble any bone with marked osteoporosis (i.e., severe cortical thinning).

Occasionally aggressive osteoporosis from disuse can mimic a permeative lesion, such as a Ewing's sarcoma or multiple myeloma, because of the severe cortical patchy or permeative pattern that projects over the medullary space and resembles a medullary permeative process (Fig. 7–5). The way to differentiate a true intramedullary permeative process from an intracortical process such as osteoporosis is to observe the cortex and see if it is solid or riddled with holes (Fig. 7–6). If it is solid, you can assume the permeative process is emanating from the medullary space (Fig. 7–7); if it has multiple small holes, you have to assume the permeative pattern is from the cortical process. I call a permeative appearance that is secondary to cortical holes a

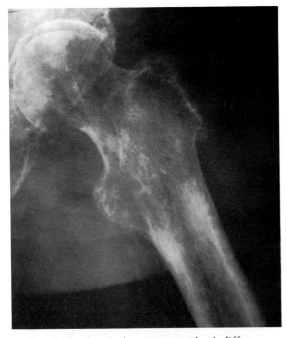

FIGURE 7–4 **Aggressive osteoporosis.** A diffuse permeative pattern throughout the proximal femur is noted in this patient, who has recently had an amputation. Note that the cortices are riddled with holes, which would indicate that this is not a true intramedullary process but an intracortical process. This is distinctive for aggressive osteoporosis and causes a pseudopermeative pattern that can be mistaken for a more sinister process.

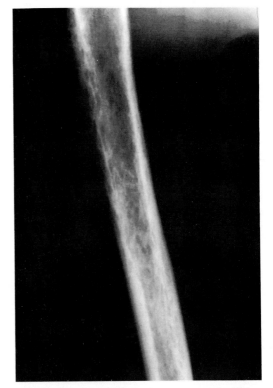

FIGURE 7–5 **Cortical holes in osteoporosis.** This patient suffered a stroke and has aggressive osteoporosis secondary to disuse. What appears to be a diffuse permeative pattern throughout the humerus is noted, on closer inspection, to be cortical holes, which in this case are due to the aggressive osteoporosis. This type of pattern, unfortunately, often leads to a biopsy to rule out multiple myeloma or other round cell tumors.

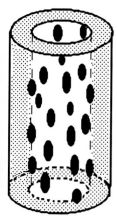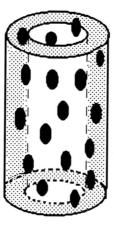

A) <u>PERMEATIVE</u>   B) <u>PSEUDOPERMEATIVE</u>

FIGURE 7–6 **Schematic of cortical holes.** This schematic of a permeative lesion *(A)* shows how only the endosteum is affected with the bulk of the cortex spared. A pseudopermeative lesion *(B)* has the entire cortex affected. Both processes will look permeative on a plain film; however, the true permeative process will have an uninvolved cortex.

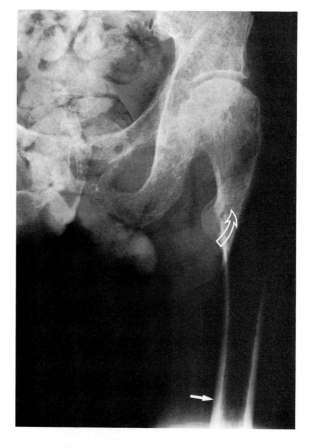

FIGURE 7–7 **Pathologic fracture in multiple myeloma.** This patient has multiple myeloma, which has caused a diffuse permeative pattern throughout his pelvis. He suffered an intertrochanteric fracture of his left hip (curved arrow), which was believed to be due either to the osteoporosis present or to the infiltration of myeloma in this region. If myeloma were the cause of the fracture, radiation treatment before pinning was being considered. If, however, the fracture were due to osteoporosis, radiation would not be given. A close look at the cortex in the proximal third of the femur (straight arrow) showed that it is not riddled with holes as it would be with osteoporosis; therefore, this was believed to be a pathologic fracture in an area of myelomatous involvement. Surgery confirmed this.

pseudopermeative process to distinguish it from a true permeative process.

Another cause for a pseudopermeative process is a hemangioma. It can cause cortical holes in two ways: from focal increased blood flow or hyperemia, causing focal osteoporosis, or by the blood vessels themselves tunneling through the cortex (Figs. 7–8 and 7–9). I have seen more than one hemangioma operated on inadvertently because the lesion was thought to be a Ewing's sarcoma—they bleed a lot.

Radiotherapy can cause cortical holes in bone and mimic a permeative pattern (Fig. 7–10). These holes are often large and would not be

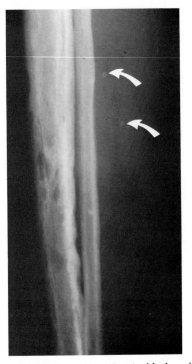

FIGURE 7–8 **Hemangioma.** Cortical holes of varying sizes are seen throughout the tibia in this patient with a large hemangioma of the tibia. Also note the phleboliths present in the soft tissues (arrows). It would be unlikely for osteoporosis to cause cortical holes of this size.

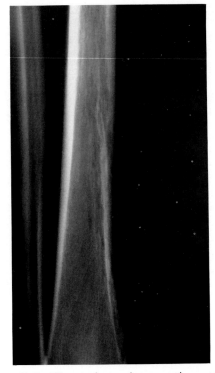

FIGURE 7–9 **Hemangioma.** A permeative pattern in the distal tibia was seen in this child with pain and an associated soft tissue mass. It was presumed to be a Ewing's sarcoma, and a biopsy was done with great loss of blood. A close examination of the cortex shows that the medial aspect is diffusely riddled with cortical holes, as compared with the lateral aspect. Although a Ewing's sarcoma could perhaps do this, one would expect diffuse periostitis with cortical involvement of this extent.

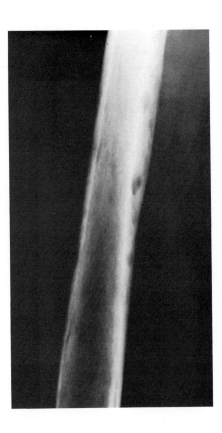

FIGURE 7–10 **Osteonecrosis secondary to radiation.** Radiation to the femur for a soft tissue sarcoma some years before this plain film has caused large cortical holes throughout the femur. It is not likely that cortical holes of this size would be caused by osteoporosis, but they could be caused by a hemangioma.

confused with a true permeative process, but they can be small and cause confusion.

If a permeative pattern is seen in bone, the differential is usually an aggressive process such as Ewing's sarcoma, infection, or eosinophilic granuloma in a young person or multiple myeloma, metastatic carcinomatosis, or primary lymphoma of bone in an older patient. If, however, the permeative pattern is seen to be a result of cortical holes (i.e., a pseudopermeative pattern), the differential is considerably kinder: aggressive osteoporosis, hemangioma, or radiation changes. This differential does not arise often but is very useful when it does come up.[2]

OSTEOMALACIA

As mentioned earlier, osteomalacia is the result of too much nonmineralized osteoid. There are many causes for osteomalacia, with the most common today being renal osteodystrophy. The radiographic findings are almost identical to those of osteoporosis, and for the most part the two disorders are indistinguishable. The only findings that are distinctive for osteomalacia are Looser's fractures, which are fractures through large osteoid seams (Fig. 7–11). They are extremely uncommon but tend to occur in the pelvis and scapula.

In children, osteomalacia is called rickets. It causes the epiphyses to become flared and irregular, and the long bones undergo bending from the bone softening (Fig. 7–12). As in adults, the most common cause is renal disease, although other causes, such as biliary disease and dietary insufficiencies, are seen.

HYPERPARATHYROIDISM

Hyperparathyroidism (HPT) occurs from excess parathyroid hormone (PTH). PTH causes osteoclastic resorption in bone, which leads to osteoporosis and osteomalacia. The most common cause is renal disease, which leads to secondary HPT. Secondary HPT is due to the response of the parathyroids to hypocalcemia. Parathyroid adenomas and hyperplasia can cause primary HPT. Up to 40 per cent of patients with primary HPT will demonstrate skeletal abnormalities radiographically.

The radiographic sign that is pathognomonic for HPT is subperiosteal bone resorption. It is seen most commonly on the radial aspect of the

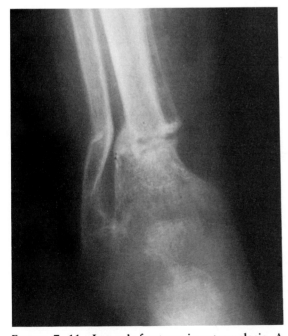

FIGURE 7–11 **Looser's fractures in osteomalacia.** A horizontal fracture of the tibia and the fibula is present in this child with osteomalacia (rickets). Fractures of this type are called Looser's fractures and are virtually pathognomonic for osteomalacia; however, they are rarely seen.

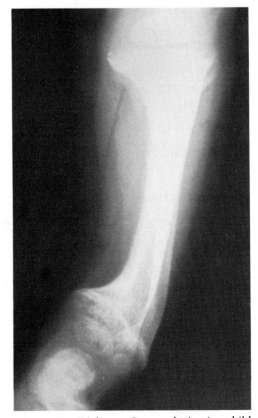

FIGURE 7–12 **Rickets.** Osteomalacia in children causes fraying and splaying of the epiphyses as well as bending of the bone secondary to bone softening. This condition has been termed rickets and is most commonly seen in renal disease.

middle phalanges of the hand (Fig. 7–13) but can be seen in any long bone in the body. It is commonly seen on the medial aspect of the proximal tibia (Fig. 7–14), in the distal clavicles, and in the sacroiliac (SI) joints where it resembles bilateral sacroiliitis (Fig. 7–15).

Other radiographic findings include osteosclerosis, usually diffuse, but often involving the spine in a manner resembling the stripes on rugby jerseys, hence the name "rugger jersey spine"

(Fig. 7–16). Brown tumors are cystic lesions that are often expansile and aggressive in appearance (Fig. 7–17). They were once said to be more common in primary HPT but are seen most commonly associated with secondary HPT today because of the overwhelming preponderance of patients with secondary disease as compared with primary. They are only rarely seen without other evidence of HPT, such as subperiosteal resorption; therefore, I will not include a brown tumor

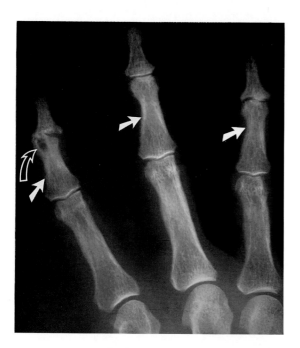

FIGURE 7–13 Hyperparathyroidism. Subperiosteal bone resorption is noted along the radial aspect of the middle phalanges (arrows), which is pathognomonic for hyperparathyroidism. The lytic lesion seen in the distal part of the middle phalanx (curved arrow) may represent a brown tumor or a geode.

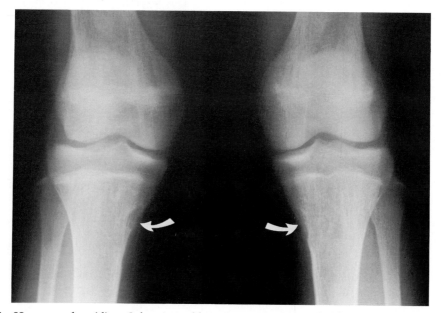

FIGURE 7–14 Hyperparathyroidism. Subperiosteal bone resorption is noted along the medial aspect of the proximal tibias (arrows), which is a characteristic location. This is pathognomonic for hyperparathyroidism.

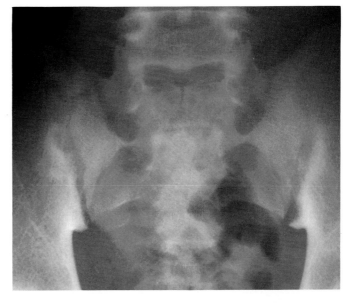

FIGURE 7–15 Hyperparathyroidism with SI joint subperiosteal erosion. Bilateral SI joint widening and erosions can be seen in this patient with renal disease. This is due to subperiosteal resorption and is a frequent finding in children with hyperparathyroidism.

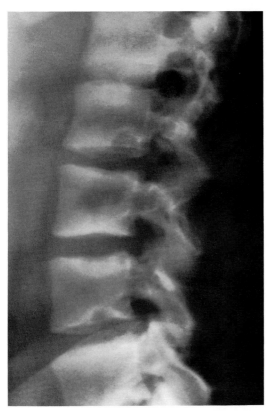

FIGURE 7–16 Hyperparathyroidism. Sclerotic bands are seen along the vertebral body end-plates. This has been termed a "rugger jersey spine" and is characteristic for hyperparathyroidism. Note how the sclerotic bands in the rugger jersey spine such as this are much less distinct than the sclerotic bands seen in osteopetrosis in Figure 7–23.

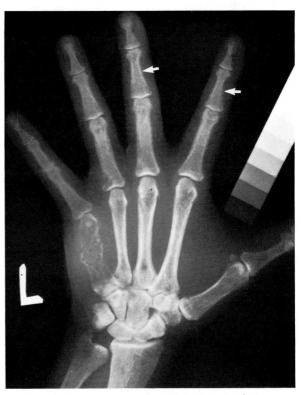

FIGURE 7–17 Hyperparathyroidism. Lytic lesions are seen in the fifth metacarpal and at the base of the fourth proximal phalanx in this patient with hyperparathyroidism. Note the subperiosteal bone resorption seen along the radial aspect of the middle phalanges (arrows). Any cystic lesion in a patient with hyperparathyroidism must be considered a brown tumor until proved otherwise.

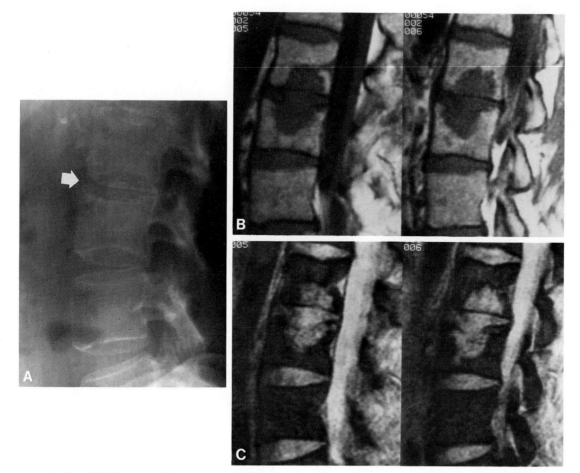

FIGURE 7–18   PTH discitis. *(A)* A lateral plain film of the lumbar spine reveals disc space narrowing with erosion of the end-plates at the L2-3 level (arrow). This is a typical appearance of disc infection. *(B)* A sagittal T1-weighted image of the lumbar spine reveals disc space narrowing and low signal extending into the end-plates and vertebral bodies adjacent to the L2-3 disc. *(C)* A T2-weighted image shows high signal in the L2-3 disc and in the tissue extending into the vertebral bodies. This is the classic magnetic resonance imaging appearance of disc infection with involvement of the vertebral bodies. However, this patient has renal osteodystrophy, and hyperparathyroidism can cause changes in the joints and the disc spaces identical to infection. Clinical correlation must be used to avoid an unnecessary biopsy.

in my differential diagnosis of a cystic lesion if the remainder of the bones are normal. A brown tumor can have a variety of appearances, so the only thing characteristic about it is that it is associated with subperiosteal bone resorption.

PTH can have an accelerating effect on bone which is undergoing slow change. In DJD, especially in the spine, PTH can cause the affected joint or disc space to mimic infection (Fig. 7–18). PTH makes the usually sclerotic end-plates fuzzy and eroded, and the narrowed disc space, which is a part of the degenerative disc disease, makes infection seem more likely. Therefore, patients with renal disease who have a presumed radiographic diagnosis of joint or disc space infection should not have an aspiration or biopsy unless strong clinical suspicion for infection is present.

How often is HPT present without subperiosteal resorption also being present? Not often, but it undoubtedly occurs. I am willing to miss all the cases of HPT that do not have associated subperiosteal resorption.

What causes the osteosclerosis in HPT? No one really knows. Several theories have evolved to explain it, but none are totally satisfactory and are best left to others to worry about.

OSTEOSCLEROSIS

The radiographic finding of diffuse increased bone density, osteosclerosis, is somewhat uncommon, yet every radiologist must have a differential diagnosis for this process. Fortunately it is a rather short differential, and there are criteria to narrow down the list of possibilities.

Dealing with the differential diagnosis for osteosclerosis is a three-step process. First, one must recognize that the bones are truly increased in density. This sounds straightforward enough but is, in fact, often difficult to do. Technical factors can easily alter the apparent bone density and be misleading. Second, once it is determined that diffuse osteosclerosis is present, one merely has to list the disease entities that could be responsible. This is the easiest step because it merely requires memorization. I will supply a mnemonic to help your memory. Lastly, one must look for radiographic findings that are specific for each disorder to rule them out or in so as to narrow down the list of possibilities. The list of diseases that cause diffuse osteosclerosis is different with each textbook that you read. There are many disorders that have been reported to cause osteosclerosis, but you only need a list that is correct 95 to 98 per cent of the time. Nobody expects you to include the one reported case of hunchback midget whale syndrome in your list. If you absolutely cannot bear the thought of leaving out a possibility in your differential diagnosis, you might as well just give your clinician the index from Resnick's book—it will be all-inclusive but not really useful to the clinician.

The entities I include in the differential for diffuse osteosclerosis are the following:

- renal osteodystrophy
- sickle cell disease
- myelofibrosis
- osteopetrosis
- pyknodysostosis
- metastatic carcinoma
- mastocytosis
- Paget's disease
- athletes
- fluorosis

The mnemonic I use to remember them is "Regular sex makes occasional perversions much more pleasurable and fantastic." Hey, it's not a great mnemonic, but in the 1990s it's not politically correct to be ribald, vulgar, off-color, coarse, crude, erotic, lewd, or even, sometimes, funny. If you want a filthy mnemonic, make up your own, you insensitive pervert.

I will cover each of these topics in generalities, trying to point out the features of each that you should look for to allow including or excluding them from the differential.

Renal Osteodystrophy. Anything that causes HPT can cause osteosclerosis, but renal disease is far and away the biggest offender. As mentioned previously, the *sine qua non* of renal osteodystrophy is subperiosteal bone resorption, seen earliest and most reliably at the radial aspect of the middle phalanges of the hands. Without this finding I will not entertain osteosclerosis being caused by renal disease. About 10 to 20 per cent of the patients with renal osteodystrophy will exhibit osteosclerosis, and the reasons for it are unknown.

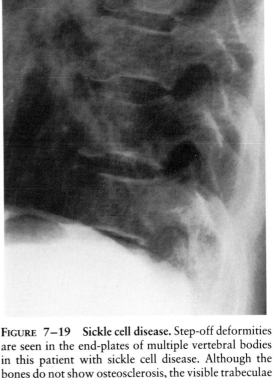

FIGURE 7–19 **Sickle cell disease.** Step-off deformities are seen in the end-plates of multiple vertebral bodies in this patient with sickle cell disease. Although the bones do not show osteosclerosis, the visible trabeculae are somewhat coarsened. The step-off deformities in the spine are characteristic for sickle cell disease. These are also called "fish vertebrae."

Sickle Cell Disease. Like renal osteodystrophy, the reason for dense bones to occur in sickle cell disease is unknown. It occurs in only a small percentage of patients. Additional signs to look for are bone infarcts and "H"-shaped or step-off deformities of the vertebral body end-plates (Fig. 7–19). These are also called "fish vertebrae" after their similarity to the vertebrae found in fish.

Myelofibrosis. Also called agnogenic myeloid metaplasia, myelofibrosis is a disease caused by progressive fibrosis of the marrow in patients over 50 years of age. It leads to anemia with splenomegaly and extramedullary hematopoiesis. Whenever osteosclerosis is seen in a patient over the age of 50, a search for a large spleen and extramedullary hematopoiesis should be made (Fig. 7–20).

Osteopetrosis. This rare hereditary abnormality results in extremely dense bones throughout the skeleton (Fig. 7–21). There is a congenita and a tarda form with different degrees of severity in each. It is not so rare that you will never see a case; therefore, I include it in this differential list. A characteristic finding is the "bone-in-bone" appearance often seen in the vertebral bodies, in which the vertebrae have a small replica of the vertebral body inside the normal one (Fig. 7–22). Also characteristic is the "sandwich vertebrae," in which the end-plates are densely sclerotic, giving the appearance of a sandwich (Fig. 7–23).

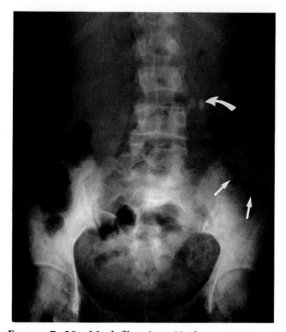

FIGURE 7–20 **Myelofibrosis.** Uniform increased bone density seen most prominently throughout the pelvis is present in this patient with myelofibrosis. Note the grossly enlarged spleen (arrows) and the opaque iron tablets (curved arrow), which are taken for the anemia often present in this disorder.

These findings do not have to be present to make the diagnosis, but their absence makes the diagnosis less likely.

Pyknodysostosis. This is the other congenital abnormality with dense bones that should be considered in the differential diagnosis for osteosclerosis. Like osteopetrosis, it is rare but is seen from time to time in busy radiology practices. These patients are typically short and have hypoplastic mandibles. The distinguishing radiographic finding that is essentially pathognomonic is that the distal phalanges often have the appearance of chalk that has been put into a pencil sharpener—they are pointed and dense (Fig. 7–24). Nothing else does this, but unfortunately pyknodysostosis does not do this in every case. Another name for this disorder is Toulouse-Lautrec syndrome; this famous artist was apparently afflicted with pyknodysostosis.

Metastatic Carcinoma. Only rarely will diffuse metastatic carcinoma cause a problem in diagnosis. I have seen only a handful of cases in which diffuse metastatic disease mimicked diffuse osteosclerosis, and in every case the primary tumor was prostate or breast carcinoma. If cortical destruction or a lytic component is present, the differential diagnosis is simplified, so these should be searched for.

Mastocytosis. This is another rare disorder that can cause uniform increased bone density. Unfortunately there are no other plain film findings that might help with the diagnosis. These patients have thickened small-bowel folds with nodules, but of course to see them an upper GI contrast study must be performed (Fig. 7–25).

FIGURE 7–21 **Osteopetrosis.** Diffuse bony sclerosis is present throughout the skeleton in this patient with osteopetrosis.

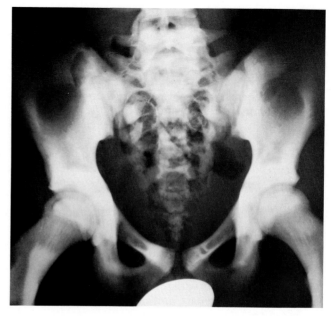

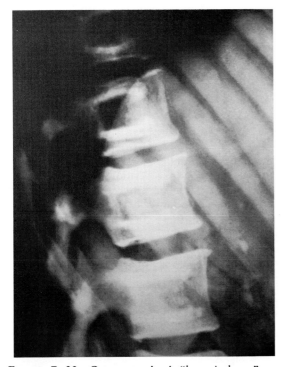

FIGURE 7–22 Osteopetrosis. A "bone-in-bone" appearance is present in the vertebral bodies in this patient with osteopetrosis. This is often seen in osteopetrosis and is occasionally seen in other disorders.

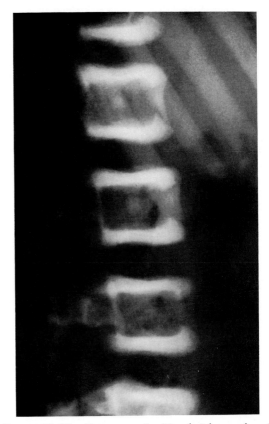

FIGURE 7–23 Osteopetrosis. "Sandwich vertebrae" are seen in the vertebral bodies in this patient with osteopetrosis. This is virtually pathognomonic for osteopetrosis when present and should not be confused with the ill-defined bands of sclerosis seen in the rugger jersey spine of hyperparathyroidism.

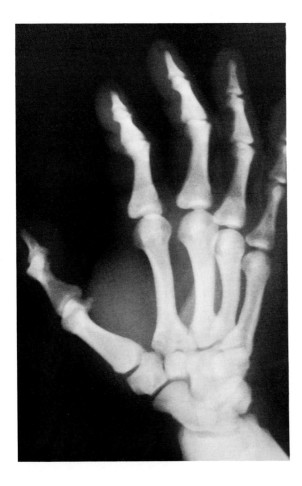

FIGURE 7–24 Pyknodysostosis. Dense sclerosis is seen throughout the hand in this patient with pyknodysostosis. A pathognomonic finding is seen in the distal phalanges, where the tufts are absent and the phalanges are pointed and sclerotic.

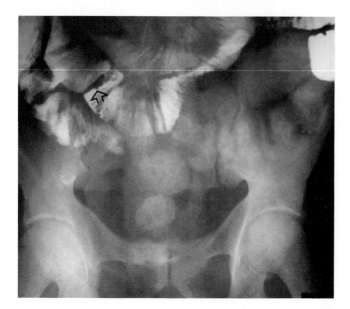

FIGURE 7–25 **Mastocytosis.** Uniform dense bones are noted throughout the pelvis in this patient with mastocytosis. Note the thickened small-bowel folds with nodules (arrow), which are often seen in mastocytosis.

Mastocytosis is rare enough that you might be justified in leaving it out of your differential—you won't miss many, but it messes up the mnemonic.

Paget's Disease. Diffuse Paget's disease that could be confused with one of the other diseases in the differential diagnosis of generalized osteosclerosis is very rare—I have seen only one or two cases ever. Paget's classically causes bony enlargement (Fig. 7–26), but this is not always present. It occurs most commonly in the pelvis (Fig. 7–27), where it has been said the iliopectineal line on the pelvic brim must be thickened if Paget's is present. In fact, the iliopectineal line is usually, but not always, thickened. Paget's can occur in any bone in the body, including the smaller bones of the hands and feet (Fig. 7–28). It has been spread through the teaching files of many institutions (I have seen many statements in teaching files that have never made the literature that have served me well and others that have misled me) that the fibula is the only bone that Paget's never affects. I must agree that the fibula is usually spared—even with profound disease all around it—but I have certainly seen exceptions to this rule.

Three distinct phases are radiographically visible in Paget's: a lytic phase, a sclerotic phase, and a mixed lytic-sclerotic phase (Fig. 7–29). The lytic phase often has a sharp leading edge, called a "flame-shaped" or "blade of grass" leading edge. In a long bone, with the sole exception being the tibia, Paget's always starts at the end of the bone; therefore, if a lesion is present in the middle of a long bone and does not extend to either end, you can safely exclude Paget's disease.

So why is Paget's in this differential if it so

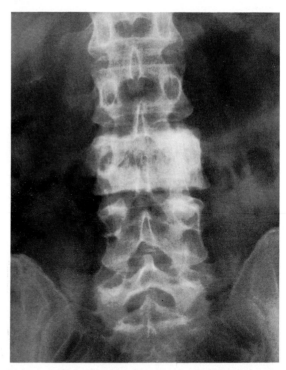

FIGURE 7–26 **Paget's disease.** Dense sclerosis with bony overgrowth is seen in the L-3 vertebral body in this patient with Paget's disease. The left L-3 pedicle is particularly dense and overgrown.

rarely fits? Good question. You can probably safely leave it out without missing too many cases, but it's good to at least think about, since it is so readily diagnosed once you do think of it. Also, it does occasionally involve a large area, such as the entire pelvis and makes the observer think that the entire skeleton might be involved.

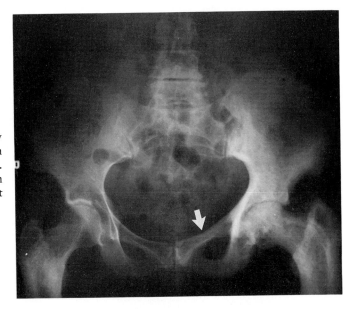

FIGURE 7–27 **Paget's disease.** Dense bony sclerosis with some bony enlargement is seen throughout the left pelvis and proximal femur. Note the thickening of the iliopectineal line on the left side (arrow) as compared with the right side.

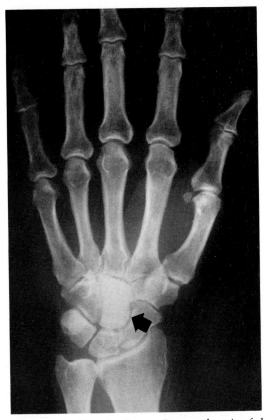

FIGURE 7–28 **Paget's disease.** Dense sclerosis of the capitate (arrow) is seen in this patient. Although no definite bony overgrowth is appreciated, it is not unusual for Paget's disease to affect a single bone uniformly such as this.

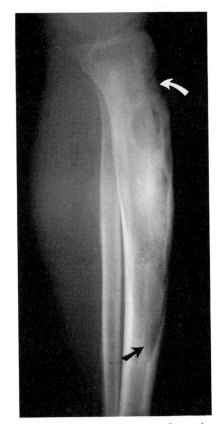

FIGURE 7–29 **Paget's disease.** A "flame-shaped" or "blade of grass" appearance is seen in the distal tibia (arrow) in this patient with Paget's disease of the tibia. The sclerotic phase of Paget's disease is seen in the mid-tibia in this patient, whereas the proximal tibia has an area of apparent cortical destruction (curved arrow), which is suspicious for sarcomatous degeneration.

Athletes. I see radiographs on professional athletes quite often and continue to be impressed by the degree of increased cortical thickness these people possess. No question about it: increased stress causes hypertrophy of bone as well as of muscle. Residents routinely question the presence of diffuse increased bone density in this set of patients, enough so that I have added normal athletes to my differential diagnosis for osteosclerosis.

Fluorosis. This is another rare disorder that could probably be left off the list without danger of missing too many cases. Fluorosis is usually a result of chronic intake in certain areas that have large amounts of fluoride present in the drinking water. It can also be a result of long-term therapy with sodium fluoride for osteoporosis. A radiographic finding that patients with fluorosis often have is ligamentous calcification. If I have a patient with dense bones and no ligamentous calcifications, I will put fluorosis lower on the list but not eliminate it. If ligamentous calcifications are present, it will go to the top of the list. Calcification of the sacrotuberous ligament is said to be characteristic for fluorosis.

CONCLUSION

There are other categories of disease that could be covered in a chapter on metabolic bone disease, but most of the remaining disorders are exceedingly rare and not likely to be seen by most radiologists on a routine basis. Excellent texts are available for additional details on the diseases I have mentioned as well as for learning about the less common entities.

REFERENCES

1. Hall FM: Bone-mineral screening for osteoporosis. Opinion. AJR 1987;149:120–122.
2. Helms C, Munk P: Pseudopermeative skeletal lesions. Br J Radiol 1990;63:461–467.

Chapter

8

Miscellaneous Conditions

There are a host of bony conditions, diseases, and syndromes that do not fit conveniently into any of the preceding chapters, yet should be given some mention in an attempted overview of musculoskeletal radiology. Many of these are simply "Aunt Minnies" and only require you to have seen them once or twice to recognize them. I have severely limited the things I have included in this chapter—it could easily have dozens of other entities, but none are very common. Besides, I need to have something to add in future editions. These are listed alphabetically for lack of a more scientific basis.

ACHONDROPLASIA

The most common cause of dwarfism is achondroplasia, a congenital, hereditary disease of failure of endochondral bone formation. The femurs and humeri are more profoundly affected than the other long bones, although the entire skeleton is abnormal. The spine typically has narrowing of the interpedicular distances in a caudal direction (Fig. 8–1), the opposite of normal where the interpedicular distances get progressively wider as one proceeds down the spine. The long bones are short but have normal width, giving them a thick appearance.

AVASCULAR NECROSIS

The term avascular necrosis (AVN) refers to the lack of blood supply with subsequent bone death and ensuing bony collapse in an articular surface. The etiology of AVN is an extensive differential that most commonly includes trauma,

TABLE 8–1 Common Causes of Avascular Necrosis

Trauma	Collagen vascular diseases
Steroids	Alcoholism
Aspirin	Idiopathic
Renal disease	

steroids, aspirin, renal disease, collagen vascular diseases, alcoholism, and idiopathic (Table 8–1).[1] The radiographic appearance ranges from patchy sclerosis (Fig. 8–2A) to articular surface collapse and fragmentation (Fig. 8–3). Just before collapse a subchondral lucency is occasionally seen (Fig. 8–4); however, this is a late and inconstant sign of AVN. Magnetic resonance (MR) imaging is extremely valuable in demonstrating the presence and extent of AVN (Fig. 8–2B and C) even when plain films are apparently normal. MR imaging is currently considered to be the most efficacious way to evaluate a joint for AVN.[2] It is useful not only in AVN of the hips but also of the knee, wrist, foot and ankle.

HYPERTROPHIC PULMONARY OSTEOARTHROPATHY

Hypertrophic pulmonary osteoarthropathy (HPO) is manifested by clubbing of the fingers and periostitis, usually in the upper and lower extremities (Fig. 8–5), which may or may not be associated with bone pain. It is most commonly seen in patients with lung cancer, but many other

161

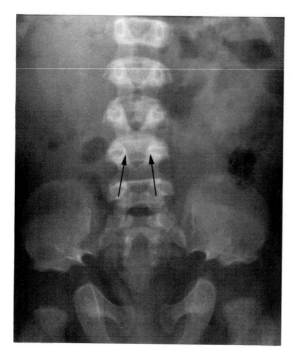

FIGURE 8–1   **Achondroplasia.** An anteroposterior (AP) plain film of the spine in this patient with achondroplasia demonstrates narrowing of the interpedicular distance (arrows) in a caudal direction, which is characteristic of this disorder. Ordinarily the interpedicular distance widens in each vertebra in a caudal direction.

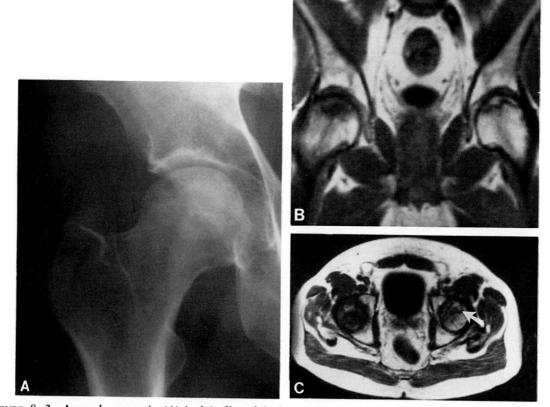

FIGURE 8–2   **Avascular necrosis.** *(A)* A plain film of the hip in this patient with avascular necrosis (AVN) shows faint patchy sclerosis throughout the femoral head. This is a relatively early plain film finding for AVN. Coronal *(B)* and axial *(C)* MR images in the same patient, which are T1 weighted (TR 500; TE 28), show typical findings in AVN. Diffuse low signal in the right hip is noted, which indicates more extensive involvement than in the left. The left hip has a low signal serpiginous rim (arrow), which is characteristic for AVN.

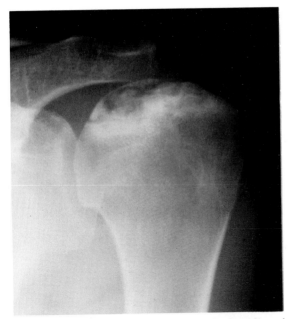

FIGURE 8–3 Avascular necrosis. An AP plain film of the shoulder reveals articular surface collapse in this patient who was treated with steroids for systemic lupus erythematosus. This is an advanced stage of AVN.

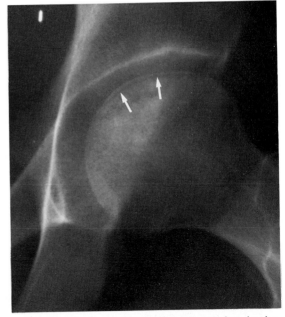

FIGURE 8–4 Avascular necrosis. An AP frog-leg lateral view of the hip in this patient with sickle cell disease shows a subchondral lucency (arrows) and patchy sclerosis in the femoral head, indicative of AVN. This is a relatively advanced stage of AVN. The subchondral lucency is often better demonstrated with the frog-leg lateral view.

FIGURE 8–5 Hypertrophic pulmonary osteoarthropathy (HPO). Periostitis can be seen along the shafts of the distal tibia and fibula (arrows) in this patient with bronchogenic carcinoma and leg pain. This is characteristic for HPO.

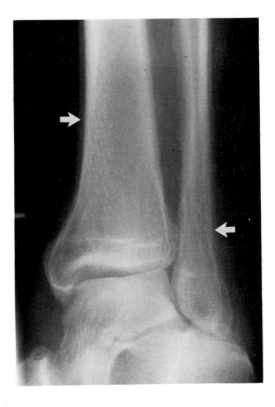

TABLE 8–2 Periostitis Without Underlying Bony Lesion

Trauma	Venous stasis
Hypertrophic pulmonary osteoarthropathy	Thyroid acropachy
	Pachydermoperiostosis

etiologies have been reported, including bronchiectasis, GI disorders, and liver disease. The actual mechanism of formation of periostitis secondary to a distant malignancy or other process is unknown. The differential diagnosis for periostitis in a long bone without an underlying bony abnormality would include HPO, venous stasis, thyroid acropachy, pachydermoperiostosis, and trauma (Table 8–2).

MELORHEOSTOSIS

Melorheostosis is a rare, idiopathic disorder characterized by thickened cortical new bone that accumulates near the ends of long bones, usually only on one side of the bone, and has an appearance likened to "dripping candle wax" (Fig. 8–6). It can affect several adjacent bones and can be symptomatic. Many feel there is some relation or overlap among melorheostosis, osteopathia striata, and osteopoikilosis (mentioned later in this chapter), all of which present with varying patterns of increased cortical bone.

MUCOPOLYSACCHARIDOSES (MORQUIO'S, HURLER'S, AND HUNTER'S SYNDROMES)

The mucopolysaccharidoses are a group of inherited diseases characterized by abnormal storage and excretion in the urine of various mucopolysaccharides such as keratan sulfate (Morquio's) and heparan sulfate (Hurler's). These patients have short stature, primarily from shortened spines, and characteristic plain film findings. In the spine, patients with Morquio's have platyspondyly (generalized flattening of the vertebral bodies) with a central anterior projection or "beak" off of the vertebral body as viewed on a lateral plain film (Fig. 8–7). Hurler's and Hunter's show platyspondyly with a "beak" that is anteroinferiorly positioned (Fig. 8–8). The pelvis in these disorders is similar in appearance to that of achondroplasts with wide, flared iliac wings and broad femoral necks. A characteristic finding in the hands is a pointed proximal fifth

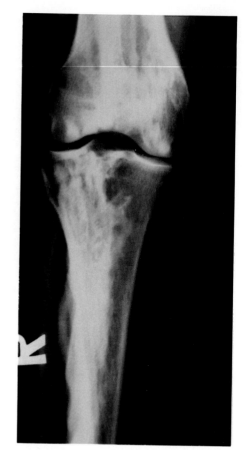

FIGURE 8–6 Melorheostosis. Dense, wavy, new bone is seen adjacent to the lateral tibial cortex, which has a "dripping candle wax" appearance that is classic for melorheostosis. A similar pattern can be seen in the medial aspect of the distal femur.

metacarpal base that has a notch appearance to the ulnar aspect (Fig. 8–9).

MULTIPLE HEREDITARY EXOSTOSES

Also known as diaphyseal aclasia, this is a not uncommon hereditary disorder that seems to affect multiple members of a family with multiple osteochondromas, or exostoses. An osteochondroma is a cartilage-capped bone outgrowth, which may be pedunculated or sessile in appearance. In the multiple hereditary form the knees are virtually always involved (Fig. 8–10). The incidence of malignant degeneration in this population has been reported to be as high as 20 per cent. As with solitary osteochondromas, the more axially situated lesions are more prone to undergo malignant degeneration, while the more peripheral lesions are less likely to do so. The proximal femurs are frequently involved and have a characteristic appearance (Fig. 8–11).

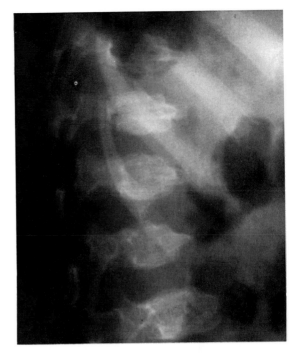

FIGURE 8–7 Morquio's. A lateral plain film of the spine reveals a central "beak" or anterior bony projection off of the vertebral bodies in this patient with Morquio's syndrome.

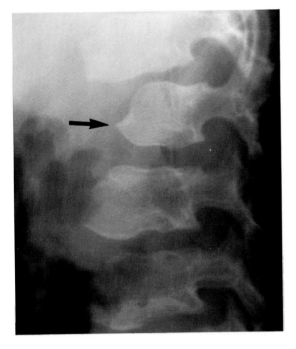

FIGURE 8–8 Hurler's. A lateral plain film of the spine in this patient with Hurler's syndrome shows an inferiorly placed bony projection extending anteriorly off of the vertebral bodies (arrow).

FIGURE 8–9 Hurler's. An AP plain film of the hand in this patient with Hurler's syndrome shows a notch (arrow) at the base of the fifth metacarpal, which is a characteristic finding in all of the mucopolysaccharidoses.

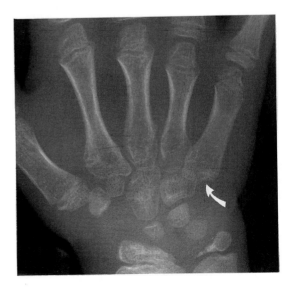

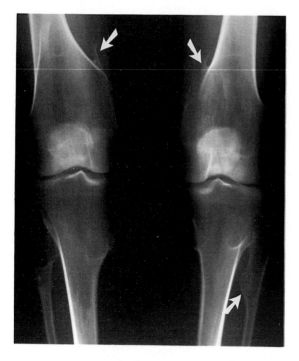

FIGURE 8–10 Multiple hereditary exostosis. The knees are involved in virtually every case of multiple hereditary exostosis. They typically show not only multiple exostoses (arrows) but also marked undertubulation in the metaphyses.

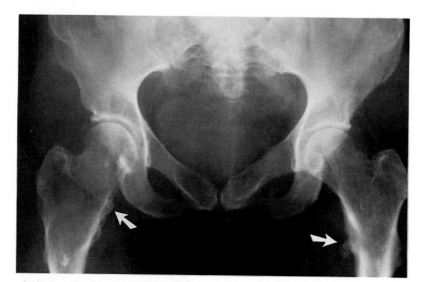

FIGURE 8–11 Multiple hereditary exostosis. The femoral necks are often involved in multiple hereditary exostosis. They will show undertubulation, as in this example, and usually have one or more exostoses (arrows).

OSTEOID OSTEOMA

The etiology of osteoid osteoma is unknown. Is it an infection (bacterial or viral), a slow growing tumor, a dessert topping? Nobody knows. It is a painful lesion that occurs almost exclusively in patients under the age of 30 that is treated successfully with surgical excision. Aspirin often gives dramatic relief of the pain and can be used for conservative treatment in lieu of surgery. A classic clinical picture for an osteoid osteoma is "night pain relieved by aspirin." However, many osteoid osteomas do not have this presentation, and most painful musculoskeletal lesions are worse at night and relieved by aspirin.

Radiographically an osteoid osteoma is said to have a typical appearance, but, in fact, it has many different appearances which can make diagnosis difficult.[3] The classically described radiographic appearance is a cortically based sclerotic lesion in a long bone that has a small lucency within it, which is called the nidus (Fig. 8–12A). It is the nidus that causes the pain and the sur-

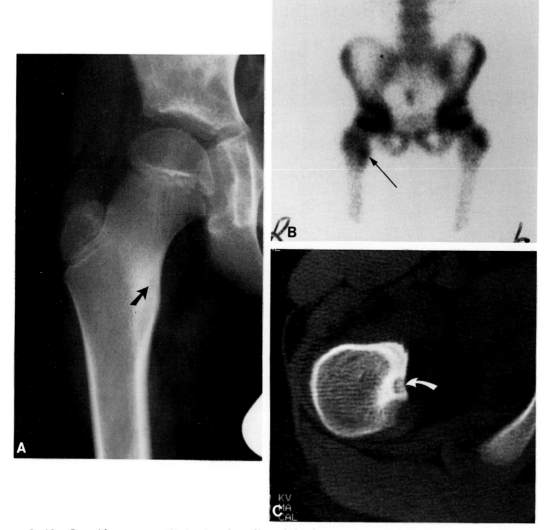

FIGURE 8–12   Osteoid osteoma. *(A)* An AP plain film of the femur in a child with hip pain shows an area of sclerosis medially near the lesser trochanter with a small lucency (arrow), which is the nidus of an osteoid osteoma. Osteomyelitis could have this identical appearance. *(B)* A radionuclide bone scan shows increased uptake in the proximal femur, which corresponds to the reactive new bone seen on the plain film. In addition, however, note the second smaller area of increased radionuclide uptake within the larger area (arrow). This corresponds to the nidus itself. This pattern on a bone scan is called the double density sign. *(C)* A CT scan of the femur shows the sclerosis medially and the lucent nidus (arrow) to better advantage. The CT and the bone scan give the surgeon a more precise anatomic location of the nidus than the plain film.

rounding reactive sclerosis. If the nidus is surgically removed, complete cessation of pain is the rule. Computed tomography (CT) and radionuclide bone scanning are often very helpful in demonstrating the exact location of the nidus (Fig. 8–12*B* and *C*).

If the nidus of an osteoid osteoma is located in the medullary rather than the cortical portion of a bone, or if it is located in a joint, there is much less reactive sclerosis present. This gives the lesion a different overall appearance than the

more common cortical lesion in that it does not appear as sclerotic. Up to 80 per cent of osteoid osteomas are located intracortically with the remainder being in the intramedullary part of a bone. Rarely an osteoid osteoma will present in the periosteum causing tremendous periostitis.

The nidus itself is usually lucent but often develops some calcification within it. It then has the appearance of a sequestrum as is seen in osteomyelitis. If the nidus calcifies completely, it blends in with the surrounding sclerosis and cannot be

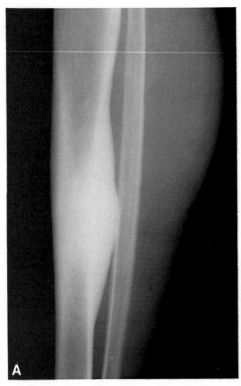

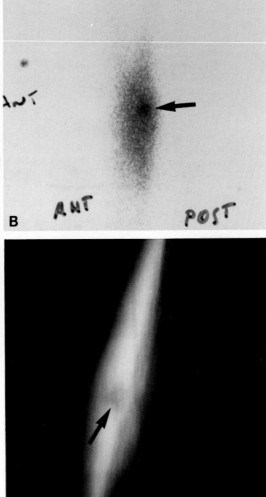

FIGURE 8–13 Osteoid osteoma. *(A)* A lateral plain film of the tibia in this child with leg pain shows cortical thickening in the posterior diaphysis. No lucency in the sclerotic area could be identified. *(B)* A radionuclide bone scan reveals uptake corresponding to the area of sclerosis in the tibia, with a more marked area of uptake centrally (arrow), which is the double density sign of an osteoid osteoma. *(C)* The surgical specimen shows the nidus (arrow) as a faint lucency within the sclerotic bone.

seen on most radiographs. Therefore, the diagnosis of an osteoid osteoma in no way is dependent on seeing a nidus.

Since an osteoid osteoma resembles osteomyelitis, regardless of the appearance of the nidus, it can be difficult to differentiate the two radiographically. In fact, it cannot be done with plain films, CT scan, or MR imaging. However, because the nidus is extremely vascular it avidly accumulates radiopharmaceutical bone scanning agents. An osteoid osteoma will have an area of increased uptake corresponding to the area of reactive sclerosis, but, in addition will demonstrate a second area of increased uptake corresponding to the nidus (Figs. 8–12 to 8–14). This has been termed the "double density" sign.[4] In

contrast, osteomyelitis has a photopenic area corresponding to the plain film lucency which represents an avascular focus of purulent material. The natural history of an osteoid osteoma is presumed to be spontaneous regression since they are rarely seen over the age of 30.

OSTEOPATHIA STRIATA

Also known as Voorhoeve's disease, this disorder is manifested by multiple 2–3 mm thick linear bands of sclerotic bone aligned parallel to the long axis of a bone (Fig. 8–15). It usually affects multiple long bones and is asymptomatic, hence it is usually an incidental finding.

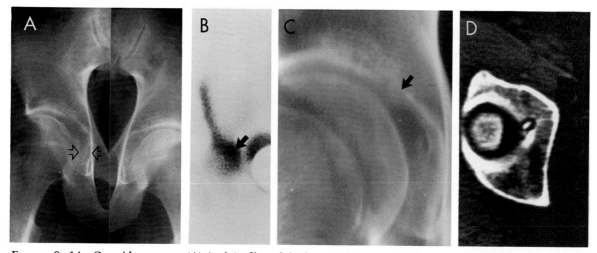

FIGURE 8–14 Osteoid osteoma. *(A)* A plain film of the hips in this 24-year-old male with right hip pain shows a widened tear drop (arrows) measurement on the right as compared to the left. This indicates a joint effusion. No other abnormality was found, so an aspiration arthrogram was performed to exclude infection. It was normal except for a joint effusion, which was culture negative. A radionuclide bone scan *(B)* was done to see if AVN or a stress fracture was the source of the pain. It revealed increased uptake throughout the acetabulum with a second area of increased uptake (arrow) corresponding to a double density sign. A conventional tomogram *(C)* showed a faint area of lucency in the location of the double density of the bone scan, but it was not convincing enough to the surgeon to be helpful. A CT scan *(D)* through the acetabulum shows a lucent nidus, which is partially calcified. This is characteristic for an osteoid osteoma; however, osteomyelitis with a sequestrum could have an identical appearance except for the bone scan double density sign.

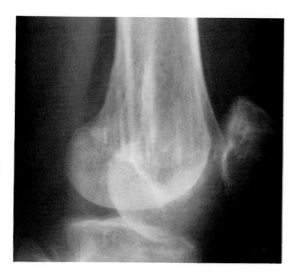

FIGURE 8–15 Osteopathia striata. Multiple linear dense streaks are seen in the distal femur, which are characteristic of osteopathia striata.

OSTEOPOIKILOSIS

Osteopoikilosis is an hereditary, asymptomatic disorder that is usually an incidental finding of multiple small (3–10 mm) sclerotic bony densities affecting primarily the ends of long bones and the pelvis (Fig. 8–16). It has virtually no clinical significance other than that it can be confused for diffuse osteoblastic metastases.

PACHYDERMOPERIOSTOSIS

Pachydermoperiostosis is a rare, familial disease that is manifested by thickening of the skin of the extremities and face and clubbing of the fingers. It seems to be more common in black people. The periosteal reaction is similar to that of hypertrophic pulmonary osteoarthropathy, but pachydermoperiostosis is rarely painful.

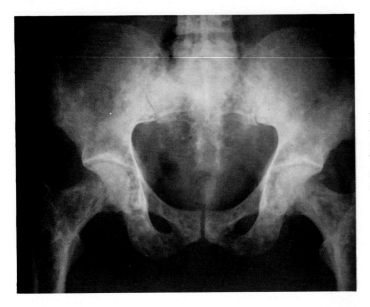

FIGURE 8–16 Osteopoikilosis. An AP of the pelvis reveals multiple small round sclerotic foci throughout the pelvis and femurs. This is diagnostic of osteopoikilosis. Metastatic disease is occasionally mistaken for this disorder.

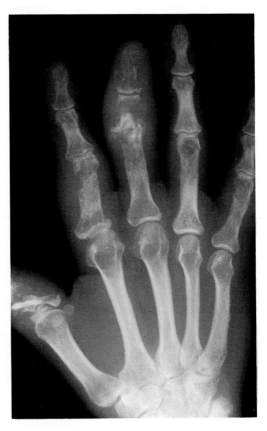

FIGURE 8–17 Sarcoid. An AP plain film of the hands in a patient with sarcoidosis shows multiple lytic lesions, many of which demonstrate a "lace-like" pattern.

SARCOID

Sarcoidosis is a noncaseating granulomatous disease that primarily affects the lungs. When the musculoskeletal system is involved, the hands are mainly affected, with the spine and long bones only infrequently involved. Sarcoid causes a characteristic "lace-like" pattern of bony destruction in the hands (Fig. 8–17). Multiple phalanges are typically affected in either one or both hands. It is so radiographically characteristic that there is almost no differential diagnosis for this pattern.

SLIPPED CAPITAL FEMORAL EPIPHYSIS

The epiphysis of the femoral head (called the capital epiphysis) has a tendency to slip medially. This is seen primarily in young teenage boys who are overweight, although it can be seen in hyperparathyroidism or idiopathically. It can be identified on an AP of the pelvis or hips by drawing a line along the lateral femoral neck and noting that in normals this line intersects about a quarter of the epiphysis (Fig. 8–18). In patients with a slipped capital epiphysis this line intersects little or none of the slipped epiphysis. This process is often found bilaterally and is treated by internally fixing the epiphysis with nails.

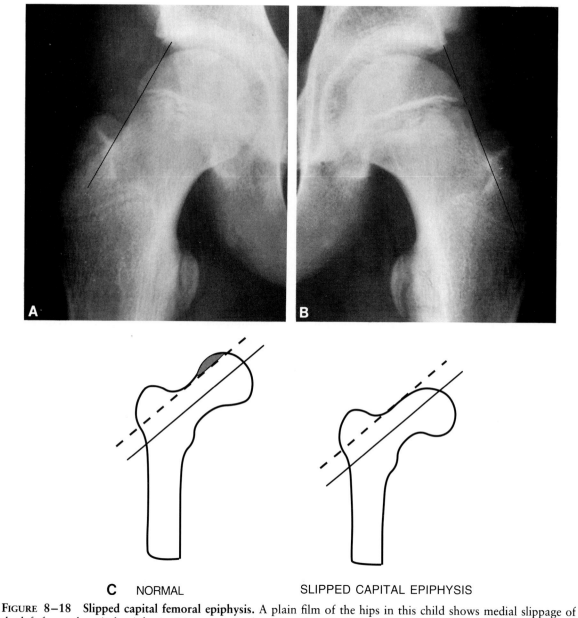

C NORMAL   SLIPPED CAPITAL EPIPHYSIS

FIGURE 8–18 **Slipped capital femoral epiphysis.** A plain film of the hips in this child shows medial slippage of the left femoral capital epiphysis *(B)* as compared to the right *(A)*. Although the amount of slippage is slight and difficult to appreciate at first glance, note that a line drawn along the lateral femoral neck on the normal side *(A)* intersects a portion of the femoral epiphysis, whereas on the left side *(B)* a similar line misses most of the epiphysis. A schematic of the normal hip and a hip with a slipped capital epiphysis *(C)* shows how a line parallel to the femoral neck (solid line) that is then moved to the lateral aspect of the femoral neck (dotted line) intersects part of the epiphysis (shaded) in the normal and misses the epiphysis in a slipped epiphysis.

REFERENCES

1. Mankin H: Nontraumatic necrosis of bone (osteonecrosis). N Engl J Med 1992;326:1473–1479.
2. Mitchell D, Kressel H, Arger P, Dalinka M, Spritzer C, Steinberg M: Avascular necrosis of the femoral head: Morphologic assessment by MR imaging, with CT correlation. Radiology 1986;161:739–742.
3. Marcove R, Heelan R, Huvos A, Healey J, Lindeque B: Osteoid osteoma. Diagnosis, localization, and treatment. Clin Orthop Relat Res 1991;267:197–201.
4. Helms CA, Hattner RS, Vogler J III. Osteoid osteoma: Radionuclide diagnosis. Radiology 1984; 151(3):779–784.

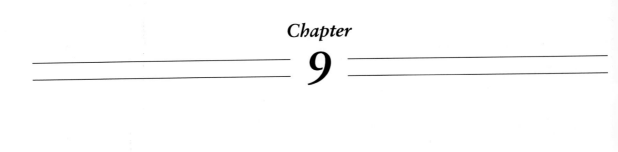

MR Imaging of the Knee

Magnetic resonance (MR) imaging of the knee has developed into one of the most frequently requested exams in radiology. This is not just because many people injure their knees but because of its high accuracy in depicting internal derangements. Accuracy reports of knee MR imaging vary from 85 to 95 per cent with many investigators feeling that MR imaging of the knee is, in fact, more accurate than arthroscopy. Very few top orthopedic surgeons will operate on a knee without an MR imaging scan to serve as a "road map." Although some surgeons feel MR imaging is too expensive for routine use in every patient, there are studies that show enormous financial savings (not to mention decreased patient morbidity) in performing an MR exam on every patient who is a candidate for knee arthroscopy. Many of these patients do not need subsequent arthroscopy and those who do benefit from a more complete preoperative assessment (not directly reflected in financial savings but clearly beneficial for surgical planning).[1] MR imaging of the knee has a very high negative predictive value; therefore, a normal MR imaging knee exam is highly accurate in excluding an internal derangement.[2,3]

Maximum diagnostic accuracy can be obtained in several ways. First, and most obvious, is to obtain high quality images. This includes using the appropriate imaging protocol. Employing an inappropriate protocol is probably the number one error committed in knee MR imaging. Second, knowing the basic MR imaging signs for internal derangements is key in achieving a high accuracy rate. Third, knowing the imaging pitfalls, such as normal variants which can mimic pathology, will further aid in diagnostic accuracy. Proper protocols, basic imaging signs, and pitfalls will be discussed in detail in this chapter.

IMAGING PROTOCOL

The proper imaging protocol is essential for a high diagnostic accuracy rate. A sagittal T1-weighted (or proton density) sequence is essential for examining the menisci. Four or 5 mm thick slices with a small (12–14 cm) field of view (FOV) and at least a 192 matrix are recommended. The knee should be imaged using a dedicated knee coil and externally rotated about 5 to 10 degrees (do not exceed 10 degrees) to put the anterior cruciate ligament in the plane of imaging. T2 spin-echo or T2* GRASS sagittal images are obtained primarily to examine the cruciate ligaments. With T2 spin-echo images meniscal tears may be difficult to see; however, they will be picked up on the proton density images. Thus the menisci and the cruciate ligaments are examined primarily on the sagittal images. Although the menisci and the cruciate ligaments can be seen on the coronal and axial images, it is rare for those images to show an abnormality that is not seen on the sagittal images.

Coronal images are obtained to examine the collateral ligaments and to look for menisco-capsular separations. These abnormalities can most often only be seen with T2-weighted images. T1 coronal images are therefore a waste of time as there is nothing to be seen on these images that cannot be equally well seen on the sagittal images. T2* GRASS coronals or repeating the sagittal spin-echo sequences in the coronal plane are imperative.

Many centers continue to use T1-weighted coronal images without realizing that they give no additional information and, in fact, can hide significant abnormalities. Why would they do this? T1-weighted coronal images were part of everyone's protocol when we first began to use MR imaging in the knee. Articles, book chapters, and speakers (including me) would give the standard protocol, not thinking enough about what each sequence was showing us. I remember reading out a knee study in the late 1980s with one of the radiology residents, and I asked him to hedge on the diagnosis of a partial tear of the medial collateral ligament and request a repeat exam with T2-weighted coronals to rule out a meniscocapsular separation. This was the second or third time that week that the resident had been so instructed, so he asked, "Why don't we just routinely do a T2 coronal—we don't see anything on the T1 coronal and we often have to hedge or repeat the exam with a T2 coronal?" I just said for him to worry about dictating the cases, I and others would take care of setting up the protocols. Well, 2 weeks later he rotated to another service, and we began doing T2 coronal images as part of our standard knee protocol. Uppity residents!

Axial images are obtained primarily for use by the technicians as a scout view. They can also be utilized for viewing the patellofemoral cartilage and for examining a medial patellar plica. As in the coronal images, to afford an opportunity to see any pathology, T2 or T2* images must be obtained. Since it takes too long to obtain another full spin-echo sequence with proton density and T2 images, a T2* GRASS sequence is recommended. The availability of fast spin-echo images affords another method of obtaining T2-weighted axials.

The protocol I currently recommend consists of a sagittal T1-weighted spin-echo series and sagittal, coronal, and axial T2* GRASS sequences (Table 9–1). Many acceptable variations of this protocol exist. Many centers, for various reasons, prefer not to use GRASS images and instead use T2 spin-echo. An acceptable protocol, avoiding GRASS images, would be sagittal and coronal proton-density and T2-weighted spin-echo sequences, with an axial image that is T1 weighted. A T1-weighted sequence in one plane is strongly recommended to examine the bone marrow. If available, fast spin-echo T2 images can be substituted for the GRASS T2* in the coronal and axial planes.

MENISCI

The normal meniscus is a fibrocartilagenous, C-shaped structure that is uniformly low in signal on both T1- and T2-weighted sequences (Fig. 9–1). With T2* sequences the menisci will usually demonstrate some internal signal. With T1-weighted images any signal within the meniscus is abnormal, except in children where some signal is normal and represents normal vascularity. Meniscal signal that does not disrupt an articular surface is representative of intrasubstance degeneration (Fig. 9–2), which is myxoid degeneration of the fibrocartilage. It most likely represents aging and normal wear and tear. It is not felt to be symptomatic and cannot be diagnosed clinically or with arthroscopy. Some choose, therefore, not to mention intrasubstance degeneration in the radiology interpretation. A grading scale for meniscal signal that is widely used is the following (Fig. 9–3): Grade 1—rounded or amorphous signal that does *not* disrupt an articular surface; grade 2—linear signal that does *not* disrupt an articular surface; grade 3—rounded or linear signal that disrupts an articular surface (Fig. 9–4). Grades 1 and 2 are intrasubstance degeneration and should not be reported as "grade 1 or 2 tears." This is a radiology grading scale, which is not known widely by orthopedic surgeons; hence, the term "tear" often leads to an unnecessary arthroscopy (arthroscopy is not indicated for intrasubstance degeneration). Only grade 3 is a meniscal tear.

When high signal in a meniscus disrupts the superior or inferior articular surface, a meniscal tear is diagnosed (Fig. 9–4). Care must be taken to be sure that the signal actually disrupts the articular surface of the meniscus before calling a tear. When high signal approaches the articular surface of the meniscus, it seems many radiologists tend to overcall it whether or not it disrupts

TABLE 9–1 Knee Protocol

	TR/TE	Nex	Matrix	Flip Angle	Thickness (mm)	FOV
Sagittal	800/15	2	192	—	4	14
Sagittal	600/20	2	192	20°	4	14
Coronal	600/20	2	192	20°	4	14
Axial	600/20	2	192	20°	4	14

Nex = number of excitations, FOV = field of view

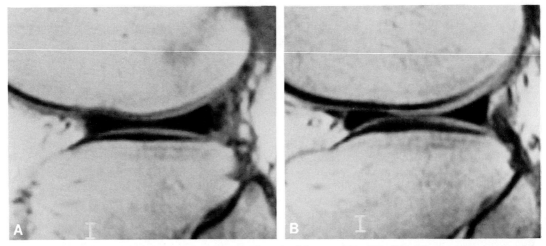

FIGURE 9–1 Normal meniscus. *(A)* A T1-weighted sagittal image (TR 600; TE 30) through a normal lateral meniscus demonstrates uniform low signal in the meniscus. This is a section through the body of the meniscus, since it has a bowtie configuration. Two sections of the body should be seen in each meniscus with 4 or 5 mm thick slices. *(B)* In the same T1-weighted sequence, this sagittal image demonstrates uniform low signal in the anterior and posterior horns of this normal lateral meniscus. (Anterior is to the left.)

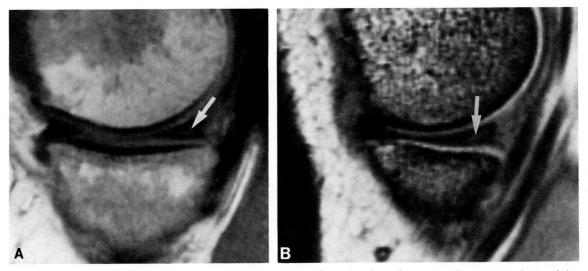

FIGURE 9–2 Intrasubstance degeneration. *(A)* Faint intermediate signal can be seen in the posterior horn of this meniscus (arrow), which does not disrupt the articular surface of the meniscus. This is intrasubstance degeneration. *(B)* Linear high signal is present in the posterior body segment of the meniscus (arrow) in this GRASS image. The signal does not disrupt the articular surface; therefore this represents intrasubstance degeneration.

the surface. This is evidenced not only from my experience of watching residents and fellows, but also by noting that most published series on accuracy of knee MR imaging have a lower specificity than sensitivity (i.e., there are more false positives than false negatives). One way to aid in avoiding false positive calls is to cover up the meniscus with a card, or your thumbnail, leaving only a thin margin of the articular surface of the meniscus visible. If this margin of articular surface of the meniscus is seen as a straight uninterrupted line, no tear of the meniscus is present. If the thin margin is interrupted, a meniscal tear is present.

Meniscal tears have many different configurations and locations with an oblique tear extending to the inferior surface of the posterior horn of the medial meniscus the most common

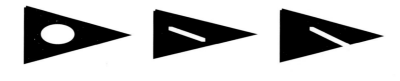

GRADE 1   GRADE 2   GRADE 3

FIGURE 9–3 **Grading scale for menisci.** A schematic of the MR imaging grading scale for meniscal abnormalities: Grade 1 has rounded or amorphous signal in the meniscus that does not disrupt an articular surface. Grade 2 has linear signal that does not disrupt an articular surface. Grades 1 and 2 represent intrasubstance degeneration. Grade 3 has signal that does disrupt an articular surface and indicates a meniscal tear.

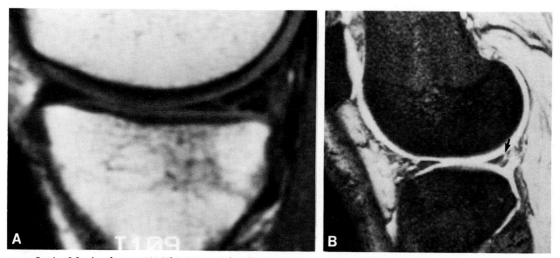

FIGURE 9–4 **Meniscal tear.** *(A)* This T1-weighted sagittal image (TR 600; TE 30) shows linear high signal in the posterior horn of the meniscus, which disrupts the inferior articular surface. This is the appearance of a meniscal tear. (Note the irregular low signal in the subarticular marrow of the tibia which is characteristic for a bony contusion.) *(B)* A vertical tear with high signal disrupting the inferior and superior articular surfaces of the posterior horn of the meniscus (arrow).

type. In a small but significant percentage of cases (around 10%) it can be virtually impossible to be certain if meniscal high signal disrupts an articular surface. In these cases it is recommended that the surgeon be advised that it is too close to call. The surgeon can then rely on his clinical expertise to decide if arthroscopy is warranted, and, if it is, the MR will guide him to where the questionable tear is located. If these equivocal cases are excluded, the remaining cases will have an extremely high accuracy rate.

Another very common meniscus tear, one that is frequently missed by radiologists, is a bucket handle tear. This is a vertical longitudinal tear that can result in the inner free edge of the meniscus becoming displaced into the intercondylar notch (Fig. 9–5). It is most easily recognized by observing on the sagittal images that only one image is present which has the bowtie appearance

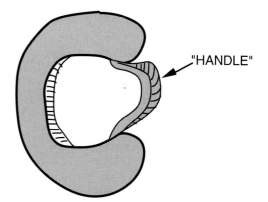

"HANDLE"

FIGURE 9–5 **Bucket handle tear.** This drawing illustrates a bucket handle tear with the torn free edge of the meniscus displaced as the "handle" of the bucket.

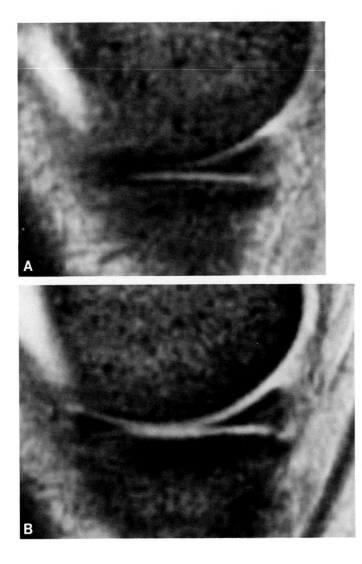

FIGURE 9–6 **Bucket handle tear.** Sagittal GRASS images through the medial meniscus at its most medial aspect reveal one bowtie, indicative of the body of the meniscus *(A)* with the adjacent image *(B)* having apparent normal anterior and posterior horns. However, since there should be two consecutive sagittal images with a bowtie configuration, this indicates a bucket handle tear. (Anterior is to the left.)

of the body segment of the meniscus (Fig. 9–6). Normally two contiguous sagittal images with a bowtie shape are seen, since the normal meniscus is 10 to 12 mm in width and the sagittal images are 4 to 5 mm in thickness. On the coronal images a bucket handle tear may reveal the meniscus to be shortened and truncated; however, often the torn meniscus remodels and truncation cannot be appreciated (Fig. 9–7). The displaced inner edge of the meniscus (the "handle" of the bucket) is often seen in the intercondylar notch on sagittal or coronal views (Fig. 9–8); however, in my experience, it can often be difficult to find the displaced meniscal fragment.

Another meniscus tear that is diagnosed by having too few bowtie segments present in the sagittal plane is a parrot beak tear. This is a radial tear of the free edge of the meniscus (Fig. 9–9), which is an uncommon tear and only rarely causes enough symptoms by itself to warrant ar-

throscopy. It should be suspected when only one bowtie segment is present and the adjacent sagittal image shows a small gap (a bucket handle tear will have a large gap) in the expected bowtie (Fig. 9–10). The apparent anterior and/or posterior horn triangles will often be rounded instead of pointed.

Use of the "bowtie sign," that is, having two consecutive sagittal images that demonstrate a bowtie configuration, is probably the most useful sign I can give beginners in evaluating a knee MR image. It will allow a bucket handle tear to virtually never be overlooked and, as the next section describes, can be used to diagnose a discoid meniscus. There are three pitfalls to be aware of in applying the bowtie sign (Table 9–2). First, if the knee and the menisci are very small, as in a child's knee, only one bowtie may be observed without a bucket handle tear being present. However, there will be only two or three sagittal im-

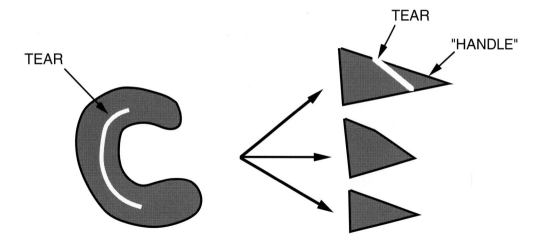

FIGURE 9–7 Schematic of bucket handle tear. This drawing shows how a vertical longitudinal tear as shown on the axial view (left) can appear on the coronal views (right). Prior to the free edge being displaced the tear may be seen (top, right); after the free edge (or "handle") displaces the remaining meniscus may appear truncated (center, right); after weight bearing the truncated meniscus smooths out to a sharp triangle that is simply decreased in width from the normal (bottom, right).

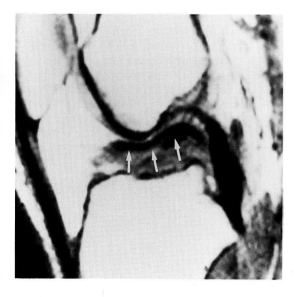

FIGURE 9–8 Displaced fragment in bucket handle tear. A sagittal T1-weighted image through the intercondylar notch in a patient with a bucket handle tear reveals the displaced free fragment or "handle" (arrows) just anterior to the posterior cruciate ligament.

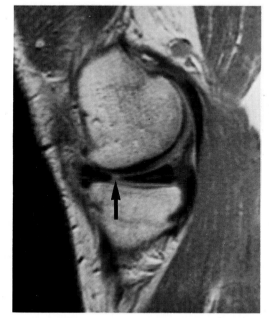

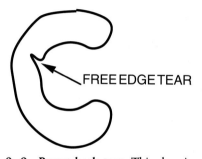

FIGURE 9–9 Parrot beak tear. This drawing shows the appearance of a radial free edge meniscal tear called a parrot beak tear.

FIGURE 9–10 Parrot beak tear. Sagittal images through the body of the medial meniscus in a patient with a parrot beak tear showed a normal bowtie configuration in the most medial image, with the next adjacent image (shown here) having a small gap (arrow), which indicates a disruption of the free edge of the meniscus. Note the rounded tip of the apparent anterior horn, which is further evidence of a torn free edge or parrot beak tear.

TABLE 9–2 Pitfalls in "Bowtie" Sign

1. Small knee with small menisci
2. Older patients (>60) who may have fraying and degeneration of free edge
3. Incomplete coverage

ages that demonstrate the anterior and posterior horns. A normal-sized knee will have two bowties and three or four images that show the anterior and posterior horns. Also, in a small knee both the medial and lateral menisci will have only one bowtie image, and bucket handle tears involving both the medial and lateral menisci are very rare.

The second pitfall in the bowtie sign is seen in older patients—over the age of 60. This is not a common age to have an internal derangement of the knee, but it does happen. Patients older than 60 often have worn down the inner free edges of their menisci so that they will only have one sagittal image of the body seen, followed by four or five images that show the anterior and posterior horns—usually a good sign for a bucket handle tear. This, unlike the pitfall described in children or small knees, does not necessarily occur in both menisci. How do I differentiate this from a real bucket handle tear? I can't. I tell the surgeon that I cannot tell if there is a bucket handle tear or not, and let them decide from a clinical standpoint.

The third pitfall to be aware of in using the bowtie sign is that the sign only works if the entire meniscus is covered with sagittal images. If the tech doesn't begin the sagittal images at the far medial or lateral aspects of the knee, the meniscus will not be imaged in its entirety. One will quickly learn to appreciate whether or not the entire meniscus is covered; nevertheless, I like to have an axial scout image with the cursors present photographed on every case (Fig. 9–11).

A discoid meniscus is a large disc-like meniscus that can have many different shapes—lens shaped, wedged, flat, and others. It is not known if it is congenital or acquired, but most are found in children or young adults. It is seen laterally in up to 3 per cent of the population, with a discoid medial meniscus being much less common. A discoid meniscus is felt to be more prone to tear than a normal meniscus and can be symptomatic even without being torn. Although they are easily identified on coronal images by noting meniscal tissue extending into the tibial spines at the intercondylar notch (Fig. 9–12), they are most reliably diagnosed by noting more than two consecutive sagittal images that show the meniscus with a bowtie appearance (Fig. 9–13).[4] Hence,

the bowtie sign can be used to diagnose a bucket handle tear (fewer than two bowties) or a discoid meniscus (more than two bowties). If thinner slices than 4 or 5 mm are used, the bowtie sign can be adjusted to whatever slice thickness is employed.

A pseudodiscoid meniscus can be encountered on coronal images through the posterior portion of the meniscus where the "C" of the meniscus curls towards the intercondylar notch (Fig. 9–14). Care should be taken to not call a discoid meniscus on the posterior coronal images, as a pseudodiscoid appearance can be found in every instance. Similarly, if one of the more posterior coronal images goes through the meniscus just anterior to the "C," it can give the appearance of a bucket handle tear with a free fragment flipped into the intercondylar notch (Fig. 9–15). This is termed a pseudobucket handle tear and is only occasionally encountered. Both of these pitfalls can be avoided by simply using the bowtie sign to make the diagnosis of a discoid or a bucket handle tear.

The lateral meniscus often has what appears to be a tear on the anterior horn near its upper margin, which is a pseudotear from the insertion of the transverse ligament (Fig. 9–16). This can easily be differentiated from a real tear by fol-

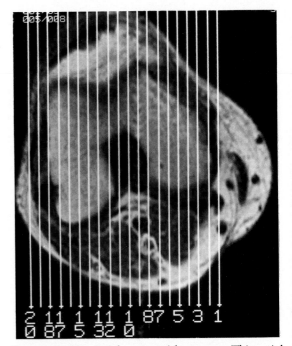

FIGURE 9–11 Axial scout with cursors. This axial scout image shows the cursors for the sagittal images. Note that they completely cover the menisci medially to laterally.

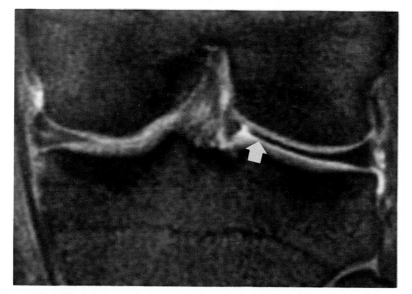

FIGURE 9–12   Discoid lateral meniscus. A coronal GRASS image through the intercondylar notch shows a large lateral meniscus with meniscal tissue extending into the notch medially (arrow).

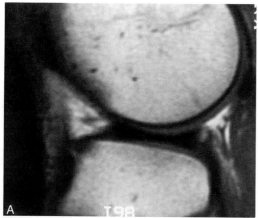

FIGURE 9–13 Discoid lateral meniscus. Three consecutive 5-mm thick T1-weighted images through the lateral meniscus, beginning with the most lateral *(A)* and extending medially *(B* and *C)*; each show the meniscus to have a bowtie configuration. Since only two images should have a bowtie shape, indicative of the body of the meniscus, this is diagnostic of a discoid lateral meniscus (Fig. 9–12 is a coronal GRASS image of the same knee). (Anterior is to the left.)

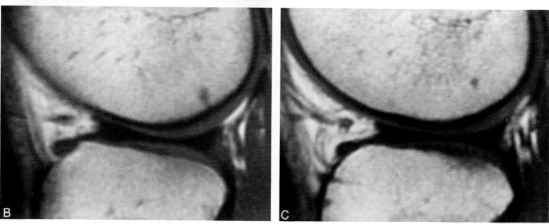

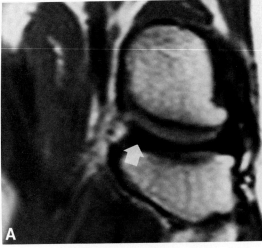

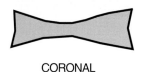

FIGURE 9–14   Pseudodiscoid meniscus. *(A)* This T1-weighted coronal image shows an apparent discoid lateral meniscus that extends into the intercondylar notch medially (arrow). *(B)* This drawing shows how a coronal image though the posterior part of the meniscus can give a normal meniscus a discoid appearance. This is called a pseudodiscoid meniscus.

B

CORONAL

Ant.

Imaging Plane

Post.

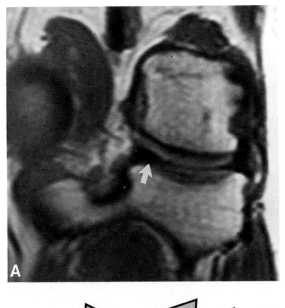

FIGURE 9–15   Pseudobucket handle tear. *(A)* This coronal T1-weighted image shows a triangular-shaped piece of meniscus (arrow), an apparent free fragment near the intercondylar notch that is often seen with a bucket handle tear that has a free fragment. *(B)* This drawing shows how a coronal image though the posterior part of a normal meniscus can give the appearance of a free fragment in the intercondylar notch. This is called a pseudobucket handle tear. The meniscus in *(A)* was normal.

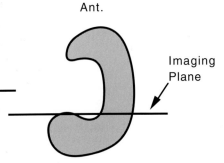

B

CORONAL

Ant.

Imaging Plane

Post.

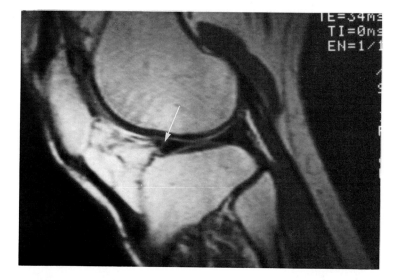

FIGURE 9–16 Pseudotear from a transverse ligament. A sagittal T1-weighted image through the lateral meniscus shows linear high signal through the upper anterior horn (arrow), which resembles a tear. This is the insertion of the transverse ligament onto the meniscus (see Fig. 9–1B for another example). (Anterior is to the left.)

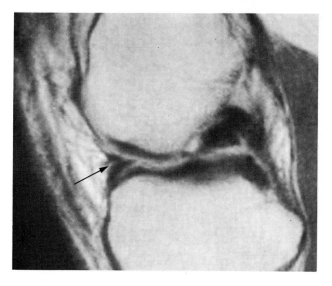

FIGURE 9–17 Pseudotear from a transverse ligament. A sagittal T1-weighted image through the medial meniscus shows linear high signal through the upper anterior horn (arrow), which resembles a tear. This is the insertion of the transverse ligament onto the medial meniscus, similar to that seen more commonly on the lateral meniscus. (Anterior is to the left.)

lowing it medially across the knee in Hoffa's fat pad to where it inserts onto the anterior horn of the medial meniscus. Although less common than on the lateral meniscus, a pseudotear from the insertion of the transverse ligament onto the anterior horn of the medial meniscus can be seen (Fig. 9–17).

CRUCIATE LIGAMENTS

The cruciate ligaments probably cause more consternation to the beginner than any other structure in the knee. I'm not sure why, but I do remember that they seemed very difficult to evaluate when I first started. In fact, MR imaging of the cruciate ligaments is more accurate than is MR imaging of the menisci, with accuracy reported near 100 per cent in several published series.[5,6]

The normal anterior cruciate ligament (ACL) is seen in the intercondylar notch as a linear, predominantly low-signal structure on T1-weighted images that often shows some linear striations near its insertion onto the medial tibial spine when viewed on sagittal images (Fig. 9–18A). T2 or T2* images are imperative for obtaining the highest accuracy in diagnosing ACL tears, as fluid and hemorrhage will often obscure the ligament on T1-weighted images (Fig. 9–18B and C).

A torn ACL is most often simply not visualized (Fig. 9–19), although sometimes the actual disruption will be seen (Fig. 9–20). Partial tears or strains of the ACL are manifested by high signal within an otherwise intact ligament. The diagnosis of a partial tear or strain is generally not critical on MR imaging as the treatment afforded the patient is dependent solely on the di-

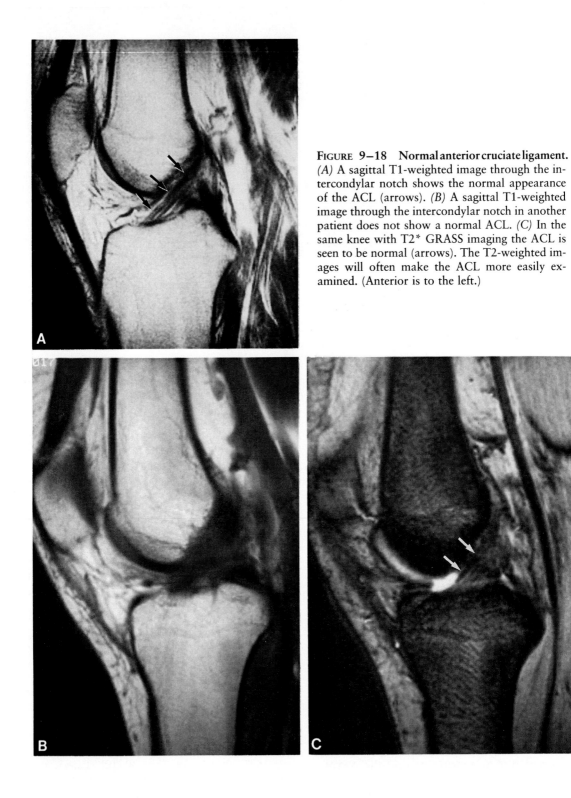

FIGURE 9–18 Normal anterior cruciate ligament. *(A)* A sagittal T1-weighted image through the intercondylar notch shows the normal appearance of the ACL (arrows). *(B)* A sagittal T1-weighted image through the intercondylar notch in another patient does not show a normal ACL. *(C)* In the same knee with T2* GRASS imaging the ACL is seen to be normal (arrows). The T2-weighted images will often make the ACL more easily examined. (Anterior is to the left.)

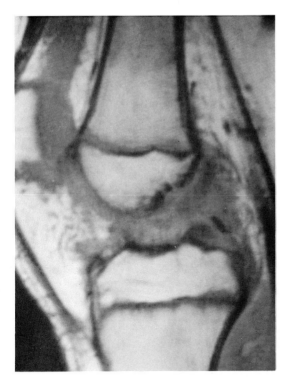

FIGURE 9–19 Torn anterior cruciate ligament. This proton density image through the intercondylar notch fails to show the ACL. This is a fairly typical example of a completely torn ACL. Care should be taken to confirm this appearance on a T2-weighted image, however. (Anterior is to the left.)

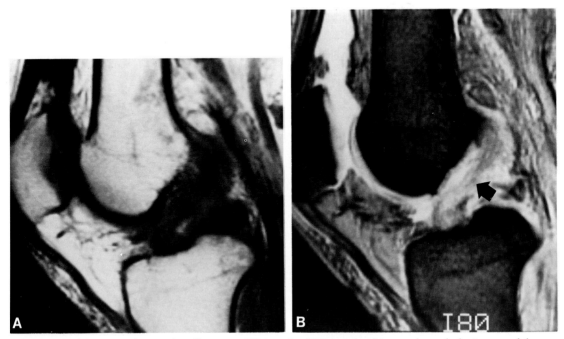

FIGURE 9–20 Torn anterior cruciate ligament. *(A)* A sagittal T1-weighted image through the intercondylar notch does not reveal a definite structure that resembles a normal ACL. This is a common MR imaging appearance of a torn ACL. *(B)* A sagittal GRASS image in the same knee shows fibers of the torn ACL, which are disrupted centrally (arrow). (Anterior is to the left.)

agnosis of a complete tear. In most instances the arthroscopist cannot tell a partial tear from an intact ACL.

The normal posterior cruciate ligament (PCL) is a gently curved, uniformly low signal structure (Fig. 9–21), which is infrequently torn and even less frequently repaired by surgeons. When torn it takes on diffuse intermediate signal throughout (Fig. 9–22). Most orthopedic surgeons do not even inspect the PCL at arthroscopy and do not repair it when torn because it rarely is a cause of instability. A former fellow I worked with tried to publish an MR imaging sign for a torn PCL. After collecting a dozen cases with torn posterior cruciates he got the operative reports from the patients' records. We were surprised to find that not one surgeon even mentioned the PCL in any of the cases! We called a few of the surgeons and each gave the same answer—they virtually never repair the PCL because it does not lead to instability; hence they don't even bother to look at it during arthroscopy. While not all surgeons subscribe to this philosophy, most do. If yours does, it's a kind of freedom you have in looking at the posterior cruciate. You can tell them it's tied in a knot and it won't matter.

A low signal round structure is often seen just anterior or posterior to the PCL on the sagittal views. A loose body or a free fragment of a piece of torn meniscus can have this appearance (Fig. 9–23), but it is most commonly due to a meniscofemoral ligament, which extends obliquely across the knee from the medial femoral condyle to the posterior horn of the lateral meniscus (Fig. 9–24). If it passes in front of the PCL it is called

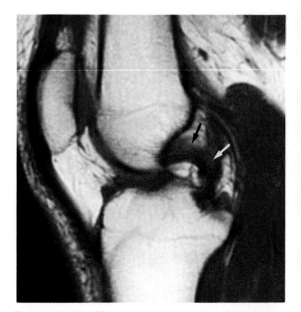

FIGURE 9–22 **Torn posterior cruciate ligament.** A sagittal T1-weighted image through the intercondylar notch reveals the PCL to have diffuse intermediate signal throughout (arrows). This is typical for a torn PCL. (Anterior is to the left.)

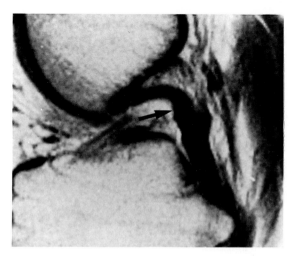

FIGURE 9–21 **Normal posterior cruciate ligament.** A sagittal T1-weighted image through the intercondylar notch shows the appearance of the normal PCL with its characteristic uniform low signal (arrow). (Anterior is to the left.)

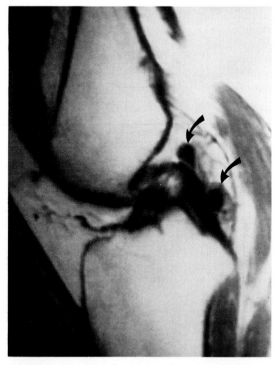

FIGURE 9–23 **Free fragment of a torn meniscus.** A sagittal T1-weighted image through the intercondylar notch in this patient with a torn meniscus shows two rounded low-signal structures (arrows), which are free fragments of meniscal tissue. A meniscofemoral ligament of Wrisberg could have the appearance of either of these loose bodies. (Anterior is to the left.)

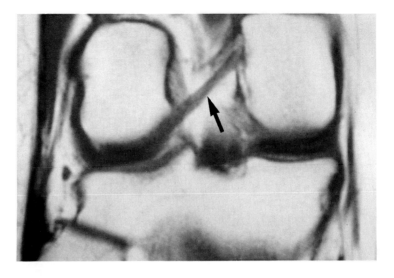

FIGURE 9–24 Ligament of Wrisberg. This coronal T1-weighted image shows an obliquely oriented structure (arrow) extending from the medial femoral condyle to the lateral meniscus. This is a normal ligament of Wrisberg.

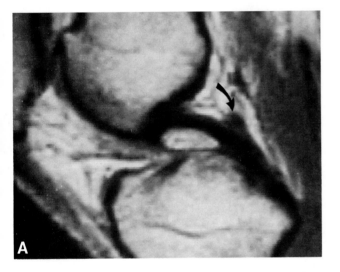

FIGURE 9–25 Ligament of Wrisberg. *(A)* A sagittal T1-weighted image through the intercondylar notch shows a rounded low-signal structure posterior to the posterior cruciate ligament, which is the meniscofemoral ligament of Wrisberg (arrow). *(B)* This drawing shows the relationship of the ligaments of Wrisberg and Humphry to the posterior cruciate ligament. (Anterior is to the left.)

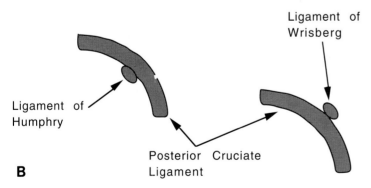

the ligament of Humphry, and if it passes behind the PCL it is the ligament of Wrisberg (Fig. 9–25). One or the other is present in up to 72 per cent of all knees. In fewer than 5 per cent of cases both will be present.

The insertion of the ligament of Humphry or Wrisberg onto the lateral meniscus can produce a pseudotear similar to that caused by the trans-

verse ligament on the anterior horn of the lateral meniscus (Fig. 9–26). Prior to calling a tear on the upper aspect of the posterior horn of the lateral meniscus, care must be taken to look for a meniscofemoral ligament to be certain it is not a pseudotear from the ligament's insertion. Similarly, prior to calling a loose body in front of or behind the PCL, care must be taken to try and

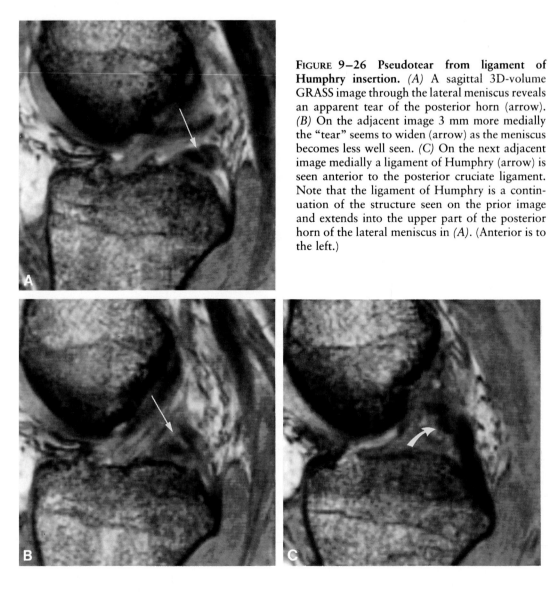

FIGURE 9–26 **Pseudotear from ligament of Humphry insertion.** *(A)* A sagittal 3D-volume GRASS image through the lateral meniscus reveals an apparent tear of the posterior horn (arrow). *(B)* On the adjacent image 3 mm more medially the "tear" seems to widen (arrow) as the meniscus becomes less well seen. *(C)* On the next adjacent image medially a ligament of Humphry (arrow) is seen anterior to the posterior cruciate ligament. Note that the ligament of Humphry is a continuation of the structure seen on the prior image and extends into the upper part of the posterior horn of the lateral meniscus in *(A)*. (Anterior is to the left.)

follow the structure across to the lateral meniscus to determine if it is a meniscofemoral ligament.

COLLATERAL LIGAMENTS

The medial collateral ligament (MCL) originates on the medial femoral condyle and inserts on the tibia. It is closely applied to the joint and is intimately associated with the medial joint capsule and the medial meniscus. The MCL is uniformly low in signal on all imaging sequences. Injuries to the MCL usually occur from a valgus stress, a blow to the lateral part of the knee. A grade 1 injury represents a mild sprain and is diagnosed on MR imaging by noting fluid or hemorrhage in the soft tissues medial to the MCL (Fig. 9–27). The ligament is otherwise normal.

A grade 2 injury is a partial tear and is seen as high signal in and around the MCL on T2 or T2* coronal sequences. The ligament is intact, although the deep or superficial fibers may show minimal disruption. A grade 3 injury is a complete disruption of the MCL. It can be best appreciated on T2 or T2* images (Fig. 9–28). It is unusual for a surgeon to operate on an MCL unless it is a complete disruption, and even then it must be accompanied by another abnormality such as an ACL tear. MCL partial tears, and even complete tears, heal quite nicely simply with immobilization.

A meniscocapsular separation occurs when the medial meniscus is torn from its attachment to the joint capsule. It occurs most commonly at the site of the MCL and often occurs concomitantly

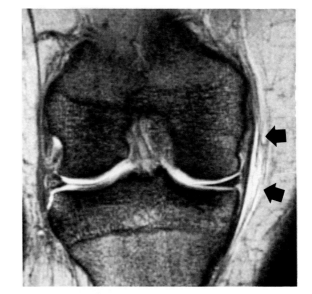

FIGURE 9–27   **Partial tear or sprain of the medial collateral ligament.** A GRASS coronal image reveals high signal in the soft tissues adjacent to the MCL (arrows), which represents edema and hemorrhage from a sprain of the MCL. The MCL is clearly intact; hence a complete tear is easily excluded.

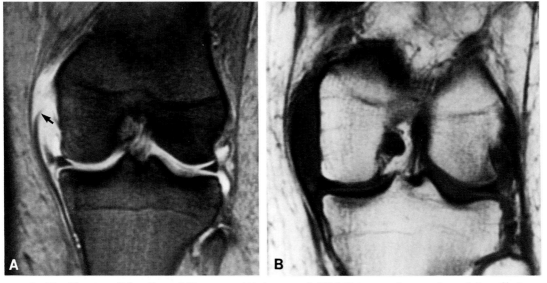

FIGURE 9–28   **Torn medial collateral ligament.** *(A)* A coronal GRASS image shows a large joint effusion with the MCL disrupted proximally (arrow). In addition, joint fluid can be seen extending between the medial meniscus and the MCL, which indicates a meniscocapsular separation. Neither of these diagnoses could be unequivocally made on the T1-weighted coronal image *(B)*.

with an MCL injury. It is easily recognized on a T2 or T2* coronal image by noting joint fluid extending between the medial meniscus and the capsule. It is essential to use T2 or T2* sequences because a T1-weighted image may not detect the fluid between the meniscus and the capsule. These injuries are often missed because T1-weighted coronal images are employed (Fig. 9–29). They can be overlooked at arthroscopy if they involve only the superficial fibers of the capsule because they

are then essentially extracapsular. It is an important diagnosis to make because it involves a very vascular portion of the meniscus; hence it will readily heal with immobilization or with suturing by the surgeon. If overlooked and continued activity occurs, it can lose the vascular interface and never heal.

The lateral collateral ligament consists of three parts. The most posterior structure is the tendon of the biceps femoris, which inserts onto the head

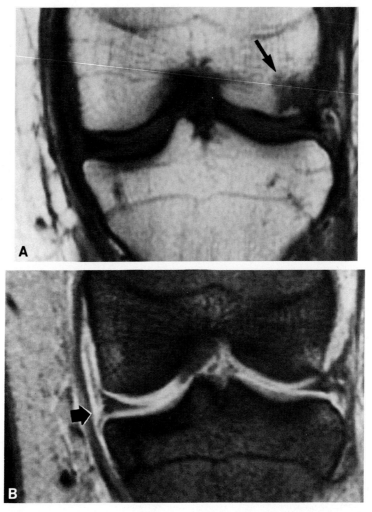

FIGURE 9–29 **Meniscocapsular separation.** *(A)* A T1-weighted coronal image reveals a contusion of the lateral femoral condyle (arrow) indicative of a valgus strain, which is often associated with an MCL tear. The MCL appears normal on this image; however, the linear low signal in the soft tissues just adjacent to the MCL is suggestive of fluid. This would indicate a partial tear or sprain of the MCL. *(B)* A coronal GRASS image in the same knee reveals fluid between the medial meniscus and the MCL (arrow), which is diagnostic for a meniscocapsular separation. Faint high signal in the MCL and adjacent to it indicate a partial tear. A T2 or T2* sequence in the coronal plane are necessary to see these abnormalities.

of the fibula. Next, anterior to the biceps, is the true lateral collateral ligament, also called the fibulocollateral ligament, which extends from the lateral femoral condyle to the head of the fibula (Fig. 9–30). The biceps and the fibulocollateral ligament usually join and insert onto the head of the fibula in a conjoined manner. Anterior to the fibulocollateral ligament is the iliotibial band, which extends into the fascia more anteriorly and blends into the lateral retinaculum on the patella. The lateral collateral ligament is infrequently torn.

PATELLA

The patellar cartilage commonly undergoes degeneration causing exquisite pain and tenderness. This is called chondromalacia patella. It can be diagnosed on sagittal images but is generally more reliably identified on axial images. Since hyaline articular cartilage has the same signal intensity as joint fluid on T1-weighted sequences, T2 or T2* sequences are necessary to diagnose chondromalacia patella in most instances.

Chondromalacia patella begins with focal

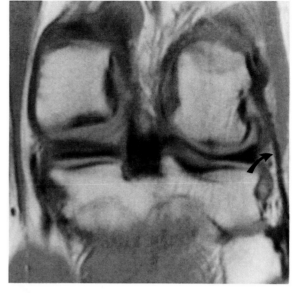

FIGURE 9–30 Normal lateral collateral ligament. This coronal T1-weighted image shows a normal fibulocollateral ligament (lateral collateral ligament) (arrow) extending from the lateral femoral condyle to the fibular head.

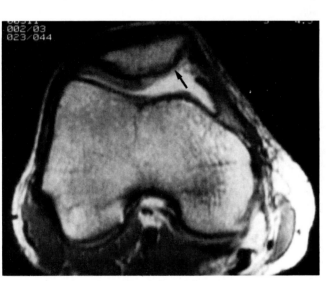

FIGURE 9–31 Chondromalacia patella. An axial T2-weighted image through the patella in a patient who dislocated his patella shows virtually no cartilage covering the medial facet (arrow). The hyaline articular cartilage was knocked off when the patella banged against the lateral femoral condyle during reduction. T2 weighting is necessary to distinguish joint fluid from cartilage.

swelling and degeneration of the cartilage. This can be seen as low- or high-signal foci in the cartilage. As it progresses it causes thinning and irregularity of the articular surface of the cartilage, and finally underlying bone is exposed. This final stage occurs more commonly from trauma than from wear and tear (Fig. 9–31).

A normal structure that is seen in over half of the population is the medial patellar plica. It is an embryologic remnant from when the knee was divided into three compartments. It is a thin fibrous band that extends from the medial capsule towards, and sometimes onto, the medial facet of the patella (Fig. 9–32). A suprapatellar and infrapatellar plica can also be present. The medial patellar plica can on rare occasions thicken and

cause clinical symptoms indistinguishable from a torn meniscus, which has been termed plica syndrome (Fig. 9–33). T2 or T2* images are necessary to visualize a plica in most instances. An abnormal plica can be easily removed arthroscopically.

An abnormality that can clinically mimic plica syndrome, as well as mimic a torn meniscus, is pes anserinus bursitis. Three tendons, the sartorius, gracilis, and semitendinosus (remembered by the mnemonic "Some Girls Stand"), insert onto the anteromedial aspect of the tibia in a fan-shaped manner that has been likened to a goose's foot, hence the name pes anserinus. A bursa lies beneath the insertion site, which can become inflamed and cause medial joint line or patellar pain

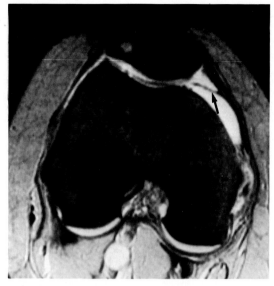

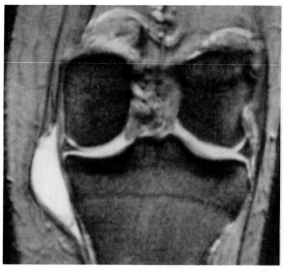

FIGURE 9–32 Plica. An axial GRASS image through the patella shows a low-signal linear structure (arrow) extending from the medial capsule towards the medial facet of the patella. This is a normal medial patellar plica. Without the joint effusion or the T2 weighting the plica would not be visualized.

FIGURE 9–34 Pes anserinus bursitus. A coronal T2* GRASS image shows a fluid collection below the medial joint line near the insertion of the pes anserinus tendons. This is pes anserinus bursitus.

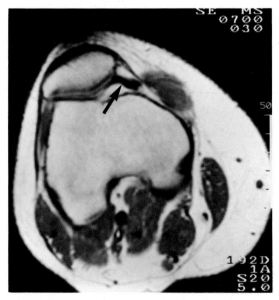

FIGURE 9–33 Thickened medial patellar plica. This axial T1-weighted image shows a thickened medial patellar plica (arrow). This could represent merely a small joint effusion; however, T2-weighted images in another plane showed no joint fluid present. This patient presented with a painful clicking knee, symptoms typical for either a torn meniscus or plica syndrome.

that can be confused with plica syndrome or a torn medial meniscus (Fig. 9–34). Making the diagnosis of pes anserinus bursitus with MR imaging can prevent an unnecessary arthroscopy procedure—one in which the pes anserinus bursitus would be overlooked since it is an extracapsular structure.

BONY ABNORMALITIES

The most frequently encountered bony abnormality seen with MR imaging is a contusion. A contusion represents micro-fractures from trauma.[7] They are also called bone bruises. They are easily identified on T1-weighted sequences as subarticular areas of inhomogeneous low signal (Fig. 9–35). With T2-weighting a contusion will show increased signal for several weeks, depending on its severity. It can be difficult to see increased signal with T2* images because of the susceptibility artifacts of the bone inherent with T2* images. Contusions can progress to osteochondritis dissecans if they are not treated with diminished weight bearing; hence an isolated bone contusion, with no other internal derangement, is a serious finding that requires treatment.

A commonly seen contusion is one that occurs on the posterior part of the lateral tibial plateau (Fig. 9–36). It is invariably associated with a torn

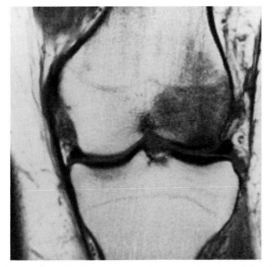

FIGURE 9–35 Contusion. A coronal T1-weighted image shows a focus of low signal in the lateral femoral condyle, which is subarticular. This is a characteristic appearance for a severe bone contusion.

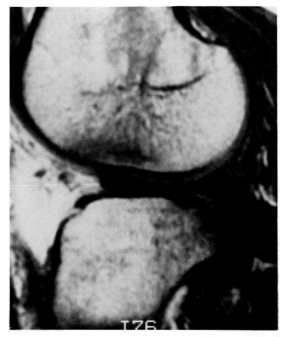

FIGURE 9–36 Contusions. A sagittal T1-weighted image through the lateral compartment shows irregular low signal in a subarticular location in the posterior tibial plateau and in the anterior part of the lateral femoral condyle. These findings are characteristic for bone contusions. This distribution of contusions in the posterior lateral tibial plateau and anterior in the lateral femoral condyle is almost always associated with a torn anterior cruciate ligament. (Anterior is to the left.)

ACL. Acute ACL tears have been reported to have this type of contusion in over 90 per cent of cases.[8]

MR imaging is useful in examining fractures about the knee. Tibial plateau fractures can be imaged precisely with computed tomography; however, MR imaging allows the soft tissues, including internal derangements, to be seen in addition to any bony abnormalities.

REFERENCES

1. Ruwe P, Wright J, Randall R, Lynch J, Jokl P, McCarthy S: Can MR imaging effectively replace diagnostic arthroscopy? Radiology 1992;183: 335–339.
2. Crues JI, Mink J, Levy T, Lotysch M, Stoller D: Meniscal tears of the knee: Accuracy of MR imaging. Radiology 1987;164:445–448.
3. Mink JH, Deutsch AL: Magnetic resonance imaging of the knee. Clin Orthop Relat Res 1989;244: 29–47.
4. Silverman J, Mink J, Deutsch A: Discoid menisci of the knee: MR imaging appearance. Radiology 1989;173:351–354.
5. Lee J, Yao L, Phelps C, Wirth C, Czajka J, Lozman J: Anterior cruciate ligament tears: MR imaging compared with arthroscopy and clinical tests. Radiology 1988;166:861–864.
6. Mink J, Levy T, Crues JI: Tears of the anterior cruciate ligament and menisci of the knee: MR imaging evaluation. Radiology 1988;167:769–774.
7. Mink JH, Deutsch AL: Occult cartilage and bone injuries of the knee: Detection, classification, and assessment with MR imaging. Radiology 1989; 170:823–829.
8. Murphy B, Smith R, Uribe J, Janecki C, Hechtman K, Mangasarian R: Bone signal abnormalities in the posterolateral tibia and lateral femoral condyle in complete tears of the anterior cruciate ligament: A specific sign? Radiology 1992;182:221–224.

Chapter

10

MR Imaging of the Shoulder

Magnetic resonance (MR) imaging of the shoulder is probably the most difficult exam to interpret that I see on a regular basis. It is a still-evolving exam so far as its diagnostic utility for abnormalities of the rotator cuff and the glenoid labrum are concerned. It has been shown by some investigators to have a high degree of accuracy,[1–4] while others report a barely acceptable rate of accuracy. Although there is currently some controversy over its utility, MR imaging of the shoulder is nevertheless replacing standard arthrography and computed tomography (CT) arthrography for examining the rotator cuff and the glenoid labrum.

ANATOMY

The rotator cuff is comprised of the tendons of four muscles that converge on the greater and lesser tuberosities of the humerus: the supraspinatus, infraspinatus, subscapularis, and teres minor (Fig. 10–1). Of these, the supraspinatus is the one that most commonly causes clinically significant problems and is almost exclusively the one that is addressed surgically.

The supraspinatus tendon lies just superior to the scapula and inferior to the acromioclavicular joint and the acromion. In inserts into the greater tuberosity of the humerus. Two to 3 cm proximal to its insertion is a section of the tendon called the "critical zone." This area is reported to have decreased vascularity and is therefore less likely to heal following trauma. It is also the area of the tendon that undergoes fibrillar and myxoid degeneration (also called tendinopathy), presumably from aging and trauma although this has not

been proved. The critical zone of the supraspinatus tendon is where the vast majority of rotator cuff tears occur.

The glenoid labrum is a fibrocartilagenous ring that surrounds the periphery of the bony glenoid of the scapula. It serves as an attachment site for the capsule and broadens the base of the glenohumeral joint to allow increased stability. Tears of the glenoid labrum most commonly occur from, and result in, humeral head instability and dislocations.

IMAGING PROTOCOL

There are many variations in the imaging protocol that are all acceptable for showing normal and pathologic findings in the shoulder. The rotator cuff, that is, the supraspinatus tendon, is best seen on oblique coronal images that are aligned parallel to the supraspinatus muscle (Fig. 10–2). Both T1- and T2-weighted sequences, or acceptable variations, are mandatory. The most commonly employed protocol is a spin-echo proton density and T2-weighted sequence. Some prefer to use a spin-echo T1-weighted image in conjunction with a GRASS or other type of T2* sequence. A more recent addition, as a substitute for more conventional T2-weighted images is a fast spin-echo T2 with fat saturation. The slice thickness should be no greater than 5 mm, and 3 mm is preferable. As with most joint imaging, a small field of view (FOV) (16–20 cm) is recommended. A dedicated shoulder coil or a surface coil placed anteriorly over the shoulder is necessary, although no particular type of shoulder coil appears to be clearly superior.

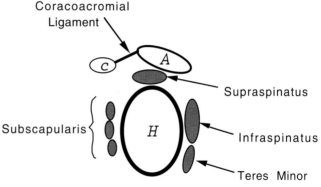

FIGURE 10–1 **Schematic of shoulder anatomy.** This drawing shows the rotator cuff muscles in a sagittal plane (C = coracoid; A = acromion; H = humeral head; anterior is on the left).

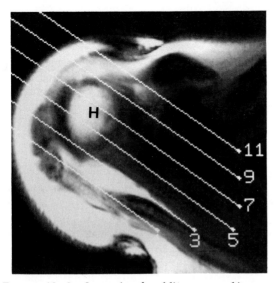

FIGURE 10–2 **Scout view for oblique coronal images.** This axial image through the supraspinatus shows the cursors angled along the plane of the supraspinatus muscle (anterior on top; H = humeral head).

The glenoid labrum is best seen on axial T2-weighted images. T1-weighted images do not give any additional information and can be eliminated. If a joint effusion is present, the labrum is easily identified. Without fluid in the joint it can be more difficult to clearly see the labrum; therefore, some radiologists will perform an MR arthrogram. Either saline alone, or saline mixed with a small amount of gadolinium (a ratio of 1:250 is recommended), can be injected into the joint followed by MR imaging. MR arthrography is not recommended as a routine part of shoulder imaging.

Most MR imaging shoulder protocols include an oblique sagittal sequence with the plane of imaging perpendicular to the oblique coronal sequence. This sequence gives very little useful information, and, in fact, we discarded it entirely for several years before recently reinstating it.

When T2 or T2* weighting is employed, fluid in the subacromial bursa can occasionally be seen to better advantage than on the oblique coronal images. Also, this is the only sequence in which the shape of the acromion can be reliably identified, although it is not critical to note the shape of the acromion.

ROTATOR CUFF

The rotator cuff commonly suffers from what has been termed impingement syndrome. This was first described by Neer, an orthopedic surgeon, who claims that 95 per cent of all rotator cuff tears occur from impingement syndrome.[5] Impingement of the critical zone of the supraspinatus tendon occurs from abduction or flexion of the humerus, which allows the tendon to be impinged between the anterior acromion and the greater tuberosity. The tendon can also be impinged by the undersurface of the acromioclavicular (AC) joint if downward pointing osteophytes or a thickened capsule are present. Other theories exist for impingement syndrome, including natural degeneration from aging and a predisposition for the critical zone to undergo degeneration due to decreased blood supply.[6] Most investigators agree that, whatever the cause, the natural course of impingement syndrome leads to a complete, or full-thickness, tear of the rotator cuff.

Treatment of impingement syndrome consists of rest, subacromial bursa steroid injections, and, if refractory to conservative care, surgery. Surgery involves removal of the anterior third of the acromion, resection of the coracoacromial ligament, and removal of any irregularities on the undersurface of the AC joint. If a tear of the supraspinatus tendon is present, it is repaired. Because the treatment for impingement syndrome is the same whether or not an actual cuff tear is present or not, the role of imaging in the diagnosis of cuff abnormalities has been questioned by some prominent surgeons.[7]

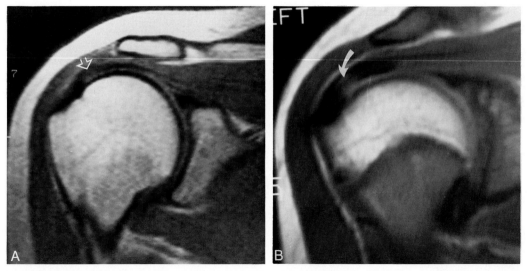

FIGURE 10–3 **Normal supraspinatus tendon.** *(A)* A T1-weighted oblique coronal image shows a normal supraspinatus tendon (arrow) with uninterrupted low signal extending from the musculotendinous junction to the insertion on the greater tuberosity. *(B)* A T1-weighted oblique coronal image in an asymptomatic 11-year-old girl shows some increased signal in the critical zone of the supraspinatus tendon (arrow). As described in the text, there are many reasons why this can be found in the normal shoulder. It is imperative to note that the high signal does not increase on T2-weighted images.

In examining the rotator cuff the anterior most oblique coronal images will show the critical zone of the supraspinatus tendon. A useful landmark for noting the supraspinatus tendon is the AC joint, which is an anterior structure and usually easily located. The infraspinatus tendon is seen on the more posterior images and can easily be mistaken for the tendon of the supraspinatus. The supraspinatus tendon can be differentiated from the infraspinatus by noting the more horizontal course of the supraspinatus as compared to the infraspinatus, which runs obliquely inferiorly to superiorly.

The normal supraspinatus tendon is said to be uniformly low in signal on all pulse sequences (Fig. 10–3A). Unfortunately, this is not always the case. In fact, it usually has some intermediate to high signal in the critical zone (Fig. 10–3B), which has caused much confusion in the evolution of interpreting shoulder MR imaging exams. We imaged around twenty "normal" volunteers (residents and fellows) in the early days of learning shoulder MR imaging, and only found one or two that had uniform low signal throughout the critical zone. This was very distressing because the literature at that time said any high signal in the critical zone meant it was abnormal. We know now that there are many causes for intermediate to high signal on T1-weighted images in the normal shoulder.

If the signal in the critical zone gets brighter on the T2-weighted images, it is abnormal and represents either tendonitis or a partial tear (severe tendonitis) (Fig. 10–4). However, if it disappears or has the same signal intensity as the adjacent muscle on T2-weighted sequences, it may represent one of many different processes:

1. Partial volume averaging of peritendinous fat can cause some high signal in the supraspinatous tendon on the oblique coronal images that does not get brighter on T2-weighted images (Fig 10–5).

2. If the plane of the oblique coronal images is slightly off of the plane of the tendon, muscle slips can be partially volume-averaged, which may appear as relatively high signal on T1-weighted images but will not get brighter with T2 images (Fig. 10–6).

3. The so-called "magic angle" effect can cause apparent high signal in a tendon that lies at 55 degrees to the bore of the magnet (as does the critical zone of the supraspinatus tendon).[8] This high signal will not be seen on T2-weighted images (or any sequence with a long TE). This is felt to be a common cause of high signal in the critical zone on T1-weighted images.

4. Myxoid and fibrillar degeneration of the supraspinatus tendon are commonly found in autopsy specimens, which increase with age. The majority of asymptomatic shoulders in patients over the age of 50 are felt to have some tendon degeneration in the supraspinatous, which has been termed

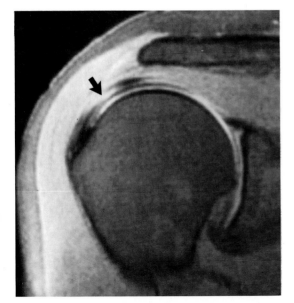

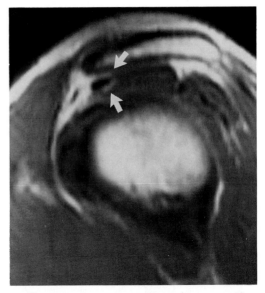

FIGURE 10–4 Partial tear of the supraspinatus. A T2-weighted oblique coronal image with fat-saturation shows high signal in the critical zone of the supraspinatus tendon (arrow) with the tendon appearing very irregular. A small amount of fluid is seen in the subacromial bursa. Arthroscopy confirmed a partial tear on the bursal side of the supraspinatus tendon.

FIGURE 10–5 Fat surrounding the supraspinatus tendon. This oblique sagittal T1-weighted image shows fat surrounding the supraspinatus tendon (arrows). It is easy to imagine some of that fat being partially volume-averaged and giving some high signal on the oblique coronal images. (Anterior is to the left.)

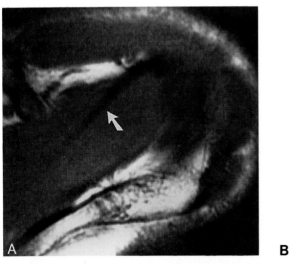

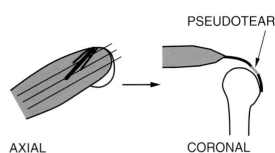

FIGURE 10–6 Steeply angled supraspinatus tendon. *(A)* An axial image through the belly of the supraspinatus muscle shows a tendon (arrow) that is steeply angled in relation to the muscle. (Anterior is to the top.) *(B)* This drawing of the supraspinatus muscle as seen in the axial plane shows a steeply angled tendon that would not be parallel to the usual plane of imaging. This can result in an apparent "gap" on the oblique coronal images.

"tendinopathy." This is seen as high signal in the critical zone on T1-weighted images that does not increase with T2 weighting.[9] Similar to the myxoid degeneration that occurs in the menisci of the knee, it has not been shown that this is symptomatic.

5. Marked internal rotation of the humeral head can cause the infraspinatus tendon to lie superior to the supraspinatus tendon and cause an apparent "gap" in the supraspinatus tendon on the oblique coronal image when both tendons are seen on the

same slice.[10] Care should be taken to study the patient with the arm in a neutral position or in external rotation.

6. Calcium deposits in the brain and lumbar spine discs have been described to occasionally cause high signal on T1-weighted images. Since calcium is often found in the critical zone of the supraspinatus tendon, it is reasonable to assume that these calcium deposits could occasionally be a source of intermediate to high signal on T1-weighted images. As in the brain and spine, the high signal on T1-weighted images would disappear or decrease on T2-weighted images.

Since high signal can be seen in the critical zone of the supraspinatus in a variety of normal situations, how can one differentiate the normal from the abnormal? So long as the T2-weighted images do not show the signal getting brighter, it probably does not matter. Tendon degeneration (tendinopathy) can be seen in asymptomatic shoulders of all ages; hence it needs to be correlated with the clinical picture. If the signal gets brighter on T2-weighted images, it must be considered pathologic—either tendonitis or a partial tear. If, in addition, fluid is present in the subacromial bursa, a small full-thickness tear should be mentioned as a possibility even if a definite

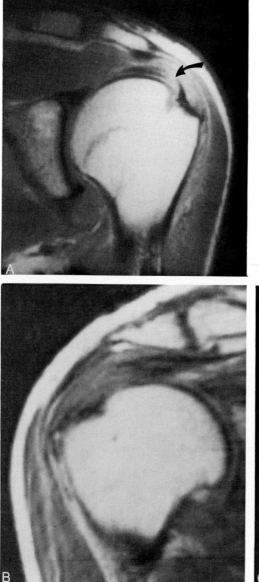

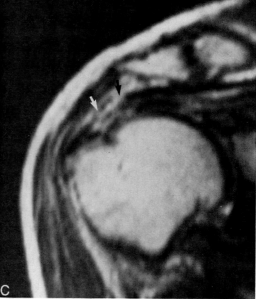

FIGURE 10–7 Torn supraspinatus. *(A)* An oblique coronal proton-density image shows disruption of the supraspinatus tendon (arrow) and a large amount of fluid in the subacromial bursa, which is seen surrounding the torn tendon. *(B)* This oblique coronal proton-density image fails to show a low signal supraspinatus tendon in the expected region of the critical zone. *(C)* In the same patient this T2-weighted image shows disruption of the supraspinatus tendon and fluid in the subacromial bursa (arrows).

tendon disruption cannot be seen. A small amount of fluid can be seen in the subacromial bursa because of a partial tear, but if a substantial amount of fluid is found, a full-thickness tear is almost certainly present.

If disruption of the supraspinatus tendon can be seen, obviously a full-thickness tear is present. In these cases fluid is invariably present in the subacromial bursa (Fig. 10–7). Care should be taken to look for retraction of the supraspinatus muscle, as marked retraction will obviate some types of surgery.

I have found that three basic categories exist for the appearance of the supraspinatus tendon:
1. *Normal*—high signal on T1-weighted images that does not get brighter on T2-weighted images. This can represent one of several processes in a normal tendon or myxoid degeneration, also called tendinopathy. This should basically be considered "normal" as it has not been proved that tendinopathy is symptomatic.
2. *Tendonitis*—high signal on T1-weighted images that gets brighter on T2-weighted sequences. Little or no fluid is present in the subacromial bursa. This represents tendonitis or a partial tear.
3. *Cuff tear*—tendon disruption and/or a large amount of fluid is present in the subacromial bursa with high signal in the critical zone on T1 and T2 images.

It is generally easy to place the MR imaging appearance of the rotator cuff into one of these three categories, and a high degree of accuracy in diagnosing the state of the rotator cuff can be expected.

BONY ABNORMALITIES

The undersurface of the anterior acromion and the AC joint should be examined for osteophytes or irregularities that can be responsible for impingement syndrome (Fig. 10–8). In the proper clinical setting an anterior acromioplasty will relieve the symptoms of impingement syndrome and prevent a more serious full-thickness cuff tear. It is imperative that the surgeon also remove any AC joint undersurface irregularity, if present, or a failed surgery can be expected.

The acromion has been classified into three types as seen on the sagittal images (Fig. 10–9). The normal appearance, type 1, is an acromion with a flat or slightly convex undersurface; a type 2 acromion has a concave undersurface; and, a type 3 has a concave undersurface with an anterior osteophyte (Fig. 10–10). Although it has been reported that a type 3 acromion is seen in up to 80 per cent of cuff tears, a type 2 is seen in 20 per cent, and a type 1 has no association

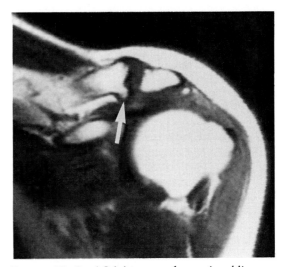

FIGURE 10–8   AC joint osteophytes. An oblique coronal T1-weighted image reveals osteophytes extending inferiorly off of the AC joint (arrow). This is a common source of impingement on the supraspinatus tendon.

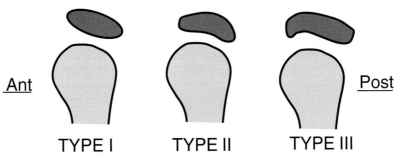

FIGURE 10–9   Schematic of types of acromion. A drawing of the acromion from a sagittal view shows the type 1 having a flat or slightly convex undersurface, a type 2 having a concave undersurface, and a type 3 having a concave undersurface and an anterior osteophyte or "hook."

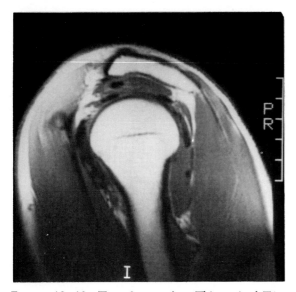

FIGURE 10–10 Type 3 acromion. This sagittal T1-weighted image shows the acromion to have a curved undersurface and an anterior "hook." This is a type 3 acromion. It is easy to imagine the supraspinatus tendon, which is just beneath the "hook," being impinged by the "hook" with abduction of the humerus. (Anterior is to the left.)

with a torn cuff, this has not been substantiated, and it is certainly not my experience. I frequently see cuff tears with a type 1 acromion, and I often see no cuff tear when a type 3 acromion is present.

Abnormalities of the humeral head include sclerosis and cystic changes about the greater tuberosity that are commonly present in patients with impingement syndrome and rotator cuff tears. Bony impaction on the posterosuperior aspect of the humeral head can be seen in patients with anterior instability of the humeral head. This is called a Hill-Sachs lesion and is best identified on the superior-most two or three axial images (Fig. 10–11). The normal humeral head should be round on the superior slices—an irregularity posteriorly is abnormal.

GLENOID LABRUM

Tears of the glenoid labrum result in glenohumeral joint instability. They are commonly caused by dislocations, but less traumatic episodes, such as repeated trauma from throwing, can result in labral tears. Torn or detached labra are often repaired arthroscopically with good results. Although the labrum is imaged exquisitely with CT arthrography, MR imaging is often preferred since it allows the rotator cuff to be seen on the same exam. Labrum and rotator cuff abnormalities often coexist and an abnormality of one can lead to an abnormality in the other.

The normal labrum is a triangular-shaped low-signal structure as viewed on an axial image, with the anterior labrum usually larger than the posterior labrum (Fig. 10–12). The anterior labrum is much more commonly involved with tears than the posterior (98 per cent and 2 per cent, respectively), and the superior labrum is said to be rarely involved. In fact the superior labrum, in my experience, is torn more often than the posterior labrum. The superior labrum is best evaluated on the oblique coronal views. Tears of the superior labrum are called SLAP lesions (Superior Labrum Anterior to Posterior). They are said to be seen mostly in throwing athletes as a result of the insertion of the long head of the biceps tendon

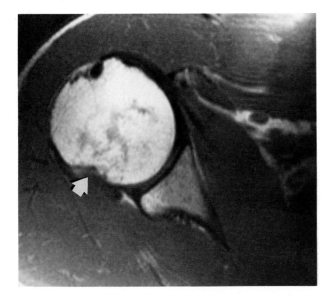

FIGURE 10–11 Hill-Sachs lesion. An axial T1-weighted image through the superior portion of the humeral head shows a posterior impaction (arrow) caused by the glenoid labrum during an anterior dislocation of the humerus. This has been termed a Hill-Sachs lesion.

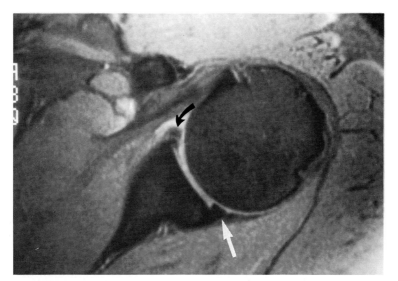

FIGURE 10–12 **Normal labrum.** An axial T2* GRASS image shows a normal anterior (curved black arrow) and posterior (straight white arrow) glenoid labrum. The anterior labrum is usually larger than the posterior.

onto the labrum avulsing part of the labrum during a forceful throwing motion.

If no joint effusion is present, a labral tear can be difficult to see unless it is extremely large. If joint fluid extends between the bony glenoid and the base of the labrum, a detached labrum is present. Tears in the body of the labrum are diagnosed by noting fluid extending into the labrum or by truncation of the labrum (Fig. 10–13). The attachment of the glenohumeral ligaments to the labrum can cause a linear high signal that can mimic a tear (Fig. 10–14), so care must be taken

to be certain high-signal fluid is actually present in the tear.[11]

A useful sign for a torn anterior labrum that has been given the unusual acronym of GLOM sign (Glenoid Labrum Ovoid Mass) is when a low-signal round structure is seen anterior to the anterior glenoid at the base of the coracoid (this is the superior aspect of the glenoid). It represents a torn anterior labrum that is retracted superiorly (Fig. 10–15). It can be the only sign of a torn labrum, meaning the appearance of the labrum is otherwise normal.[12]

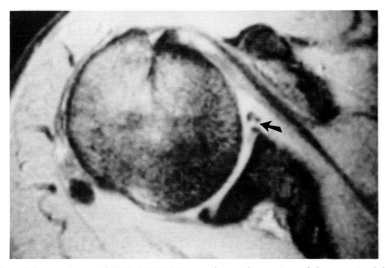

FIGURE 10–13 **Torn labrum.** An axial T2* GRASS image shows disruption of the anterior labrum (arrow). Note the normal posterior labrum for comparison.

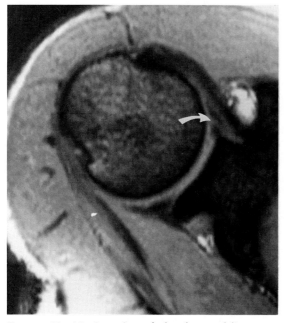

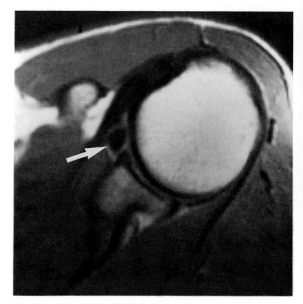

FIGURE 10–14 Insertion of glenohumeral ligament. This axial T2* GRASS image reveals linear intermediate signal extending obliquely across the anterior labrum (arrow), which simulates a tear. This is the insertion of the middle glenohumeral ligament onto the labrum.

FIGURE 10–15 GLOM sign. An axial T2 image through the glenohumeral joint at the level of the coracoid shows an ovoid mass adjacent to the anterior labrum (arrow), which is a torn anterior labrum that has been retracted superiorly.

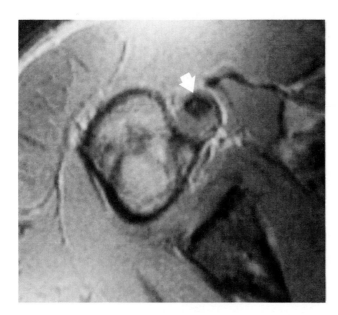

FIGURE 10–16 Biceps tendinitis. An axial T2* GRASS image shows the biceps tendon (arrow) to be swollen and filled with high signal indicating tendonitis.

BICEPS TENDON

The long head of the biceps tendon runs in the bicipital groove between the greater and lesser tuberosities and inserts onto the superior labrum. It can be impinged by an abnormal acromion in the same way the supraspinatus tendon is impinged, resulting in tenosynovitis or tendonitis.

In tenosynovitis fluid can be seen in the tendon sheath surrounding an otherwise normal tendon. Because fluid in the glenohumeral joint can normally fill the biceps tendon sheath, this diagnosis is difficult to make with MR imaging alone. If the tendon is enlarged and/or has signal within it, tendonitis is present (Fig. 10–16). If the tendon

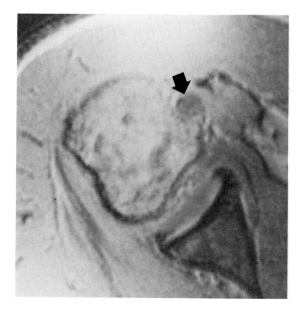

FIGURE 10–17 Ruptured biceps tendon. An axial T2-weighted image shows the biceps tendon sheath filled with fluid (arrow) but with no tendon. This indicates a torn biceps tendon.

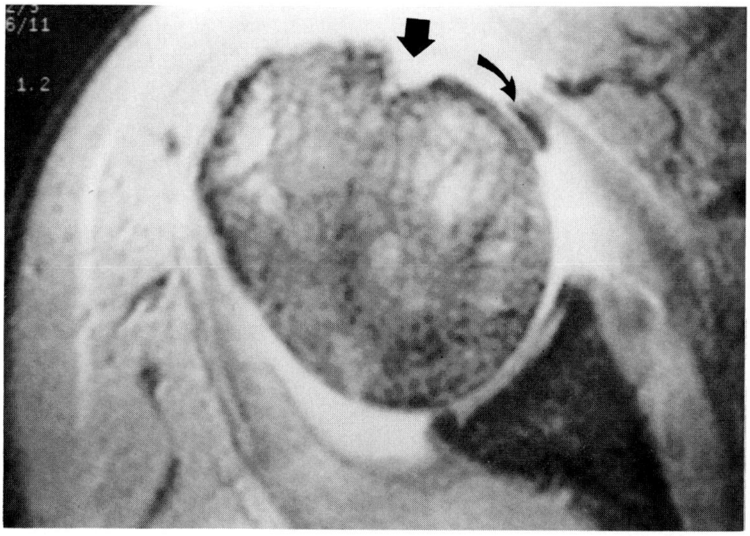

FIGURE 10–18 Dislocated biceps tendon. This axial T1-weighted image shows an empty bicipital groove (arrow), suggesting a torn biceps tendon; however, the biceps tendon is dislocated and can be seen anterior to the labrum (curved arrow).

is not seen on one or more of the axial images, it is disrupted (Fig. 10–17) or dislocated. Dislocation is uncommon, but when it occurs, the tendon can be seen to lie anteromedial to the joint (Fig. 10–18).

SUPRASCAPULAR NERVE ENTRAPMENT

The suprascapular nerve is made up of branches from the C4, C5, and C6 roots of the brachial plexus. It runs superior to the scapula, from anterior to posterior, just medial to the coracoid process. It gives off a branch that innervates the supraspinatus muscle as it courses posteriorly in the suprascapular notch. It then innervates the infraspinatus after it runs through the spinoglenoid notch in the posterior scapula. It can easily be entrapped by a tumor or a ganglion as it runs above the scapula because it is bounded superiorly by the transverse ligament both anteriorly and posteriorly. A fairly common finding is a ganglion in the spinoglenoid notch that impresses the infraspinatus portion of the nerve with resultant pain and atrophy of the infraspinatus muscle (Fig. 10–19). This has been reported almost exclusively in males who are athletic, particularly weightlifters. The ganglion can be per-

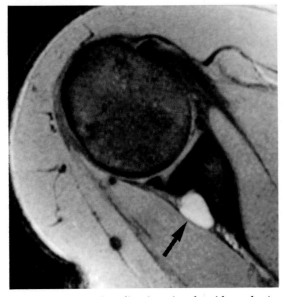

FIGURE 10–19   Ganglion in spinoglenoid notch. An axial T2 image reveals a high-signal mass posterior to the scapula in the spinoglenoid notch (arrow). This is a ganglion that has impressed the suprascapular nerve causing shoulder pain and atrophy of the infraspinatus muscle.

cutaneously drained with CT guidance or surgically removed. They can also spontaneously rupture with cessation of symptoms.[13]

REFERENCES

1. Burk DJ, Karasick D, Kurtz AB, Mitchell DG, Rifkin MD, Miller CL, Levy DW, Fenlin JM, Bartolozzi AR: Rotator cuff tears: Prospective comparison of MR imaging with arthrography, sonography, and surgery. Am J Roentgenol 1989;153:87–92.
2. Evancho AM, Stiles RG, Fajman WA, Flower SP, Macha T, Brunner MC, Fleming L: MR imaging diagnosis of rotator cuff tears. Am J Roentgenol 1988;151:751–754.
3. Farley T, Neumann C, Steinbach L, Jahnke A, Petersen S: Full-thickness tears of the rotator cuff of the shoulder: Diagnosis with MR imaging. Am J Roentgenol 1992;158:347–351.
4. Zlatkin MB, Iannotti JP, Roberts MC, Esterhai JL, Dalinka MK, Kressel HY, Schwartz JS, Lenkinski RE: Rotator cuff tears: Diagnostic performance of MR imaging. Radiology 1989;172:223–229.
5. Neer C: Anterior acromioplasty for the chronic impingement syndrome in the shoulder. A preliminary report. J Bone Joint Surg 1972;54-A:41–50.
6. Neviaser R, Neviaser T: Observations on impingement. Clin Orthop Relat Res 1990;254:60–63.
7. Rockwood C, Lyons F: Shoulder impingement syndrome: Diagnosis, radiographic evaluation, and treatment with a modified Neer acromioplasty. J Bone Joint Surg 1993;75-A:409–424.
8. Erickson S, Cox I, Hyde J, Carrera G, Strandt J, Estowski L: Effect of tendon orientation on MR imaging signal intensity: A manifestation of the "magic angle" phenomenon. Radiology 1991;181:389–392.
9. Kjellin I, Ho CP, Cervilla V, Haghighi P, Kerr R, Vangness CT, Friedman RJ, Trudell D, Resnick D: Alterations in the supraspinatus tendon at MR imaging: Correlation with histopathologic findings in cadavers. Radiology 1991;181:837–841.
10. Davis S, Teresi L, Bradley W, Ressler J, Eto R: Effect of arm rotation on MR imaging of the rotator cuff. Radiology 1991; 181:265–268.
11. Kaplan P, Bryans K, Davick J, Otte M, Stinson W, Dussault R: MR imaging of the normal shoulder: Variants and pitfalls. Radiology 1992; 184:519–524.
12. Legan J, Burkhard T, Goff W, Balsara Z, Martinez A, Burks D, Kallman D, O'Brien T, Lapoint J: Tears of the glenoid labrum: MR imaging of 88 arthroscopically confirmed cases. Radiology 1991;179:241–246.
13. Fritz R, Helms C, Steinbach L, Genant H: Suprascapular nerve entrapment: Evaluation with MR imaging. Radiology 1992;182:437–444.

Lumbar Spine: Disc Disease and Stenosis

Imaging the lumbar spine for disc disease and stenosis has evolved in the past 10 years from predominantly myelography-oriented exams to plain computed tomography (CT) and magnetic resonance (MR) imaging exams. Multiple studies have shown that myelography, in addition to being invasive, is not as accurate as CT or MR imaging,[1-3] yet myelography continues to be performed. There is little justification for a lumbar myelogram for disc disease or stenosis in this era. Telling this to a group of spine surgeons will elicit howls of protest, yet even their surgical literature does not support myelography.[4,5]

Although few differences between CT and MR imaging have been noted concerning diagnostic accuracy in the lumbar spine, MR imaging will give more information and a more complete anatomic depiction than will CT. There are a host of things that can be seen on an MR imaging study that cannot be seen with CT, yet it remains to be seen if the additional information afforded by an MR imaging exam will prove to be clinically useful. For example, MR imaging can determine if a disc is degenerated by showing loss of signal on T2-weighted images (Fig. 11-1). CT cannot give this information, but it hardly matters since no treatment is currently given solely for a degenerated disc. In fact, degenerative discs have been reported in asymptomatic children who deny a past history of back pain.[6]

Currently, the only area in which MR imaging is clearly superior to CT in imaging the lumbar spine is in evaluating the post-operative back. The use of gadolinium has greatly aided the differentiation of post-op fibrosis from recurrent disc protrusion. The single area in which CT has been shown to be superior to MR imaging in the lum-bar spine is in diagnosing spondylolysis. Pars defects can be very difficult to appreciate with MR imaging, yet they are easily seen with CT. Other than spondylolysis and the post-op spine, CT and MR imaging are seemingly diagnostically equivalent.

IMAGING PROTOCOLS

To achieve a high degree of accuracy it is imperative that the proper imaging protocol be observed. Thin section axial images should be obtained from the mid-body of L-3 to the mid-body of S-1. Angling of the plane of imaging to be parallel to the discs is not necessary (Fig. 11-2), and contiguous images without skip areas are considered mandatory (Fig. 11-3). Even though sagittal images will be obtained, free fragments and areas of stenosis are often seen on the axial images to better advantage than on the sagittal. Both T1- (or proton-density) weighted and T2- (or T2*-) weighted images should be obtained in both the sagittal and the axial planes. Attempts to shorten the study by foregoing one of the T2 sequences are not recommended. The addition of T2 axial images will increase the diagnostic accuracy as well as the confidence of many diagnoses.

DISC DISEASE

Terminology plays a large role in how radiologists describe disc bulges or protrusions. Since the advent of CT in the 70s, disc bulges have been described by their morphology. A broadbased disc bulge has been said to be a bulging annulus fibrosus, while a focal disc bulge is a herniated

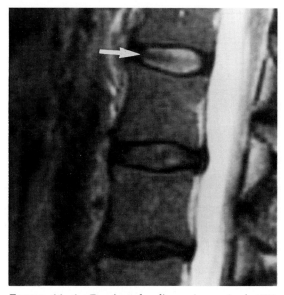

FIGURE 11–1 Dessicated disc. A sagittal T2-weighted image shows the L2-3 and L3-4 discs to be abnormally low in signal indicating disc dessication and degeneration. Compare with the normal L1-2 disc (arrow), which has high signal.

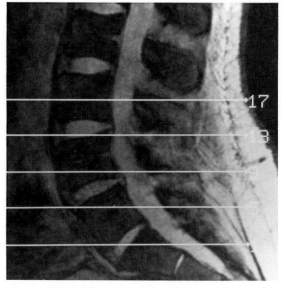

FIGURE 11–3 Proper MR imaging technique. This MR imaging scout with cursors placed contiguously from the body of L-3 to S-1 allows complete coverage of the lower lumbar spine in the axial plane.

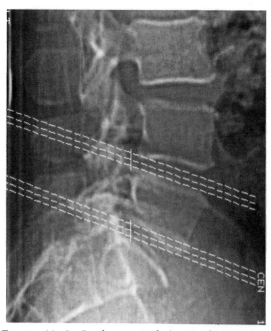

FIGURE 11–2 Inadequate technique—skip areas. A CT scout film with cursors placed through the L4-5 and L5-S1 disc spaces. This allows large gaps or skip areas that can result in missed free fragments of discs. Also, the L3-4 disc space should be imaged.

nucleus pulposus (HNP) (Fig. 11–4). This is no more than 90 per cent accurate. More significantly, most surgeons do not care what name is applied to a disc bulge—they do not treat a bulging annulus any differently than an HNP. They treat the patient's symptoms and have to decide if the disc bulge is responsible for those symptoms. It has been shown in multiple studies that from 10 to 25 per cent of asymptomatic young people have disc protrusions,[7] hence just seeing a disc bulge on CT or MR imaging does not mean it is clinically significant.

MR imaging has a high degree of accuracy in delineating disc protrusions and showing if neural tissue is impressed (Fig. 11–5). MR imaging can also show if annular fibers of the disc are disrupted—a so-called extrusion. Although CT cannot diagnose extrusions, clinicians do not currently treat extrusions any differently than protrusions (annular fibers intact). It is true that an extrusion must be present before a sequestration (free fragment) can occur; however, an extrusion without a free fragment has no more significance than a mere disc bulge. The key question is whether or not the bulging disc material is impressing neural tissue and causing the patient's symptoms.

Free Fragments

A type of disc extrusion that is critical to diagnose is the free fragment or sequestration.

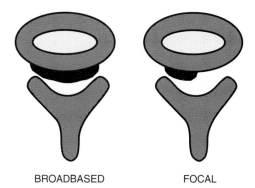

FIGURE 11–4 Schematic of types of disc protrusions. The broadbased disc bulge (left) is typical for a bulging annulus fibrosus. A focal disc bulge (right) is more consistent with a herniated nucleus pulposus.

BROADBASED   FOCAL

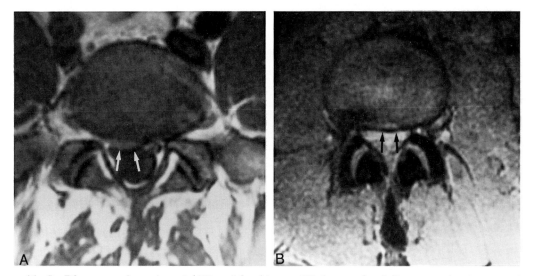

FIGURE 11–5 Disc protrusions. An axial T1-weighted image *(A)* shows a focal disc protrusion (arrows). An axial GRASS image *(B)* shows a broadbased disc protrusion (arrows). Either of these could be a herniated disc or a bulging annulus fibrosis. Since these are both showing impression of the thecal sac, they could each cause symptoms.

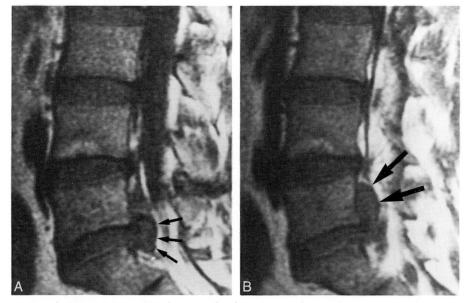

FIGURE 11–6 Free fragment. *(A)* A sagittal T1-weighted MR image shows a large amount of disc material bulging posteriorly at the disc space (arrows). *(B)* The adjacent slice shows disc material that has migrated cephalad (arrows) and now lies posterior to the L-5 vertebral body. This is a large free fragment.

Missed free fragments are one of the most common causes of failed back surgery.[8] The preoperative diagnosis of a free fragment contraindicates chymopapain, percutaneous discectomy, and, for many surgeons, microdiscectomy. At the very least it means the surgeon needs to explore more cephalad or caudal during the surgery in order to remove the free fragment. As free fragments can be very difficult to diagnose clinically, imaging is critical in the evaluation of the spine for any patient contemplating surgery. At times it can be difficult to be absolutely certain as to whether or not a disc that lies above or below the disc space is still attached to the parent disc or is really "free." So long as disc material is above or below the level of the disc space it really does not matter if it is attached or not—chymopapain and percutaneous discectomy would still be contraindicated and many surgeons would not perform a microdiscectomy. The key element is recognizing that disc material is present away from the level of the disc space.

Free fragments are diagnosed on MR imaging by noting disc material cephalad or caudal to the disc space (Fig. 11–6). Up to 80 per cent of free fragments will have high signal on T2-weighted images even though the parent disc may be of low signal.[9] Free fragments may migrate either

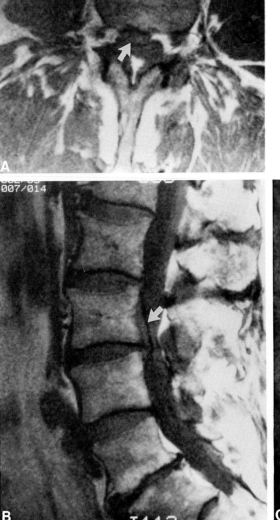

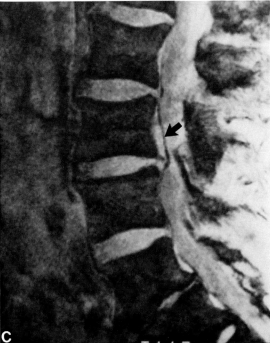

FIGURE 11–7 **Free fragment more evident on axial images.** The axial image *(A)* reveals an obvious large free disc fragment (arrow), which is causing an obvious distortion of the thecal sac. It is not as conspicuous on the T1- *(B)* or T2-weighted *(C)* sagittal images. The free fragment can be seen posterior to the L-3 vertebral body (arrow) and is displacing the posterior longitudinal ligament.

cranially or caudally with no apparent preference.

Axial images often show the free fragment more conspicuously than the sagittal images (Fig. 11–7); therefore, contiguous axial images without large skip areas or gaps are imperative in order to not miss free fragments.

A conjoined root, which is a normal variant of two roots exiting the thecal sac together or in an anomalous manner (seen in 1 to 3 per cent of the population)[10] (Fig. 11–8), or a Tarlov cyst, a normal variant in which a nerve root sleeve is dilated, can have a similar appearance to a free fragment but can almost always be differentiated from disc material by their signal staying isointense to the thecal sac on both T1 and T2 sequences. It is critical to identify a conjoined root or a Tarlov cyst and not confuse them for a free fragment. A surgeon will often change his procedure and certainly his amount of surgical exploration if he thinks there is a free fragment present. Many surgeons have inadvertently damaged conjoined or anomalous nerve roots thinking they were free fragments. Obviously, a free fragment should be removed and a conjoined nerve root should be left alone—the imaging study is where that difference should be ascertained, not during surgery.

Lateral Discs

Discs will occasionally protrude in a lateral direction causing the nerve root that has already exited the central canal to be stretched (Fig. 11–9). Although not common (less than 5 per cent of cases), these are frequently overlooked and are known to be a source of failed back surgery.[11] Since they affect the previously exited root they can clinically mimic symptoms of a disc protrusion from one level more cephalad (Fig. 11–10). For example, in a patient with multi-level disc disease and symptoms referable to the L3-4 disc, the disc protrusion is usually a posterior L3-4 bulge that impresses the L4 nerve root. However, a lateral disc at L4-5 could impress the L4 nerve root and cause the same symptoms. If not noticed, surgery could be performed at the L3-4 disc—the wrong level. Also, it is important to notify the surgeon that the disc is lateral to the neuroforamen, as a standard surgical approach through the lamina might not allow removal of a lateral disc.

Lateral discs are best identified on axial images. Sagittal images will often show a lateral disc occluding a neuroforamen, but many times a lateral disc will not extend into the foramen and the sagittal images will appear normal.

STENOSIS

By definition, spinal stenosis is encroachment of the bony or soft tissue structures in the spine on one or more of the neural elements with resulting symptoms. These symptoms are often indistinguishable from those of disc disease, and, in fact, disc disease often coexists with spinal

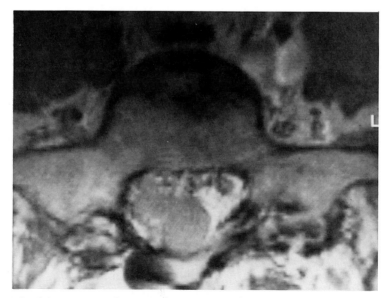

FIGURE 11–8 Conjoined root. An axial proton-density image shows a mass in the right lateral recess that had signal characteristics identical to the thecal sac on all sequences. This is a conjoined nerve root. A free fragment would not have signal identical to the thecal sac on all sequences.

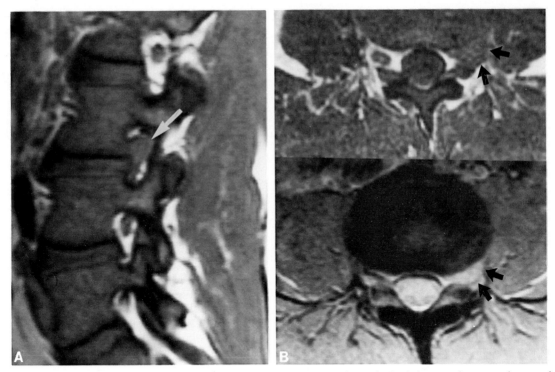

FIGURE 11–9 Lateral disc. *(A)* A sagittal T1-weighted MR image through the left neuroforamen shows a low signal structure in the L-4 neuroforamen (arrow), which is a lateral disc protrusion. *(B)* Axial T1 (upper) and T2* (lower) show the lateral disc (arrows) in the left neuroforamen.

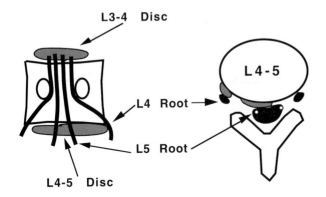

FIGURE 11–10 Schematic of lateral disc. This schematic illustrates how a posterior L4-5 disc protrusion affects the L5 nerve root, yet a lateral L4-5 disc affects the L4 root.

stenosis. Patients with spinal stenosis classically present with back pain and bilateral sciatica, intermittent claudication, pain with hyperextension and relief with flexion, and pain with standing that is relieved by lying down.

Spinal stenosis is classically divided into congenital and acquired types; however, even the most severe forms of congenital stenosis do not cause symptoms unless a component of acquired stenosis (usually degenerative disease of the facets and the discs) is present. A more useful classification of stenosis is on an anatomic basis: central canal, neuroforaminal, and lateral recess. It is important to realize that stenosis and disc disease are often present concomitantly, and it can be very difficult to clinically differentiate the two. As with disc disease, it is imperative that any imaging findings be matched with the clinical picture. It is not unusual to have a patient with severe stenosis on an imaging study and no clinical symptoms.

Central Canal Stenosis

Although at one time measurements were considered very useful in the determination of central

FIGURE 11–11 **Central canal stenosis.** An axial T1-weighted image shows compression of the thecal sac in an anteroposterior direction, diagnostic of central canal stenosis.

→

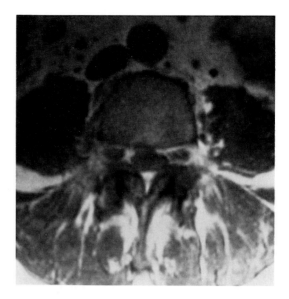

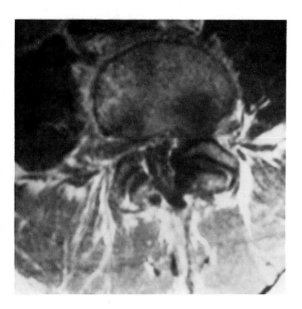

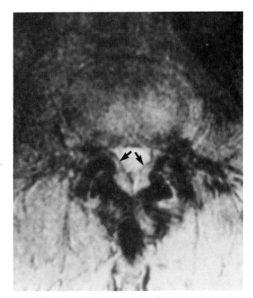

FIGURE 11–12 **Facet hypertrophy causing stenosis.** This MR image shows marked facet degenerative disease with hypertrophy of the facets causing lateral recess and central canal stenosis.

←

canal stenosis, they are no longer felt to be a valid indicator of disease. Instead, simply noting whether the thecal sac is compressed or round will reliably serve for determining central canal stenosis (Fig. 11–11). A subjective assessment as to whether the compression (usually in an anteroposterior direction) is mild, moderate, or severe is all that is necessary for evaluating the central canal. It is quite common to note mild or moderate central canal stenosis with flattening of the thecal sac in a patient who is asymptomatic.

The most common cause of central canal stenosis is degenerative disease of the facets with bony hypertrophy which encroaches on the central canal (Fig. 11–12). This is also the most common cause of lateral recess stenosis. When the facets undergo DJD they often have some slippage which results in buckling of the ligamentum flavum. Although a misnomer, this has been termed ligamentum flavum hypertrophy, and is a common cause of central canal stenosis (Fig. 11–13). Frequently, mild disc bulging is associated with minimal facet hypertrophy and ligamentum flavum hypertrophy. This combination can result in severe focal central canal stenosis.

FIGURE 11–13 **Ligamentum flavum hypertrophy.** Inward bulging of the ligamentum flavum (arrows) is shown on this MR image. Central canal stenosis from ligamentum flavum hypertrophy is common.

Less common causes of central canal stenosis include bony overgrowth from Paget's disease, achondroplasia, posttraumatic changes, and severe spondylolisthesis.

Neuroforaminal Stenosis

Degenerative joint disease (DJD) of the facets with bony hypertrophy is the most common cause of neuroforaminal stenosis; however, encroachment on the nerve root in the neuroforamen can be seen with free disc fragments, post-operative scar, and from a lateral disc protrusion.

The neuroforamen is best evaluated on axial images just cephalad to the disc space. The disc space lies at the inferior portion of the neuroforamen, and the exiting nerve root lies in the superior or cephalad portion of the neuroforamen. Although the neuroforamen can be clearly seen on sagittal MR images (Fig. 11–14), care must be taken to evaluate the entire neuroforamen and not just the 4 or 5 mm of one sagittal image. A normal appearing neuroforamen on a sagittal image does not exclude neuroforaminal stenosis (the axial images must be evaluated), whereas a stenotic foramen seen on a sagittal image (Fig. 11–15) can be counted on as being reliable for pathology.

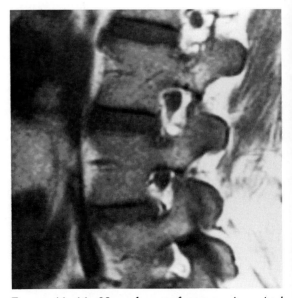

FIGURE 11–14 Normal neuroforamen. A sagittal T1-weighted image through the neuroforamen shows the nerve roots surrounded by fat with no evidence of foraminal stenosis. This does not exclude, however, a focus of foraminal stenosis that is medial or lateral to this sagittal image.

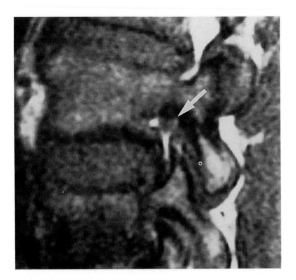

FIGURE 11–15 Neuroforaminal stenosis. Marked narrowing of the neuroforamen (arrow) is seen on this sagittal T1-weighted image.

Lateral Recess Stenosis

The lateral recesses are the bony canals in which the nerve roots lie after they leave the thecal sac and before they enter the neuroforamen. The lateral recesses are bounded by the neuroforamen caudally and cranially. They are triangular in shape when viewed on axial images, and the nerve root can be identified as a low-signal rounded structure on all imaging sequences. Hypertrophy of the superior articular facet from DJD is the most common cause of encroachment on the lateral recesses (Fig. 11–16), although, as with the neuroforamen, disc fragments and post-operative scarring can cause nerve root impingement.

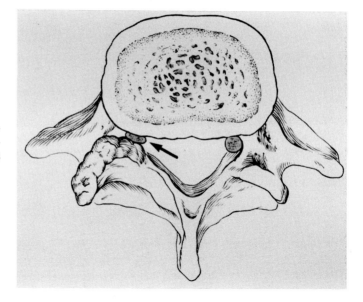

FIGURE 11–16 Lateral recess stenosis. Hypertrophy of the right-sided facet with encroachment into the lateral recess (arrow) is seen on this drawing.

POST-OPERATIVE CHANGES

Failed back surgery, unfortunately, is common. It can occur from many causes including inadequate surgery (including missed free disc fragments), post-operative scarring, failure of bone grafting for fusion, and recurrent disc protrusion. CT is useful in evaluating bone grafts but is not reliable for differentiating post-operative scarring from disc material. MR imaging has been shown to be particularly useful in distinguishing scar from disc material.[12]

The use of intravenous gadolinium (Gd-DTPA) will allow virtual certainty in distinguishing scar from disc. Scar tissue will be enhanced following administration of gadolinium, whereas disc material will have only some minimal peripheral enhancement, presumably due to inflammation (Fig. 11–17).

BONY ABNORMALITIES
Spondylolysis and Spondylolisthesis

Defects in the bony pars interarticularis (spondylolysis) are commonly found in asymptomatic individuals, yet they can be a source of low back pain and instability. Prior to disc surgery or other back surgery it is imperative that any spondylolysis be identified. Since spondylolysis can mimic back pain from other pathology, it is important to assess it preoperatively. If necessary it can then be surgically addressed at the same time as the other surgery. Failure to note and evaluate spondylolysis is a known source of failed back surgery.

CT is superior to MR imaging at identifying spondylolysis.[13] Although MR imaging will show spondylolysis defects, they can be very difficult to see at times. As previously mentioned, this is the only area in which CT is reported to be clearly superior to MR imaging in evaluating the lumbar spine. Spondylolysis is identified on the axial images through the mid-vertebral body as a break in the normally intact bony ring of the lamina (Fig. 11–18). Care must be used in calling spondylolysis on the sagittal views as the normal pars often has a low signal area that resembles spondylolysis. If the pars appears normal on the sagittal view, it can be considered a reliable finding; however, if the pars appears abnormal on the sagittal view, the axial view must be used to determine if a break is really present or not.

Spondylolisthesis (forward slippage of one vertebral body on a lower one) occurs from either slippage of two vertebral bodies following bilateral spondylolysis or from DJD of the facets with slippage of the facets. Bilateral spondylolysis can result in a large amount of slippage, whereas facet DJD will usually result in only minimal slippage.

A grading scale that is widely used to describe the degree of spondylolisthesis is the Meyerding grading scale. The more caudal vertebral body is divided into fourths, and the posterior corner of the more cephalad vertebral body is marked at the position where it has slipped forward. If it has slipped forward only into the first quarter of the more caudal vertebral body, it is a grade 1 spondylolisthesis; slippage into the second quarter is a grade 2, and so on (Fig. 11–19).

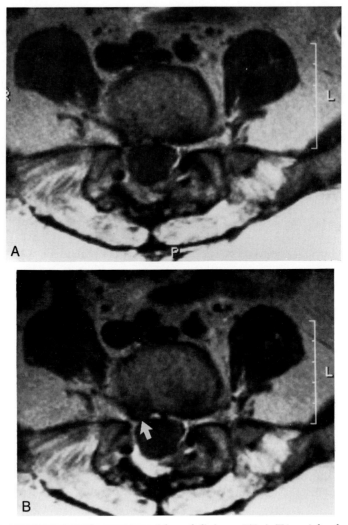

FIGURE 11–17 Post-operative scar enhancement with gadolinium. *(A)* A T1-weighted axial image shows soft tissue around the thecal sac in this post-operative patient that could represent scar but makes evaluation for recurrent disc protrusion difficult. *(B)* A T1-weighted axial image through the same level following administration of Gd-DTPA intravenously shows enhancement of the scar tissue surrounding the thecal sac. In addition, a focal right-sided disc protrusion can be identified (arrow).

If spondylolisthesis is severe it can result in central canal stenosis, neuroforaminal stenosis, or both.

End-plate Changes

Parallel bands of high or low signal adjacent to the vertebral body end-plates are often seen in association with degenerative disc disease. The most common appearance is of high signal bands on T1-weighted images that remain high on T2-weighted images (Fig. 11–20). This represents fatty marrow conversion. It was seen in 16 per cent of cases in the first report by Modic, et al.,[1] and was termed type 2 changes (generally referred to as "Modic type 2"). Modic type 1 changes are seen as low signal bands parallel to the end-plates on T1-weighted images that get brighter on T2-weighted images. This represents an inflammatory or granulomatous response to degenerative disc disease. The type 1 changes were reported in 4 per cent of cases and must be distinguished from disc space infection (Fig. 11–21). In disc space infection the disc should get bright on the

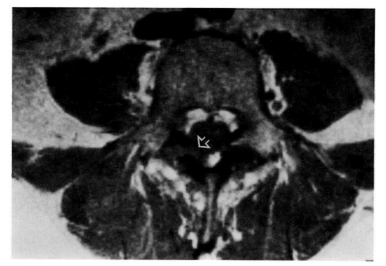

FIGURE 11–18 **Spondylolysis.** An axial T1-weighted image through the mid-vertebral body reveals a break in the right bony lamina (arrow), which indicates spondylolysis.

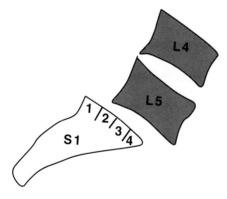

FIGURE 11–19 **Schematic of spondylolisthesis grading scale.** This schematic shows the grading scale used to gauge the degree of spondylolisthesis. This example would be a grade 2 spondylolisthesis since the posterior edge of the slipped L5 vertebral body lies above the second quadrant of the S1 vertebral body.

FIGURE 11–20 **Type 2 marrow changes.** A sagittal T1-weighted image in a patient with degenerative disc disease shows bands of fatty marrow parallel to the L4-5 end-plates (arrows), which are type 2 marrow changes seen often with degenerative disc disease.

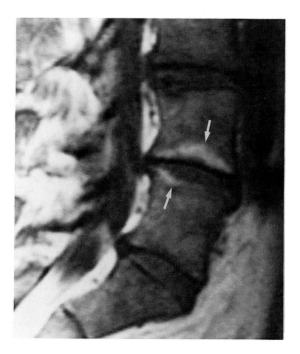

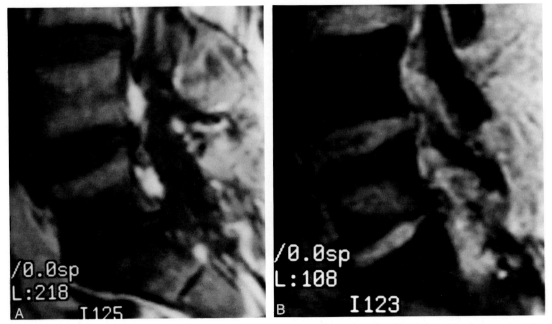

FIGURE 11–21   **Disc infection.** *(A)* A sagittal T1-weighted image shows bands of low signal in the vertebral bodies adjacent to the L5-S1 end-plates. On a T2-weighted image *(B)* the vertebral body/end-plate signal increases. This would simply represent Modic type 1 disc degeneration changes; however, the disc itself also gets bright with T2 weighting. This indicates a disc infection but must be correlated clinically.

T2-weighted images, whereas it is unusual for a degenerative disc to have high signal on T2-weighted images. Modic type 3 changes are parallel bands of low signal adjacent to the end-plates on both T1- and T2-weighted images. Type 3 changes represent bony sclerosis seen on plain films.

REFERENCES

1. Modic M, Masaryk T, Ross J, Carter J: Imaging of degenerative disk disease, Radiology 1988;168:177–186.
2. Hesselink J: Spine imaging: History, achievements, remaining frontiers. AJR 1988;150:1223–1230.
3. Sartoris DJ, Resnick D: Computed tomography of the spine: An update and review. Crc Crit Rev Diagn Imaging 1987;27(4):271–296.
4. Jackson R, Becker G, Jacobs R, Montesano P, Cooper B, McManus G: The neuroradiographic diagnosis of lumbar herniated nucleus pulposus (I): A comparison of computed tomography, myelography, CT-myelography, discography, and CT-discography. Spine 1989;14:1356–1361.
5. Jackson R, Cain J, Jacobs R, Cooper B, McManus G: The neuroradiographic diagnosis of lumbar herniated nucleus pulposus (II): A comparison of computed tomography, myelography, CT-myelography, and magnetic resonance imaging. Spine 1989;14:1362–1367.
6. Tertti M, Salminen J, Paajanen H, Terho P, Kormano M: Low-back pain and disk degeneration in children: A case-control MR imaging study, Radiology 1991;180:503–507.
7. Boden S, Davis D, Dina T, Patronas N, Wiesel S: Abnormal magnetic-resonance scans of the lumbar spine in asymptomatic subjects. J Bone Joint Surg 1990;72-A:403–408.
8. Onik G, Mooney V, Maroon J, Wiltse L, Helms C, Schweigel J, et al: Automated percutaneous discectomy: A prospective multi-institutional study. Neurosurgery 1989;26:228–233.
9. Masaryk T, Ross J, Modic M, Boumphrey F, Bohlman H, Wilber G: High-resolution MR imaging of sequestered lumbar intervertebral disks. AJR 1988;150:1155–1162.
10. Helms CA, Dorwart RH, Gray M: The CT appearance of conjoined nerve roots and differentiation from a herniated nucleus pulposus. Radiology 1982;144:803–807.
11. Winter DDB, Munk PL, Helms CA, Holt RG: CT and MR of lateral disc herniation: Typical appearance and pitfalls of interpretation. J Can Assoc Radiol 1989;40:256–259.
12. Ross J, Masaryk T, Schrader M, Gentili A, Bohlman H, Modic M: MR imaging of the postoperative spine: Assessment with gadopentetate dimeglumine. AJR 1990;155:867–872.
13. Grenier N, Kressel HY, Schiebler ML, Grossman RI: Isthmic spondylolysis of the lumbar spine: MR imaging at 1.5 T. Radiology 1989;170:489–494.

MR Imaging of the Foot and Ankle

I have always found topics on the foot and ankle to be exceedingly boring. This is mainly because I was never called on to use any of the information I learned; hence I quickly forgot all that I was told. I learned early in my residency that during lectures on the foot and ankle I could find better use of my time—like running or playing golf. That has changed now that magnetic resonance (MR) imaging is being used in the foot and ankle. MR imaging is playing an increasingly important role in examining the foot and ankle. Orthopedic surgeons and podiatrists are learning that critical diagnostic information can be obtained in no other way and are relying on MR imaging for many therapeutic decisions.

When most of us first encounter an ankle MR image, we get out a cross-sectional atlas and start trying to determine where all the tendons, muscles, vascular structures, and so on lie. I can assure you this will be unnecessary after reading this chapter. Although the anatomy of the foot and ankle can be complex, the significant anatomy, that is, the anatomy that must be learned because it is affected by disease, is fairly straightforward and easily learned.[1] There is no need to memorize tendons, ligaments, and muscles that are only rarely seen to be abnormal; therefore this chapter will dwell only on the pathologically significant areas.

TENDONS

One of the more common reasons to perform an MR imaging exam on the foot and ankle is to examine the tendons. Although multiple tendons course through the ankle, only a few are routinely affected pathologically. These are primarily the flexor tendons, located posteriorly in the ankle. The extensor tendons, located anteriorly, are rarely abnormal.

Tendons can be directly traumatized or be injured from overuse. Either etiology can result in *tenosynovitis,* which is seen on MR imaging as fluid in the tendon sheath with the underlying tendon appearing normal; *tendonitis* or a partial tear, which is seen as focal or fusiform swelling of the tendon with signal within the tendon that gets bright on T2 or T2* images; thinning or attenuation of the tendon is a more severe form of tendonitis, often presaging a tendon rupture; and *tendon rupture,* which is best identified on axial images by noting absence of a tendon on one or more images.

Making the distinction between tenosynovitis and tendonitis is not crucial since the treatment is similar for both entities. However, it is important to distinguish between tendonitis and a complete disruption because surgical repair is often warranted for the latter and not for the former. It is often difficult to make the distinction clinically.

Complete tendon disruption can be difficult to see on sagittal or coronal images because of the tendency for tendons to course obliquely to the plane of imaging. An exception to this is the Achilles tendon, which is usually best seen on a sagittal image.[2] The imaging protocol for the foot and ankle must include axial images with T1 (or proton density) and T2 (or T2*) sequences. Usually it is not recommended that both ankles be studied together. An extremity coil around one ankle with a small field of view (FOV) will give the highest image quality. A sagittal image with both T1 and T2 weighting is also performed but can be replaced with images in the coronal plane in some cases depending on the preference of the radiologist.

Achilles Tendon

The Achilles tendon does not have a sheath associated with it; therefore, tenosynovitis does not occur. Tendonitis is commonly seen in the Achilles; however, it is such an easy clinical diagnosis that MR imaging is usually not necessary. Complete disruption is commonly seen in athletes and in males around the age of 40. It is also commonly associated with other systemic disorders that cause tendon weakening, such as rheumatoid arthritis, collagen vascular diseases, crystal deposition diseases, and hyperparathyroidism.

Achilles tendon disruption can be treated surgically or by placing the patient in a cast with equinus positioning (marked plantar flexion) for several months. It is very controversial as to which treatment is superior, with both methods of treatment seemingly working well. I have known two surgeons who were dogmatic in their approach to always recommending surgery for torn Achilles tendons until they ruptured their own and opted for nonsurgical treatment.

MR imaging is being used by many surgeons to help decide if surgery should be performed. If a large gap is present (Fig. 12–1), some surgeons feel surgery should be performed to re-appose the torn ends of the tendon. Whereas, if the ends of the tendon are not retracted, nonsurgical treatment is preferred. No papers have been published to show that this is, in fact, scientifically valid.

Posterior Tibial Tendon

The posterior tibial tendon is the most medial and the largest, with the exception of the Achilles, of the flexor tendons (Fig. 12–2). The flexor tendons are easily remembered and identified by using the mnemonic "Tom, Dick, and Harry," with Tom representing the posterior Tibial tendon, Dick the flexor Digitorum longus, and Harry the flexor Hallucis longus. The posterior tibial tendon inserts onto the navicular, second to fourth cuneiforms, and the bases of the second to fourth metatarsals. As it sweeps under the foot, it provides some support for the longitudinal arch; hence, problems in the arch or plantar fascia can sometimes lead to stress on the posterior tibial tendon with resulting tendonitis or even rupture. Rupture of the posterior tibial tendon results clinically in a flat foot due to the loss of arch support given by this tendon. Posterior tibial tendonitis and rupture are commonly encountered in rheumatoid arthritis.

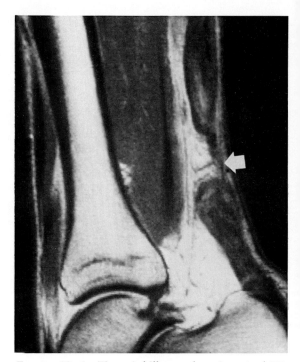

FIGURE 12–1 Torn Achilles tendon. A sagittal T1-weighted image reveals the Achilles to be torn with a 2 cm gap. Only a thin remnant of the tendon remains intact across the gap (arrow). Note the high signal in the swollen ends of the separated tendon, indicative of hemorrhage and edema.

Differentiation of tendonitis from tendon rupture can be difficult clinically, and MR imaging has become very valuable for making this distinction.[3] Most surgeons will operate on a disrupted posterior tibial tendon, whereas nonoperative therapy is usually preferred for tendonitis.

Posterior tibial tendonitis is seen on axial T1-weighted images as swelling and/or signal within the normally low signal tendon on one or more images (Fig. 12–3). T2 or T2* images show the signal in the tendon getting brighter. Tendon disruption is diagnosed by noting the absence of low signal tendon on one or more axial images (Fig. 12–4). This typically occurs just at or above the level of the tibiotalar joint.

Flexor Hallucis Longus

The flexor hallucis longus (FHL) tendon is easily identified near the tibiotalar joint because it is usually the only tendon at that distal level that has muscle still attached. In the foot the FHL is easily identified beneath the sustentaculum talus, which it uses as a pulley to plantar flex the foot.

The FHL is known as the Achilles tendon of the foot in ballet dancers because of the extreme

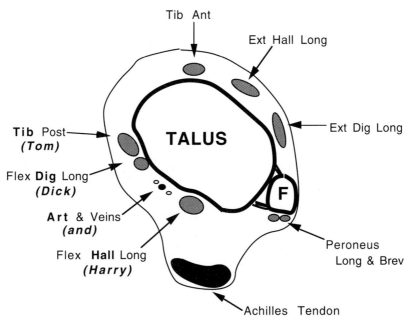

FIGURE 12–2 Schematic of ankle anatomy. This drawing of the tendons around the ankle at the level of the tibiotalar joint shows the relationship of the flexor tendons posteriorly and the extensor tendons anteriorly.

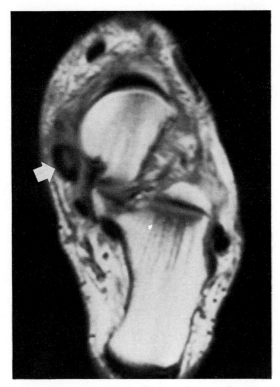

FIGURE 12–3 Posterior tibial tendon tendonitis. A proton-density axial image through the ankle at the level of the mid-calcaneus shows the posterior tibial tendon (arrow) swollen and containing high signal. This is the appearance of marked tendonitis.

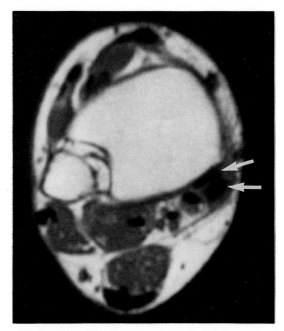

FIGURE 12–4 Torn posterior tibial tendon. An axial T1-weighted image through the ankle in this patient with chronic pain reveals two posterior tibial tendons (arrows) where there should only be one. This is a longitudinal tear of the tendon, which usually must be surgically repaired.

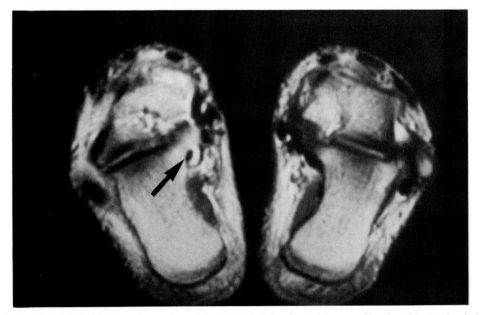

FIGURE 12–5 Flexor hallucis longus tenosynovitis. A T2-weighted axial image of both ankles in this ballet dancer with a painful right ankle reveals fluid in the tendon sheath around the FHL (arrow). This needs to be correlated with the clinical exam because fluid can normally extend into the tendon sheath of the FHL from the tibiotalar joint in up to 20 per cent of normal people.

flexion position they frequently employ. Ballet dancers often will have tenosynovitis of the FHL, seen on MR imaging as fluid in the sheath surrounding the tendon (Fig. 12–5). Care must be taken to have clinical correlation, as up to 20 per cent of normal people have a communication between the ankle joint and the FHL tendon sheath; therefore, fluid can be seen in the FHL tendon sheath from a connection to an ankle joint, which has an effusion. Rupture of the FHL is rare.

Peroneal Tendons

The peroneus longus and brevis tendons can be seen posterior to the distal fibula, to which they are bound by a thin fibrous structure, the superior retinaculum. The fibula serves as a pulley for the tendons to work as the principal everter of the foot. The tendons course close together adjacent to the lateral aspect of the calcaneus until a few centimeters below the lateral malleolus where they separate, with the peroneus brevis inserting onto the base of the fifth metatarsal and the peroneus longus crossing under the foot to the base of the first metatarsal. Avulsion of the base of the fifth metatarsal from a pull by the peroneus brevis is known as a "dancer's fracture" or a Jones fracture.

Disruption of the superior retinaculum, often seen in skiing accidents,[4] can result in displacement of the peroneal tendons (Fig. 12–6), which

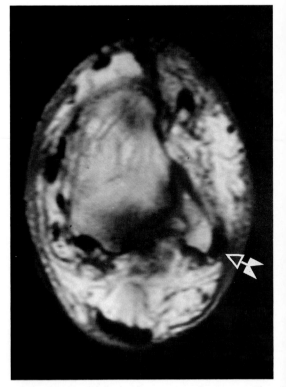

FIGURE 12–6 Dislocated peroneus longus tendon. An axial T1-weighted image in this skier who injured his ankle in a fall shows a low-signal rounded structure (arrow) lateral to the lateral malleolus. This is a dislocated peroneus longus tendon.

must be surgically corrected. It often occurs with a small bony avulsion, called a flake fracture, off of the fibula caused by the avulsed superior retinaculum.

Entrapment of the peroneal tendons in a fractured calcaneus or fibula can occur, and is easily diagnosed with MR. This can be a difficult diagnosis to make clinically. Complete disruption of the peroneals is uncommon, but is easily noted with MR.

AVASCULAR NECROSIS

Avascular necrosis (AVN) commonly occurs in the foot and ankle. The talar dome is the second most common location of osteochondritis dissecans (the knee is the most common site). MR imaging is useful in identifying and staging osteochondritis dissecans. Even when not apparent on plain films, MR imaging can show osteochondritis dissecans as a focal area of low signal in the subarticular portion of the talar dome on T1-weighted images. On T2 or T2* images if high signal is seen surrounding the dissecans fragment, in the bone at the bed of the fragment, or throughout the fragment (Fig. 12–7), it is most likely an unstable fragment. If the fragment has become displaced and lies in the joint as a loose body, MR imaging can sometimes be useful in localizing it; however, loose bodies in any joint can be exceedingly difficult to find.

Diffuse low signal throughout a tarsal bone on T1-weighted images is typical for AVN. This occasionally occurs in the tarsal navicular (Fig. 12–8). MR imaging can be useful in making this diagnosis when plain films are normal or equivocal. AVN in the tarsal navicular can result from continued weight bearing on a fracture that was not diagnosed. This is often seen in athletes, especially basketball players, and can be a career-ending injury in a professional athlete.

TUMORS

There are a few tumors that have a predilection for the foot and ankle.[5] Up to 16 per cent of synovial sarcomas occur in the foot. Desmoid tumors are commonly seen in the foot. Giant cell tumors of tendon sheath (also called xanthomas and pigmented villonodular synovitis [PVNS]) are often found in the tendon sheaths of the foot and ankle (Fig. 12–9). They are characterized by marked low signal in the synovial lining and in the tendons on T1 and T2 images, similar to the appearance of PVNS in a joint.

The differential diagnosis for calcaneal tumors is similar to that of the epiphyses: giant cell tumor, chondroblastoma (Fig. 12–10), infection—and, in addition, a unicameral bone cyst (Fig. 12–11).

Soft tissue tumors in the medial aspect of the foot and ankle can press on the posterior tibial

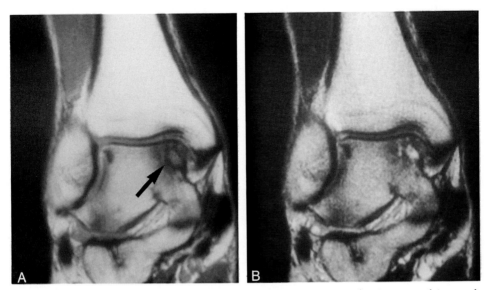

FIGURE 12–7 Unstable osteochondritis dissecans of the talus. *(A)* A proton-density coronal image through the talus shows a focus of low signal in the medial subarticular part of the talus (arrow). This is a characteristic appearance for osteochondritis dissecans. *(B)* A T2-weighted image shows high signal throughout the focus of osteochondritis dissecans, which indicates an unstable fragment.

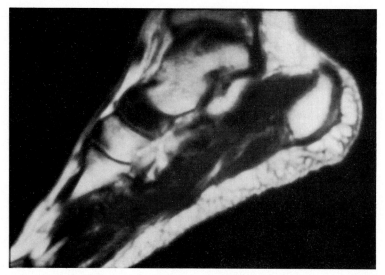

FIGURE 12–8 **Avascular necrosis of the tarsal navicular.** A T1-weighted sagittal image of the ankle in this patient with pain on the dorsum of the foot shows diffuse low signal throughout the tarsal navicular. This is a characteristic appearance for avascular necrosis and will often precede any plain film findings.

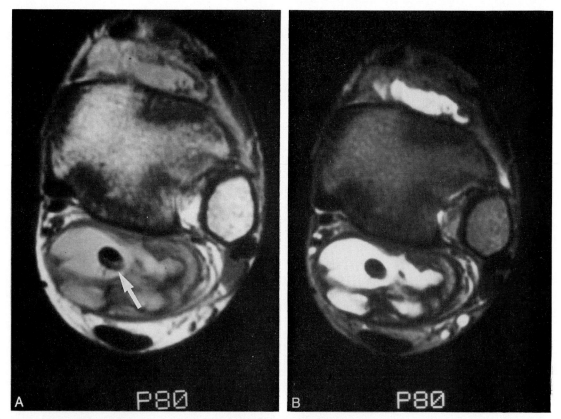

FIGURE 12–9 **Giant cell tumor of tendon sheath.** Axial proton density *(A)* and T2-weighted *(B)* images reveal a mass surrounding the flexor hallucis longus tendon (arrow), which is confined by the tendon sheath. Although high signal fluid is present, large amounts of low signal material is lining the distended tendon sheath. This low signal is hemosiderin, which is typically found in a giant cell tendon of tendon sheath. PVNS in a joint has an identical appearance.

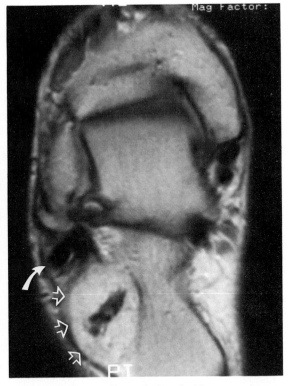

FIGURE 12–10   Calcaneal chondroblastoma. An axial T1-weighted image through the calcaneus shows an expansile lesion (arrows) with some low signal structures within which were areas of calcification on the plain film. This is a chondroblastoma. It was impinging on the peroneal tendons (curved arrow) causing pain with eversion of the foot.

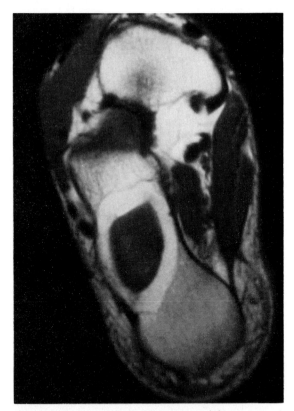

FIGURE 12–11   Calcaneal unicameral bone cyst. A T1-weighted axial image through the calcaneus reveals a typical unicameral bone cyst. Note that some fatty material is present in the periphery and fluid is present in the central portion. Biopsy of the peripheral portion could lead to an erroneous diagnosis of an intraosseous lipoma. Unicameral bone cysts will occasionally have fatty elements within as well as serous fluid.

nerve resulting in tarsal tunnel syndrome.[6] Clinically, patients with tarsal tunnel syndrome present with pain and paresthesia in the plantar aspect of the foot. In the aforementioned mnemonic, "Tom, Dick, and Harry," the "and" is for Artery, nerve, and vein. It is the position of the posterior tibial nerve. The nerve is easily compressed in the tarsal tunnel, which is bounded medially by the flexor retinaculum—a strong fibrous band that extends across the medial ankle joint for about 5 to 7 cm in a superior to inferior direction. Ganglions and neural tumors, both of which can look similar on T1- and T2-weighted images, often lie in the tarsal tunnel (Fig. 12–12) and compress the posterior tibial nerve, resulting in pain and paresthesia on the plantar aspect of the foot extending into the toes. Tarsal tunnel syndrome often occurs secondary to trauma, fibrosis, or idiopathically, all of which may not respond to surgical intervention; hence, MR imaging is valuable in delineating a treatable lesion in many cases. An MR imaging exam for tarsal

tunnel syndrome is becoming increasingly requested as surgeons learn how valuable it can be in identifying the source of the symptoms.

Anomalous muscles in the foot or ankle are reported to be present in up to 6 per cent of the population. These can be mistaken for a tumor and biopsied unnecessarily. MR imaging will show these "tumors" to have imaging characteristics identical to normal muscle (Fig. 12–13) and to be sharply circumscribed. Accessory soleus and peroneus brevis muscles are the most common accessory muscles encountered around the foot and ankle.

LIGAMENTS

MR imaging is not the best way to diagnose ankle ligament abnormalities. The clinical evaluation is usually straightforward, and no diagnostic imaging of any type is necessary. Never-

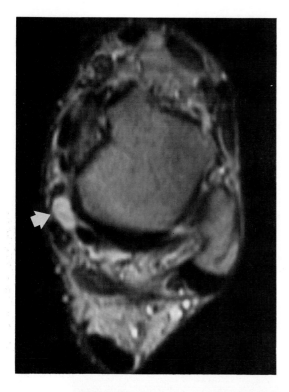

FIGURE 12–12 **Ganglion causing tarsal tunnel syndrome.** A T2-weighted axial image of the ankle in a patient complaining of pain and paresthesia on the plantar aspect of the foot shows a high signal mass (arrow) lying between the flexor digitorum tendon anteriorly and the flexor hallucis longus tendon posteriorly. This is the position of the posterior tibial nerve that can be impinged by a mass, such as in this case, resulting in tarsal tunnel syndrome. This was a small ganglion. (Case courtesy of Dr. Rick Mitchell.)

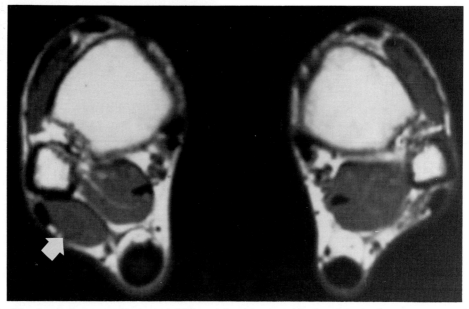

FIGURE 12–13 **Anomalous muscle.** An axial T1-weighted image of both ankles in this patient complaining of a mass in the right ankle shows an anomalous muscle (arrow) lateral to the flexor hallucis longus muscle, which is responsible for the mass the patient feels.

theless, in clinically equivocal cases or when the exam is ordered for other reasons, the ligaments can be clearly evaluated with high quality MR imaging in most instances.[7]

The deltoid ligament lies medially as a broad band beneath the medial flexor tendons. Although it is often seen on coronal images deep to the posterior tibial tendon, it has a variable an-atomic position and is not well studied with MR imaging.

The lateral collateral ligament complex is responsible for over 80 per cent of all ankle ligament injuries. It is made up of two parts: a superior group, the anterior and posterior tib-fib ligaments that make up part of the syndesmosis (Fig. 12–14); and an inferior group, the anterior

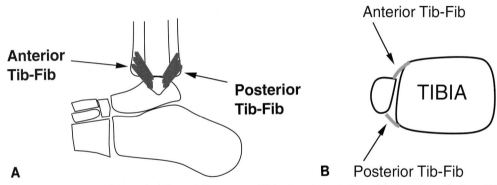

FIGURE 12–14 Schematic of lateral collateral ligaments. This drawing of the ankle in a lateral view *(A)* shows how the anterior and posterior tib-fib ligaments extend off of the fibula and course superiorly to the tibia. A drawing in the axial plane *(B)* shows that the fibula has a flat or convex surface at the origin of these ligaments.

and posterior talofibular ligaments and the calcaneofibular ligament (Fig. 12–15). The anterior and posterior tib-fib ligaments can be seen on axial images at or slightly above the tibiotalar joint. The anterior and posterior talofibular ligaments are seen on the axial images just below the tibiotalar joint and emanate from a concavity in the distal fibula called the malleolar fossa (Fig. 12–15*B*). The most commonly torn ankle ligament is the anterior talofibular ligament. It is easily identified when a joint effusion is present because it makes up the anterior capsule of the joint (Fig. 12–16). The anterior talofibular ligament is usually torn without other ligaments being involved; however, if the injury is severe enough, the next ligament to tear is the calcaneofibular ligament. Finally, with very severe trauma, the posterior talofibular ligament will tear. The calcaneofibular and posterior talofibular ligaments will not be torn without a tear of the anterior talofibular ligament.

On sagittal T2 or T2* images the posterior tib-fib ligament can mimic a loose body in the joint. A round, low signal structure at the posterior tibiotalar joint line should be considered a normal structure rather than a loose body (Fig. 12–17). This pitfall is probably the most clinically important piece of ankle ligament information in this section, as unnecessary surgery for a presumed loose body can occur because of failure to recognize the normal anatomy.

Sinus Tarsi Syndrome

An entity that has a high association with torn lateral collateral ligaments in the ankle is sinus tarsi syndrome. Clinically these patients have lateral ankle pain and a feeling of hindfoot instability. Up to 70 per cent of these patients have torn lateral collateral ligaments and up to one third of patients who tear their lateral collateral

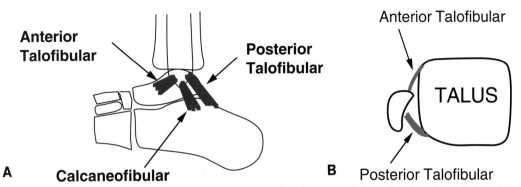

FIGURE 12–15 Schematic of lateral collateral ligaments. This drawing of the ankle in a lateral view *(A)* shows how the anterior and posterior talofibular ligaments and the calcaneofibular ligament extend off of the fibula and course inferiorly. These ligaments arise off of the fibula more distally than the anterior and posterior tib-fib ligaments. A drawing in the axial plane *(B)* shows that the anterior and posterior talofibular ligaments arise from the level of the distal fibula, which has a concave medial surface, the malleolar fossa.

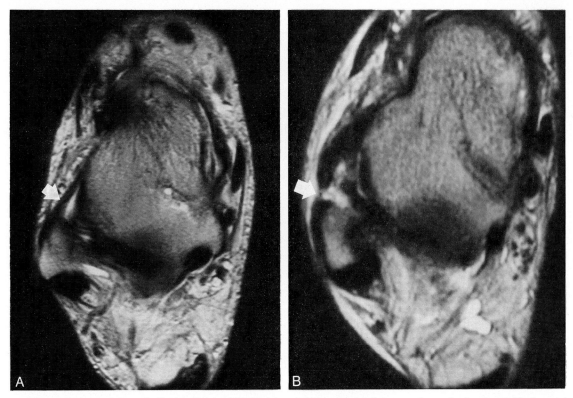

FIGURE 12–16   Anterior talofibular ligament. *(A)* An axial T2-weighted image through the distal fibula at the level of the malleolar fossa (the concave medial surface of the fibula) shows an intact anterior talofibular ligament (arrow), which makes up part of the joint capsule at this level. Note the high signal joint fluid adjacent to the ligament. *(B)* This axial T2-weighted image at the level of the malleolar fossa reveals a thickened anterior talofibular ligament that has a disruption (arrow). The marked thickening of the ligament indicates a chronic process. (Case courtesy of Dr. Jerrold Mink.)

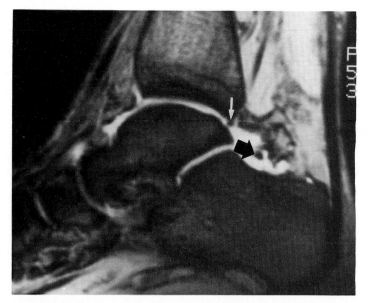

FIGURE 12–17   Posterior tib-fib ligament and loose body. A sagittal T2* GRASS image through the mid-ankle in a patient with occasional locking and a plain film that shows a calcified loose body near the posterior talus reveals two apparent loose bodies. The more posterior one (large arrow) matches the calcified loose body on the plain film. The other one (small arrow) is not a loose body but is the posterior tib-fib ligament, which often resembles a loose body on sagittal T2 images.

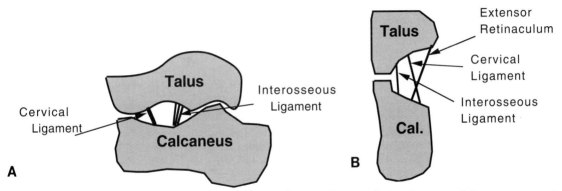

FIGURE 12–18 Schematic of the sinus tarsus. A sagittal *(A)* and an axial *(B)* schematic of the sinus tarsus show the positions of the cervical and the interosseous ligaments. The cervical ligament lies more anteriorly and laterally in relation to the interosseous ligament.

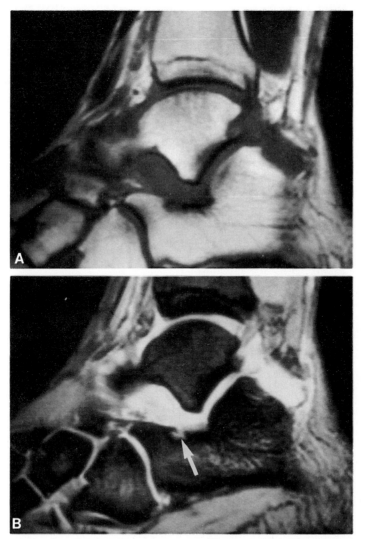

FIGURE 12–19 Sinus tarsi syndrome. A sagittal T1-weighted image *(A)* shows obliteration of the normal fat in the sinus tarsus. No ligaments are visualized. A sagittal T2-weighted image *(B)* reveals no evidence of the normal cervical or interosseous ligaments and a small subchondral cyst (arrow) where the cervical ligament should insert on the calcaneous. The high signal throughout the sinus tarsus represents either fluid or fibrosis. These findings are classic for sinus tarsi syndrome.

ligaments have been reported to have sinus tarsi syndrome.[8] In the past diagnosis has relied on clinical suspicion and injection of xylocaine into the sinus tarsus, which causes resolution of the pain. Treatment is varied but can include a joint fusion.

The sinus tarsus is the space that lies between the talus and the calcaneus and opens up in a cone-like configuration to the lateral aspect of the ankle beneath the lateral malleolus. It is filled with fat and several ligaments that give some hindfoot stability. The most lateral of these ligaments are slips of ligaments from the lateral extensor retinaculum. Medial to these are the cervical ligament, and the most medial ligament is the interosseous ligament (Fig. 12–18). In sinus tarsi syndrome the fat in the sinus tarsus is obliterated and one or more of the ligaments are disrupted (Fig. 12–19). This syndrome is causing an increasing amount of MR imaging requests as surgeons and podiatrists recognize that a definitive diagnosis of sinus tarsi syndrome can be made with imaging.

BONY ABNORMALITIES

Tarsal coalition is a common cause of a painful flat foot. It occurs most commonly at the calcaneonavicular joint and the middle facet of the talocalcaneal joint (Fig. 12–20). Up to 80 per cent of patients with tarsal coalition have bilateral coalition. It can be difficult (or impossible) to see the coalition on plain films; however CT and MR imaging will show bony coalition with a high degree of accuracy. The coalition, however, can also be fibrous or cartilaginous. In these cases, secondary findings, such as joint space irregularity at the affected joint or DJD at nearby joints that are subjected to accentuated stress, can be seen. For now, MR imaging does not appear to have superiority to CT for diagnosing tarsal coalition.

Fractures of the foot and ankle are usually well documented with plain films. Stress fractures, however, can be difficult to radiographically or clinically diagnose and can mimic more sinister abnormalities. MR imaging will show stress fractures as linear low signal on T1-weighted images with high signal on T2 weighting (Fig. 12–21).

MR imaging has had mixed reviews when used for diagnosing osteomyelitis in the foot. In diabetics with foot infections it is important to diagnose osteomyelitis, as the treatment is often much more aggressive, including amputation, than if the bone is not involved. Unfortunately, MR imaging is not highly accurate in this regard. If the marrow appears normal, MR imaging is useful in predicting no osteomyelitis; however, if low signal is present in the marrow around a joint, osteomyelitis may or may not be present. Low signal can be caused by edema or hyperemia without infection. MR imaging is therefore very sensitive but not very specific in diagnosing osteomyelitis in the foot and ankle.[9]

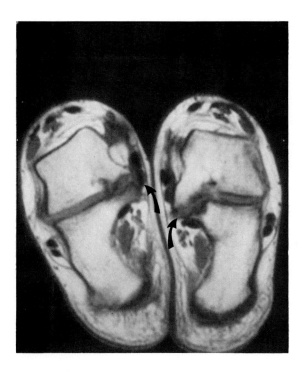

FIGURE 12–20 Tarsal coalition. An axial T1-weighted image in a patient with painful flat feet shows bilateral talocalcaneal coalition (arrows), which is primarily fibrous. The joint space is irregular and widened bilaterally. In cases of suspected coalition both ankles should be imaged because coalition often occurs bilaterally.

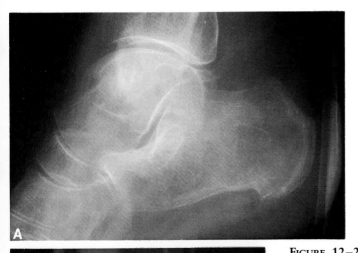

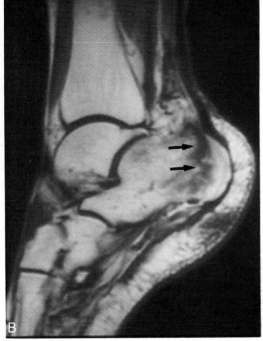

FIGURE 12–21   Calcaneal stress fracture. A 70-year-old woman with a prior history of lung cancer presented with heel pain and a normal plain film *(A)*. A bone scan showed diffuse increased radionuclide uptake throughout the posterior calcaneus. A sagittal T1-weighted MR image *(B)* revealed a linear area of low signal (arrows), which is characteristic for a stress fracture. Metastatic disease would not have this appearance.

REFERENCES

1. Kneeland J, Macrandar S, Middleton W, Cates J, Jesmanowicz A, Hyde J: MR imaging of the normal ankle: Correlation with anatomic sections. AJR 1988;151:117–126.
2. Quinn S, Murray W, Clark R, Cochran C: Achilles tendon: MR imaging at 1.5 T. Radiology 1987;164:767–770.
3. Rosenberg Z, Cheung Y, Jahss M, Noto A, Norman A, Leeds N: Rupture of posterior tibial tendons: CT and MR imaging with surgical correlation. Radiology 1988;169:229–236.
4. Oden R: Tendon injuries about the ankle resulting from skiing. Clin Ortho 1987;216:63–69.
5. Keigley B, Haggar A, Gaba A, Ellis B, Froelich J, Wu K: Primary tumors of the foot: MR imaging. Radiology 1989;171:755–759.
6. Erickson S, Quinn S, Kneeland J, Smith J, Johnson J, Carrera G, Shereff M, Hyde J, Jesmanowicz A: MR imaging of the tarsal tunnel and related spaces: Normal and abnormal findings with anatomic correlation. AJR 1990;155:323–328.
7. Erickson S, Smith J, Ruiz M, Fitzgerald S, Kneeland J, Johnson J, Shereff M, Carrera G: MR imaging of the lateral collateral ligament of the ankle. AJR 1991;156:131–136.
8. Klein M, Spreitzer A: MR imaging of the tarsal sinus and canal: Normal anatomy, pathologic findings, and features of the sinus tarsi syndrome. Radiology 1993;186:233–240.
9. Erdman W, Tamburro F, Jayson H, Weatherall P, Ferry K, Peshock R: Osteomyelitis: Characteristics and pitfalls of diagnosis with MR imaging. Radiology 1991;180:533–539.

Chapter

13

Miscellaneous MR Imaging

There are several additional areas in which magnetic resonance (MR) imaging is useful but not well enough developed or of enough widespread use to have an entire chapter devoted to them. Included in this group are MR of the temporomandibular joint (TMJ), wrist, and the hip.

TEMPOROMANDIBULAR JOINT

Diagnostic imaging of the TMJ is performed for so-called internal derangements. I say "so-called" because there is really only one abnormality, for the most part, that makes up the internal derangement—an anteriorly displaced disc. For years disc displacement was diagnosed by arthrography, a painful and somewhat technically demanding study. Some centers replaced arthrography of the TMJ with CT scanning, and now MR imaging has virtually eliminated all other imaging studies for internal derangements.[1]

Anatomy

The TMJ is a sliding-hinge joint that opens by both hinging and sliding forward (translation). It has a fibrous disc or meniscus that sits on the apex of the condyle and is made up of two thickened portions: the anterior and posterior bands (Fig. 13–1). The thin intermediate zone lies between the anterior and posterior bands. The normal disc has an asymmetric bowtie configuration on sagittal images, with the posterior band larger than the anterior band. The disc is relatively low in signal on all MR imaging sequences (Fig. 13–2), although some intermediate signal, representing normal hydration, can be seen in the normal posterior band on high resolution images.

The intermediate zone is an important anatomic landmark because in a normal joint it will always be situated between the two most closely apposed cortical surfaces of the articular eminence of the temporal bone and the condylar head, regardless of whether the mouth is open, closed, or partially open. By using this landmark the disc can be diagnosed as normal in position or anteriorly displaced.

Imaging Technique

Thin section (3 mm), sagittal T1-weighted images in both a closed and a partially open-mouth position with a small field of view (FOV) and a surface coil are all that are necessary to properly image the TMJ. It is one of the few areas in musculoskeletal imaging in which only one plane of imaging is required.

The partial open-mouth position (mouth open about 10 to 15 mm with gauze or something soft between the teeth to avoid motion) is obtained because occasionally the disc cannot be easily identified on the closed mouth images since it is crowded into the low signal glenoid fossa. With partial mouth opening the condyle is not pressing the disc into the glenoid fossa as much, allowing easy identification (Fig. 13–2). Why not just image only in the partial open-mouth position? Because often the disc reduces to a normal position with minimal mouth opening, and the diagnosis of an anteriorly displaced disc would be missed. If the partial open-mouth images are examined first, the size and shape of the disc can be determined and then the closed mouth images can be examined to determine the disc position.

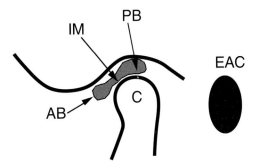

FIGURE 13–1 Schematic of normal TMJ. (Anterior is to the left.) This drawing shows how the normally positioned TMJ disc lies between the head of the mandibular condyle (C) and the eminence of the temporal bone. The disc has three portions: the anterior band (AB), the larger posterior band (PB), and the thin intermediate zone (IM). The posterior band is over the apex of the condyle in the closed mouth position, as in this example. (EAC = external auditory canal.)

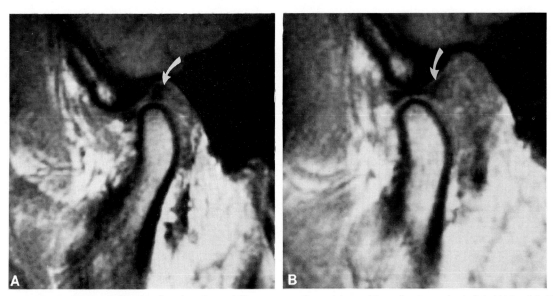

FIGURE 13–2 Normal disc in closed and partial open-mouth positions. (Anterior is to the left.) *(A)* In this T1-weighted sagittal image in the closed-mouth position the disc can be seen as a low signal, bowtie-shaped structure with the posterior band (arrow) superior to the apex of the condyle and the anterior band just anterior to the condylar head. *(B)* In the open-mouth position the disc is more easily identified and the posterior band (arrow) is noted to have some intermediate signal, indicative of normal hydration.

Pathology

In patients with internal derangements of the TMJ the disc can be found in an anterior position in relation to the condylar head (Fig. 13–3). If the patient is able to open the mouth and the disc slides back into a normal position, it usually does so with a click or pop that can be painful. This is usually what brings the patient to the dentist or physician. As the process worsens, the disc cannot be returned to the normal position with mouth opening. These patients have some limitation of mouth opening and usually have more severe pain. This has been termed an anteriorly displaced disc without reduction. It has a high incidence of osteoarthritis of the TMJ and often requires surgery to repair or remove the disc.

Since it is easily determined whether or not the disc reduces (a click or pop is apparent when the disc reduces), I do not spend imaging time trying to determine whether or not the disc reduces with full mouth opening. Also, reduction of the disc can change from day to day—it may be reducing when the patient is having MR imaging performed and not when the patient is being examined by his referring doctor. This can lead to some confusion for the referring doctor. In addition, these patients have pain when they open their mouths widely, therefore 10 to 15 minutes in the magnet in a full open-mouth position can be very uncomfortable, which can lead to patient motion and a nondiagnostic study. Since the full open-mouth position is painful and doesn't give the referring physician any information they can't easily determine clinically, I don't obtain such images. The reason I am expounding on this is because most radiologists have recommended im-

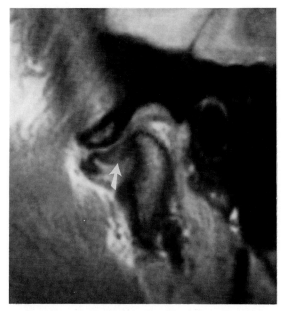

FIGURE 13–3 **Anteriorly displaced disc.** (Anterior is to the left.) A sagittal T1-weighted image in a partial open-mouth position shows the disc clearly anteriorly displaced with some high signal in the posterior band (arrow). Although it is slightly folded downward, it still has a bowtie shape.

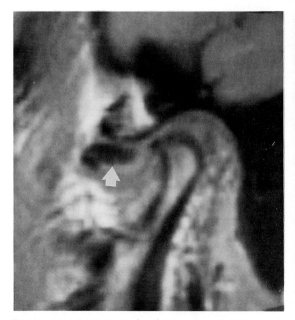

FIGURE 13–4 **Anteriorly displaced and misshaped disc with degenerative joint disease.** This sagittal T1-weighted image in a patient with advanced TMJ disease shows an anteriorly displaced disc (arrow) that has lost its normal bowtie shape and is low in signal throughout, indicative of dessication. Note the anterior osteophyte on the condyle, indicative of DJD, a common association with advanced TMJ dysfunction.

aging the TMJ with the patient's mouth fully open and closed. There appears to be no justification for this.

If the disc is anteriorly displaced and has lost its usual asymmetric bowtie shape (Fig. 13–4), this should be reported. This represents a more severely damaged disc, one that usually cannot be repaired. It has a high association with joint osteoarthritis.

Although other imaging sequences (T2 weighting, motion studies), and other imaging planes can be obtained, they offer little additional information to the referring physician or dentist and are therefore not recommended on a routine basis. I usually image both joints simultaneously because we have bilateral coupled coils, but only the symptomatic side needs to be imaged. In the days of arthrography of the TMJ we did not perform bilateral studies routinely. A bilateral study is sometimes useful to get a feel for the anatomy since there is usually some symmetry, but other than that it's not necessary—especially if it's going to cost the patient more than a unilateral study.

WRIST

MR imaging of the wrist has been slower to develop than that of other joints for several rea-sons. Technical demands to obtain thin-section, high resolution images have only recently been met. The main reason, however, is due to the confusion and controversy surrounding the wrist amongst the clinicians. This is the reason wrist arthrography has not enjoyed the same popularity as that of the knee or shoulder. Nevertheless, MR imaging of the wrist has some definite utility. It is useful in evaluating the carpal bones for fractures and avascular necrosis. It seems to have some use for evaluating the triangular fibrocartilage (TFC) and the intercarpal ligaments[2] and can be used for carpal tunnel syndrome.

Imaging Techniques

Thin section (2 to 3 mm) T1- and T2-weighted images in both an axial and a coronal plane are usually employed with a dedicated wrist coil or a small surface coil. A small FOV (5 to 8 cm) should be used for maximal resolution. Three-D volumetric images with thin (1 to 2 mm) slices are used in many centers to replace the T2-weighted images. These are especially useful for examining the TFC and the intercarpal ligaments.[3]

Pathology

Triangular Fibrocartilage. The TFC lies between the distal ulna and the carpal bones and is thought to have some shock-absorbing function. It can tear or become detached and cause significant wrist pain and dysfunction. Tears of the TFC can be diagnosed with arthrography or with MR imaging, although it is somewhat controversial as to the significance of a torn TFC. That is because torn TFCs (and torn intercarpal ligaments, for that matter) are found with a high frequency in older patients who do not have wrist pain or dysfunction. Nevertheless, in a young patient with a painful, torn TFC, most hand surgeons would surgically intervene if conservative care was ineffective. For this reason imaging may play a role.

The normal TFC is predominantly low signal on all imaging sequences and seen to be triangular in shape with the base attaching to the ulna and the apex attaching onto the radius (Fig. 13–5). A detached or torn TFC is best seen in the coronal plane and is usually accompanied by joint fluid in both the distal radioulnar and the proximal carpal joints (Fig. 13–6).

Avascular Necrosis (AVN). The wrist has several bones that have a propensity to undergo AVN. The lunate is commonly affected and is known as Kienböck's malacia. It is seen as uniform low signal on T1-weighted images (Fig. 13–7). As is found with AVN in other joints, MR imaging can be useful in showing AVN when plain films are normal.

The proximal pole of the navicular often un-

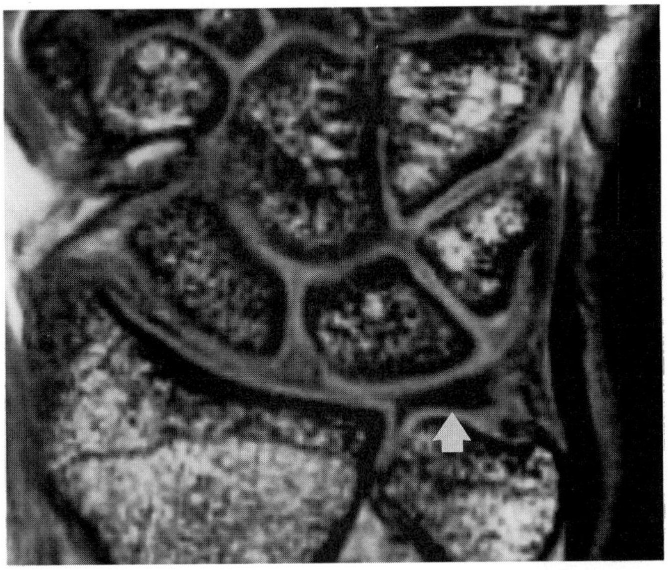

FIGURE 13–5 Normal TFC. A coronal 3D-volume thin section image of a normal wrist shows the TFC (arrow) with its attachment to the radius separated by a thin layer of cartilage.

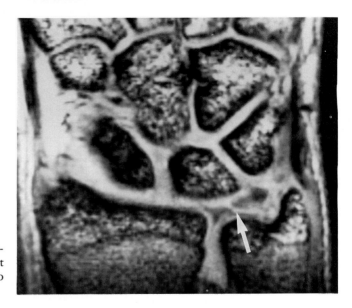

FIGURE 13–6 Torn TFC. A coronal 3D-volume thin section image of a wrist in a patient with ulnar-sided wrist pain shows the TFC to be torn in its midsubstance (arrow).

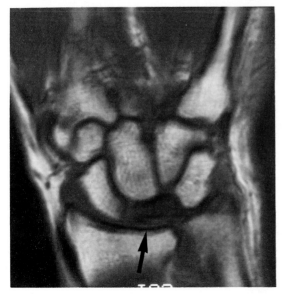

FIGURE 13–7 Kienböck's malacia. A coronal T1-weighted image shows the lunate (arrow) to be devoid of the normal high signal from fatty marrow. This is diagnostic of AVN, called Kienböck's malacia when it occurs in the lunate.

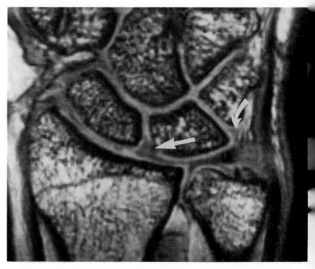

FIGURE 13–8 Scapholunate ligament. A coronal 3D-volume thin section image of a normal wrist shows the appearance of the scapholunate ligament (arrow). A normal lunatotriquetral ligament (curved arrow) can also be seen, although it is not always identified.

FIGURE 13–9 Carpal tunnel syndrome secondary to mass. *(A)* An axial T2-weighted image through the carpal tunnel at the level of the hook of the hamate shows the median nerve (arrow) to be high in signal and somewhat flattened. *(B)* A more proximal axial image reveals the median nerve (large arrow) to be somewhat enlarged as well as high in signal. The high signal mass superficial to the median nerve and flexor tendons (small arrows) is a ganglion that was extending into the carpal tunnel causing the median nerve to be compressed.

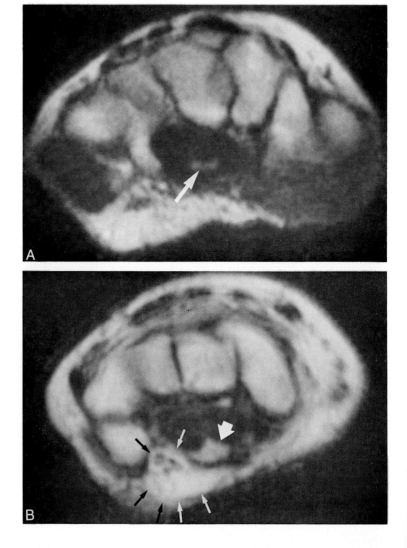

dergoes AVN following a fracture. MR can demonstrate the AVN earlier than plain films, allowing earlier treatment. Subtle or occult fractures of the navicular (or any other carpal bone) can be identified with MR. MR should be considered when clinical suspicion of a fracture is high and plain films are negative since a missed fracture of the navicular can lead to AVN.

Intercarpal Ligaments. The intercarpal ligaments can tear and cause pain and instability in the wrist. They are usually diagnosed arthrographically; however MR imaging is beginning to play a role in their evaluation. The scapholunate ligament is the most commonly torn intercarpal ligament. It should be identified at the proximal part of the scapholunate joint in every wrist unless it is torn (Fig. 13–8). The next most common intercarpal ligament to tear is the lunatotriquetral ligament, which is found at the proximal portion of the joint. Unfortunately it is not always visualized, even with excellent images; hence, it is difficult to diagnose a torn lunatotriquetral ligament with any certainty.

Further complicating the diagnosis of torn intercarpal ligaments is the fact that they can be torn as a matter of aging and wear and tear without being symptomatic. Hence, diagnosing a torn ligament may have no clinical significance whatsoever. Cadaver studies have reported torn intercarpal ligaments in up to 80 per cent of older people.

Carpal Tunnel Syndrome. The median nerve can become impinged in the carpal tunnel by a variety of processes and result in paresthesia in the hand and fingers. Surgical removal of the offending agent (if any—it is most often idiopathic or due to overuse of the hands in stressful positions, such as typing) and excision of the flexor retinaculum is usually curative if conservative treatment fails. MR imaging is useful in identifying tumors, ganglia, swollen flexor tendon sheaths, or other masses in the carpal tunnel. The median nerve will have increased signal on T2-weighted images due to the edema; it can be seen to be flatter than normal in the carpal tunnel, with swelling of the nerve often present more proximally (Fig. 13–9).

Many hand surgeons dispute the need for imaging the carpal tunnel because of the ease with which the diagnosis of carpal tunnel syndrome is made. If surgery is performed, it is easy to inspect the entire carpal tunnel, making preoperative imaging unnecessary.

HIP

The main use of MR imaging of the hip is to diagnose AVN. It is also used to diagnose hip fractures when plain films are equivocal.[4] (Hip fractures have been discussed in Chapter 5, Trauma.)

AVN can be diagnosed with great sensitivity with MR imaging.[5] It has a characteristic appearance with involvement of the anterosuperior portion of the femoral head. The area of AVN typically is surrounded by a low signal serpiginous border (Fig. 13–10). AVN can be diagnosed earlier and more reliably using MR imaging than with plain films or nuclear medicine.

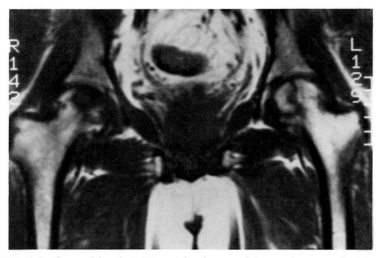

FIGURE 13–10 **AVN of the femoral head.** A T1-weighted coronal image shows marked low signal in the right femoral head, which indicates advanced hip AVN. The left hip has AVN that shows some high signal surrounded by a low signal serpiginous border. This is characteristic for AVN.

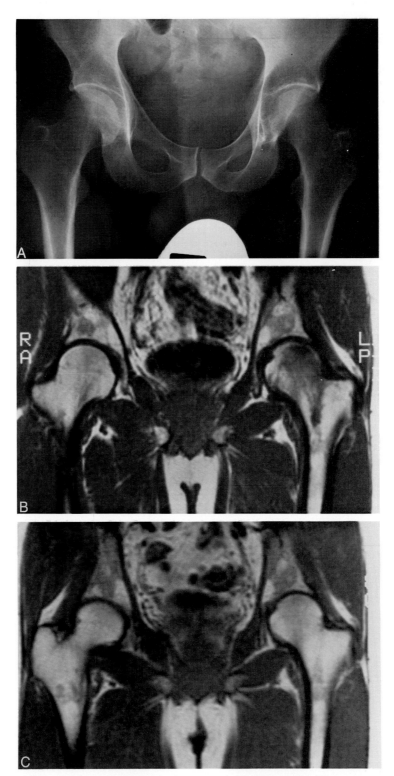

FIGURE 13–11 **Idiopathic transient osteoporosis of the hip.** *(A)* A plain film of a 40-year-old male with left hip pain shows osteoporosis involving the left hip, with no other abnormalities seen. *(B)* A T1-weighted (TR 700; TE 12) coronal MR exam done at the same time as the plain film shows low signal in the superior portion of the left femoral head. This is a characteristic appearance for AVN but is a nonspecific finding. Clinically this patient had no underlying causes for AVN, and he was treated conservatively. *(C)* Seven months later, after near total cessation of the hip pain, a repeat MR exam (TR 600; TE 20) shows no abnormality in the hip. This is consistent with idiopathic transient osteoporosis of the hip.

Transient Osteoporosis of the Hip

This poorly understood disorder is an idiopathic process that begins with a painful hip and no underlying disorder or other findings other than osteoporosis, which is limited to the painful hip. Some feel it is early AVN; however, this has not been conclusively proved. Its appearance on MR imaging is similar to early AVN[6] in that low signal on T1-weighted images, which is high signal on T2-weighted images, is seen throughout the femoral head and neck (Fig. 13–11). Transient osteoporosis of the hip invariably is self-limited with full resolution. It tends to occur more often in males.

REFERENCES

1. Kaplan PA, Helms CA: Current status of temporomandibular joint imaging for the diagnosis of internal derangements. AJR 1989;152:697–705.
2. Kang H, Kindynis P, Brahme S, Resnick D, Haghighi P, Haller J, Sartoris D: Triangular fibrocartilage and intercarpal ligaments of the wrist: MR imaging. Cadaveric study with gross pathologic and histologic correlation. Radiology 1991;181:401–404.
3. Totterman S, Miller R, Wasserman B, Blebea J, Rubens D: Intrinsic and extrinsic carpal ligaments: Evaluation by three-dimensional Fourier transform MR imaging. AJR 1993;160:117–123.
4. Rizzo P, Gould E, Lyden J, Asnis S: Diagnosis of occult fractures about the hip. MRI compared with bone-scanning. J Bone Joint Surg 1993;75-A:395–401.
5. Mitchell D, Kressel H, Arger P, Dalinka M, Spritzer C, Steinberg M: Avascular necrosis of the femoral head: Morphologic assessment by MR imaging, with CT correlation. Radiology 1986;161:739–742.
6. Takatori Y, Kokubo T, Ninomiya S, Nakamura T, Okutsu I, Kamogawa M: Transient osteoporosis of the hip. Magnetic resonance imaging. Clin Orthop Relat Res 1991;271:190–194.

Index

Note: Page numbers in *italics* refer to illustrations; page numbers followed by t refer to tables.